Springer-Verlag Italia Srl.

P. Caione • L. R. Kavoussi • F. Micali (Eds)

Retroperitoneoscopy and Extraperitoneal Laparoscopy in Pediatric and Adult Urology

Springer

EDITORS

Prof. Paolo Caione
Ospedale Pediatrico Bambino Gesù
U.O. Chir. Urologica
Piazza S. Onofrio, 4
00165 Roma

Prof. Louis R. Kavoussi
John Hopkins Bayview
Medical Center
4940 Eastern Avenue Baltimore
Maryland 21224, USA

Prof. Francesco Micali
Department of Urology
Tor Vergata University
Via della Ricerca Scientifica
00133 Roma, Italy

COORDINATING EDITOR

Dr. Salvatore Micali
Department of Urology
Tor Vergata University
Via della Ricerca Scientifica
00133 Roma, Italy

Originally published by Springer-Verlag Italia, Milano in 2003

ISBN 978-88-470-2925-5 ISBN 978-88-470-2923-1 (eBook)
DOI 10.1007/978-88-470-2923-1

Library of Congress Cataloging-in-Publication Data: applied for

Typesetting: Compostudio, Cernusco sul Naviglio (Milano)

Cover design: Simona Colombo (Milano)

SPIN: 10859451

To our wives and sons,
for constant love and support.
To our patients and their families,
for stimulating challenges and a measure of insight.

Preface

Urology has been a leader in minimally invasive surgical sciences. Procedures, such as transurethral resection of the prostate, ureteroscopy and extracorporeal shock wave lithotripsy have revolutionized urologic practice and served as a model for other disciplines. The most recent advances in surgery have come in the arena of laparoscopy. As the majority of urologic organs are in a retroperitoneal location, the natural evolution has been towards the realm of retroperitoneoscopy. Over the past decade, great strides have been made in standardizing access and dissection techniques when approaching retroperitoneal organs. As such, we believe the time is right for a text in this area. Although there are many textbooks regarding laparoscopic urologic surgery, this is a unique compilation dedicated to the retroperitoneoscopic approach.

We have been very fortunate to recruit a renowned group of authors to contribute to these efforts. Of note, laparoscopic surgical techniques and retroperitoneoscopy are not static. Indeed, each week we are seeing rapid advances in our specialty. It is our hope that this text will serve as a constant basic reference for urologists interested in novel endoscopic approaches to treat pathology of the urinary tract. Attempts have been made to organize the text in a logical fashion and be as thorough as possible. Topics are presented in a progressive fashion. The initial chapters deal with basic instrumentation and access techniques and specific applications are discussed further on in the text. Care is taken to alert readers to pitfalls with discussions of complications throughout the book.

To create such a thorough textbook on a focused subject requires significant efforts from many individuals. We would like to thank all the authors for all their wonderful contributions. Indeed, this textbook could only be possible through their hard work and brilliance. We also would like to express our thanks to Springer-Verlag Italia and specifically to Antonella Cerri, for her invaluable guidance in producing this textbook.

June, 2002

The Editors

Table of Contents

List of Contributors

Marco Bitelli
Department of Urology
Tor Vergata University
Via della Ricerca Scientifica
00133 Rome, Italy

Renaud Bollens
Erasme Hospital
University Clinics of Brussels
Department of Urology
Route de Lennik 808
1070 Brussels, Belgium

Pierluigi Bove
Department of Urology
Tor Vergata University
Via della Ricerca Scientifica
00133 Rome, Italy

Patrizia Bozza
Pediatric Hospital "Bambin Gesù"
Anaesthesia and Intensive Care
Department
Piazza S. Onofrio, 4
00165 Rome, Italy

Guglielmo Breda
Division of Urology/Department
of Surgery
Ospedale Nuovo
V. dei Lotti, 40
36031 Bassano del Grappa (VI), Italy

Jeffrey A. Cadeddu
The Clinical Center for
Minimally Invasive
Urologic Cancer Treatment
Department of Urology
The University of Texas
Southwestern Medical
Center at Dallas
5323 Harry Hines Blv.
Dallas, Texas 75235-9110, USA

Paolo Caione
Division of Pediatric Urology
Pediatric Hospital "Bambin Gesù"
Piazza S. Onofrio, 4
00165 Rome, Italy

Nicola Capozza
Division of Pediatric Urology
Pediatric Hospital "Bambin Gesù"
Piazza S. Onofrio, 4
00165 Rome, Italy

Adara Caruso
Division of Urology
Ospedale Nuovo
Via dei Lotti, 40
36061 Bassano del Grappa (VI), Italy

Eduardo F. Carvalhal
Minimally Invasive Surgery Center
and Urological Institute,
The Cleveland Clinic Foundation
9500 Euclid Avenue, A100
Cleveland, OH, 44195, USA

Filadelfo Coniglione
Anaesthesia and Intensive Care
Institute
Tor Vergata University
S. Eugenio Hospital
Piazzale dell'Umanesimo, 10
00144 Rome, Italy

A. Damoun
Erasme Hospital
University Clinics of Brussels
Department of Urology
Route de Lennik 808
1070 Brussels, Belgium

M. Dauri
Anaesthesia and Intensive Care Institute
Tor Vergata University
S. Eugenio Hospital
Piazzale dell'Umanesimo, 10
00144 Rome, Italy

Vincenzo Disanto
Ecclesiastical Institution
Regional General Hospital "F. Miulli"
Via delle Vittime di Via Fani, 1
70021 Acquaviva delle Fonti (BA), Italy

Steven G. Docimo
Children's Hospital of Pittsburgh
4A424 DeSoto Wing
3705 Fifth Avenue
Pittsburgh, PA 15213, USA

Michael Franks
Children's Hospital of Pittsburgh
4A424 DeSoto Wing
3705 Fifth Avenue
Pittsburgh, PA 15213, USA

S. Ekane
Erasme Hospital
University Clinics of Brussels
Department of Urology
Route de Lennik 808
1070 Brussels, Belgium

Flavio Forte
Department of Urology
Tor Vergata University
Via della Ricerca Scientifica
00133 Rome, Italy

Oscar Eduardo Fugita
John Hopkins Bayview Medical Center
4940 Eastern Avenue Baltimore
Maryland 21224, USA

Durga D. Gaur
Department of Urology
Bombay Hospital
Institute of Medical Sciences
19 Marine Lines
Bombay 400 020, India

Inderbir S. Gill
Section of Laparoscopy and Minimally Invasive Surgery
Urological Institute
The Cleveland Clinic Foundation
9500 Euclid Avenue, A100
Cleveland, OH, 44195, USA

N. Heffawi
Anaesthesia and Intensive Care Institute
Tor Vergata University
S. Eugenio Hospital
Piazzale dell'Umanesimo, 10
00144 Rome, Italy

P. Hoffmann
Erasme Hospital
University Clinics of Brussels
Department of Urology
Route de Lennik 808
1070 Brussels, Belgium

Thomas W. Jarrett
Division of Endourology
James Buchanan Brady Urological Institute
John Hopkins Medical Institutions
Baltimore, Maryland, USA

Louis R. Kavoussi
Johns Hopkins Bayview Medical Center
4940 Eastern Avenue Baltimore
Maryland 21224, USA

Daniela Marconi
Department of Obstetrics and Gynaecology
Fatebenefratelli Hospital
Isola Tiberina
Piazza Fatebenefratelli, 2
00186 Rome, Italy

Ennio Matarazzo
Division of Pediatric Urology
Pediatric Hospital "Bambin Gesù"
Piazza S. Onofrio, 4
00165 Rome, Italy

Francesco Micali
Department of Urology
Tor Vergata University
Via della Ricerca Scientifica
00133 Rome, Italy

Salvatore Micali
Department of Urology
Tor Vergata University
Via della Ricerca Scientifica
00133 Rome, Italy

Robert G. Moore
Minimally Invasive Surgery
Scott Department of Urology
Baylor college of Medicine
Houston, Texas 77030, USA

Kenneth Ogan
The Clinical Center for Minimally Invasive
Urologic Cancer Treatment
Department of Urology
The University of Texas
Southwestern Medical
Center at Dallas
5323 Harry Hines Blv.
Dallas, Texas 75235-9110, USA

John G. Pattaras
Minimally Invasive Surgery
Department of Urology
Emory University School
of Medicine
Atlanta, GA, USA

Craig A. Peters
Children's Hospital
Department of Urology
300 Longwood Avenue
Boston, MA 02115, USA

Nicola Piazza
Division of Urology
Ospedale Nuovo
Via dei Lotti, 40
36061 Bassano del Grappa (VI), Italy

Peter A. Pinto
Division of Endourology
James Buchanan Brady Urological Institute
Johns Hopkins Medical Institutions
Baltimore, Maryland, USA

Carlo Romanini †
Deparment of Obstetrics and Gynaecology
Fatebenefratelli Hospital
Isola Tiberina
Piazza Fatebenefratelli, 2
00186 Rome, Italy

Thierry Roumeguere
Erasme Hospital
University Clinics of Brussels
Department of Urology
Route de Lennik 808
1070 Brussels, Belgium

Gino A. Scalese
Ecclesiastical Institution
Regional General Hospital "F. Miulli"
Via delle Vittime di Via Fani, 1
70021 Acquaviva delle Fonti (BA), Italy

Francis X. Schneck
Children's Hospital of Pittsburgh
4A424 DeSoto Wing
3705 Fifth Avenue
Pittsburgh, PA 15213, USA

Claude C. Schulman
Erasme Hospital
University Clinics of Brussels
Department of Urology
Route de Lennik 808
1070 Brussels, Belgium

J. S. Valla
Department of Pediatric Surgery
Lenval Hospital
57, Avenue de la Californie
06200 Nice, France

Marc Vanden Bossche
Erasme Hospital
University Clinics of Brussels
Department of Urology
Route de Lennik 808
1070 Brussels, Belgium

Antonio Villani
Pediatric Hospital "Bambin Gesù"
Anaesthesia and Intensive Care Department
Piazza S. Onofrio, 4
00165 Rome, Italy

Guido Virgili
Department of Urology
Tor Vergata University
Via della Ricerca Scientifica
00133 Rome, Italy

Alexandre Zlotta
Erasme Hospital
University Clinics of Brussels
Department of Urology
Route de Lennik 808
1070 Brussels, Belgium

Errico Zupi
Department of Obstetrics and Gynaecology
Fatebenefratelli Hospital
Isola Tiberina
Piazza Fatebenefratelli, 2
00186 Rome, Italy

Chapter 1

Retroperitoneal Laparoscopy in Adult and Pediatric Patients

Paolo Caione

Introduction

We are living in a special era, one in which tremendous scientific progress and technological advances have been made that also affect the field of urology. Concerning the future of surgical procedures, minimally invasive surgery and video-assisted surgery are novel steps in this process of change. Laparoscopy is expected to play a primary role in both adult and pediatric urology, but its efficacy and safety in the different indications, as are continuously being proposed in the medical literature, still need to be verified.

As we discuss urological indications, retroperitoneal access in laparoscopic surgery seems, theoretically, to be the best way to approach the organs of the urogenital tract, as they are located in the extraperitoneal space. Most open urological procedures were carried out via an extraperitoneal approach in the past five decades of surgical history; however, retroperitoneal access will probably now gain favor in laparoscopic procedures, as compared to the transperitoneal ones.

Since the pioneering experience reported by Wittmoser [1] in 1973 for lumbar sympathecotomy and the first urological attempt carried out by Wickham [2] in 1979 for retroperitoneoscopic ureterolithotomy, retroperitoneal laparoscopic surgery began to be applied clinically in urology less than one decade ago. Gaur [3] presented in 1972 the inflated glove balloon technique to create the working space for his first experience in conducting retroperitoneal laparoscopic procedures and, shortly thereafter, published his first case report of retroperitoneal laparoscopic nephrectomy [4]. Almost 1 year before, Claymann and colleagues [5] had published the first report of transperitoneal laparoscopic nephrectomy in an adult patient. From that point, the reports on retroperitoneal laparoscopic procedures have progressively increased in number and retroperitoneoscopy has gained more popularity, but its acceptance is not yet universal.

Although the interest of the urological community has increased greatly recently, only a few centers worldwide have adopted retroperitoneal laparoscopy as the standard surgical access for their patients as of yet. The lack of working space behind the peritoneum, as well as the difficulty in orientation and in identifying the anatomical components within the virtual extraperitoneal space are the problems most frequently encountered by the surgeon who attempts to utilize the retroperitoneal laparoscopic access [6]. These concerns are often considered as deterrents for beginners or for surgeons who are not experts in video-assisted endourological techniques, in combination with the fear of any of the major operative complications that have been reported during urological laparoscopic procedures [7—9].

Nevertheless, retroperitoneal laparoscopic procedures have been considered a safe and reliable surgical technique in several contributions published in the last few years, with results similar to the corresponding open procedures in terms of complication rates [10—12]. The less operative invasiveness and the reduced postoperative morbidity have been reported as specific advantages for the patient, but single contributions on personal clinical experience are often not enough to provide ultimate conclusions about the safety and efficacy of retroperitoneal laparoscopy [6]. Renal surgery and adrenal surgery have been demonstrated as reliable for a progressively larger number of surgical indications, even for malignancies. Patient age is not considered a real problem anymore, as retroperitoneal laparoscopic procedures have been successfully reported in both elderly [13] and pediatric patients, even those younger than 1 year [14].

The reduced invasiveness of the retroperitoneal or extraperitoneal laparoscopic procedures has been demonstrated to offer a significant advantage, if compared with corresponding open surgery. The advantage was greater in elderly patients [6, 13], who benefited from quicker recovery and fewer postoperative complications. A universal consensus has not yet been reached regarding the utility of these minimally invasive procedures in the pediatric age group, and mainly in infancy and in younger children. M. Franks, F.X. Schneck, and S.G. Docimo (see Chap. 11, this volume) present in this book their point of view on pediatric retroperitoneoscopy, with which we mostly agree. Our opinion is that further advancements in technology and more appropriate instrumentation will facilitate the current use of both transperitoneal and retroperitoneal laparoscopy in pediatric urology. The continuous increase in experience is paramount to correctly extend the clinical indications and to reduce the risk of possible complications.

The question of whether laparoscopic surgery in the urogenital organs is better performed via a transperitoneal or via a retroperitoneal/extraperitoneal approach is still being debated. The pros and cons are extensively presented and discussed by two experts in this field and their collaborators, Inderbir S. Gill (Chap. 21, this volume) and Louis A. Kavoussi (Chap. 22, this volume).

From a theoretical point of view, the concept of avoiding entering the peritoneal cavity is a well-accepted principle in urology, for any surgical procedure being performed on extraperitoneal organs. The bowel is not manipulated or mobilized via the extraperitoneal access and there is no risk of intraperitoneal hematoma or urinoma (Chap. 21, this volume). No long-term peritoneal adhesions occur. Urologists are commonly confident with the flank position of the patient and with the extra- or retroperitoneal open access. Retroperitoneal laparoscopy can therefore easily be converted to a retroperitoneal open procedure, if needed, without violation of the abdominal cavity.

Another point in favor of retroperitoneal laparoscopy in renal surgery is that the renal vessels are directly and promptly controlled by this access, allowing the correct surgical procedure for radical nephrectomy in adult oncological diseases.

Conversely, the lack of a wide working space and the difficult definition of anatomical landmarks represent the most significant problems that may be encountered using the retroperitoneal laparoscopic access.

The need for adequate experience is crucial in retroperitoneal laparoscopy. There is clear evidence that fewer complications arise in laparoscopic procedures when performed by well-trained surgeons with extensive clinical experience in both adults [8] and children [15]. Results of retroperitoneoscopic surgery presented recently by a single center [16] show a similar trend, with a strong influence of clinical experience. As urologists become more familiar with these procedures, the complication rates decrease.

As a consequence, one of the critical points in laparoscopy, and for all innovative surgical techniques, as retroperitoneal or extraperitoneal laparoscopy represents, is the possibility of participating in a valid training program for beginners or nonexpert surgeons. Adequate training is essential to shorten the learning curve and reduce significantly the operating time. The most important goal of a training program, however, is to tremendously reduce the risk of severe complications that may occur during retroperitoneoscopic surgery in complex cases. Retroperitoneal laparoscopic procedures involve many technological innovations that require continuous, practical refresher courses of any surgeon who desires to undertake this. Moreover, some practical difficulties in performing retroperitoneoscopic surgery, as represented by the lack of wide working space and the more difficult identification of the traditional anatomical landmarks, represent a further reason to devote special attention to training programs in laparoscopy and retroperitoneoscopy, both with the use of simulators (pelvic trainers) and with increasing clinical experience. The constant introduction of new technologies and advancements in instrumentation, in combination with the perspective of robotic surgery (Chap. 21, this volume [17—19]), will increase the need for well-trained urological staff for this novel aspect of minimally invasive urology.

Acknowledgments. I wish to thank the co-editors and particularly each of the authors very much for their timely and innovative contributions to this work. Their adherence to the requests and to deadlines has been most admirable. Many thanks are also addressed to the publisher, Springer-Verlag International, for being willing to accept our wishes in terms of quality of printing and for respecting the editors' wishes.

References

1. Wittmoser R (1973) Die Retroperitoneoskopie als neue Methode der lumbalen Sympathikotomie. Fortschr Endoskop 4:219-223
2. Wickham JEA (1979) The surgical treatment of renal lithiasis. In Wickham IEA (ed) Urinary calculus disease. Churchill Livingstone, New York, pp 145-198
3. Gaur DD (1992) Laparoscopic operative retroperitoneoscopy: Use of a new device. J Urol 148:1137-1139
4. Gaur DD, Agarwal DK, Purohit KC (1993) Retroperitoneal laparoscopic nephrectomy: initial case report. J Urol 149:103-105

5. Clayman RV, Kavoussi LR, Soper NJ et al (1991) Laparoscopic nephrectomy: an initial case report. J Urol 146:278-282
6. Gaur DD, Rathi SS, Ravandale AV, Gopichand M (2001) A single-centre experience of retroperitoneoscopy using the balloon technique. BJU Int 87:602-606
7. Adams JB, Micali S, Moore RG, Babayan RK, Kavoussi RL (1996) Complications of extraperitoneal balloon dilation. J Endourol 10:375-378
8. Fahlenkamp D., Rassweiler J, Fornara P, Frede T. Loening SA (1999) Complications of laparoscopic procedures in urology: experience with 2407 procedures at 4 German Centers. J Urol 162:765-771
9. Keeley FX, Tolley DA (1998) A review of our first 100 cases of laparoscopic nephrectomy: defining risk factors for complications. Br J Urol 82: 615-618
10. McDougall EM, Clayman RV, Fadden PT (1994) Retroperitoneoscopy: the Washington University Medical School experience. Urology 43:446-452
11. Mandressi A, Buizza C, Antonelli D, Chisena S, Servadio G (1995) Retroperitoneoscopy. Ann Urol (Paris) 29:91-96
12. Gasman D, Saint F, Barthelemy Y, Antiphon P, Chopin D, Abbou CC (1996) Retroperitoneoscopy: a laparoscopic approach for adrenal and renal surgery. Urology 47:801-806
13. Hsu TH, Gill IS, Fazeli-Matin S et al (1999) Radical nephrectomy and nephoureterectomy in the octogenarian and nonagenarian: comparison of laparoscopic and open approaches. Urology 53:1121-1125
14. Valla JS, Guilloneau B., Montupet P et al (1996) Retroperitoneal laparoscopic nephrectomy in children: preliminary report of 6 cases. J Laparoendosc Surg 6:S55-S59
15. Peters CA (1996) Complications in pediatric urological laparoscopy: results of a survey. J Urol 155:1070-1073
16. Kumar M, Kumar R, Hemal AK, Gupta NP (2001) Complications of retroperitoneoscopic surgery at one centre. BJU Int 87:607-612
17. Kavoussi LR, Moore RG, Partin JB et al (1995) Comparison of robotic versus human laparoscopic camera control. J Urol 54:2134-2136
18. Sung GT, Gill IS, Hsu TH (1999) Robotic-assisted laparoscopic pyeloplasty: a pilot study. Urology 53:1099-1103
19. Docimo SG (2001) Robotics in urology: new toys or new era? Dialog Pediatr Urol 24:3-4

Chapter 2

Inception, Progress and Future Perspectives of Retroperitoneal Laparoscopy

DURGA D. GAUR

Inception

In 1969 Bartel first performed endoscopic visualization of the pelvic retroperitoneum using a mediastinoscope and 4 years later using a similar technique; Wittmoser even performed a retroperitoneal endoscopic lumbar sympathectomy [1,2]. Sommerkamp soon extended the use of this simple gasless direct vision technique for exposing the kidney for a renal biopsy and called it 'lumboscopy' [3]. Following his publication, there were numerous reports on endoscopic exposure of the pelvic and the lumbar retroperitoneal space. Retroperitoneal laparoscopy in a real sense, however, was only started by Wickham (1979), who performed a ureterolithotomy using pneumoinsufflation and a standard laparoscope [4].

Not much progress could be made in laparoscopic urology for more than a decade as most workers in this field, trying to replicate the steps of transperitoneal laparoscopy in the retroperitoneal space, failed to create a satisfactory pneumoretroperitoneum. Disheartened by the poor results of retroperitoneoscopy in the past, even a laryngoscope and an Amplatz sheath were used by Bay-Nielsen and Schultz (1982) and Clayman et al. (1985), respectively, to perform a retroperitoneal endoscopic ureterolithotomy [5,6]

Overview of Laparoscopic Urology in the Past Decade

Although there was hardly any laparoscopic activity in the field of urology during the decade preceding 1991, the following decade saw a meteoric rise in the activity and there was hardly any urological procedure which was not performed laparoscopically. This sudden surge in urological laparoscopic activity was the result of two historical events: one was the publication of the first laparoscopic nephrectomy by Clayman et al. in 1991 and the other the publication of the balloon technique of retroperitoneoscopy by Gaur the following year [7,8]. This is shown by the fact that about 40 times more urological laparoscopic articles were published in the world literature during the last decade than in the previous decade (Fig. 1). Nevertheless, the urologists could not compete with the general surgeons and the gynecologists, as so far their contribution has been a mere 6% of the total number of articles pertaining to laparoscopy published in the medical literature worldwide (Fig. 2).

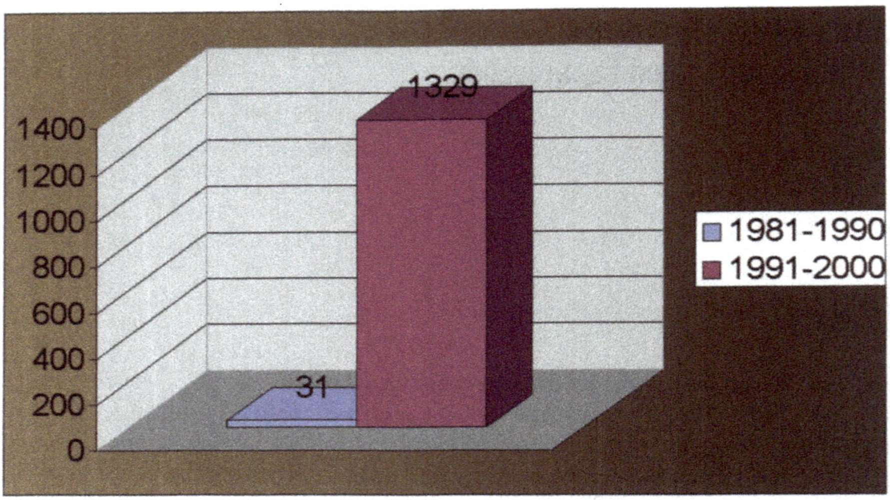

Fig. 1. The laparoscopic urological articles published during the last two decades

There were two main reasons for this gross disparity between the urological and the nonurological laparoscopic activity. One was that most urological laparoscopic procedures have a steep learning curve, more so if performed by the retroperitoneal approach. Unless one has performed a relatively larger number of procedures, one cannot have the same degree of confidence as one's counterparts in the other specialties, in which the bulk of the work consists of simpler procedures on the appendix, gall bladder, and the fallopian tubes. The other was that

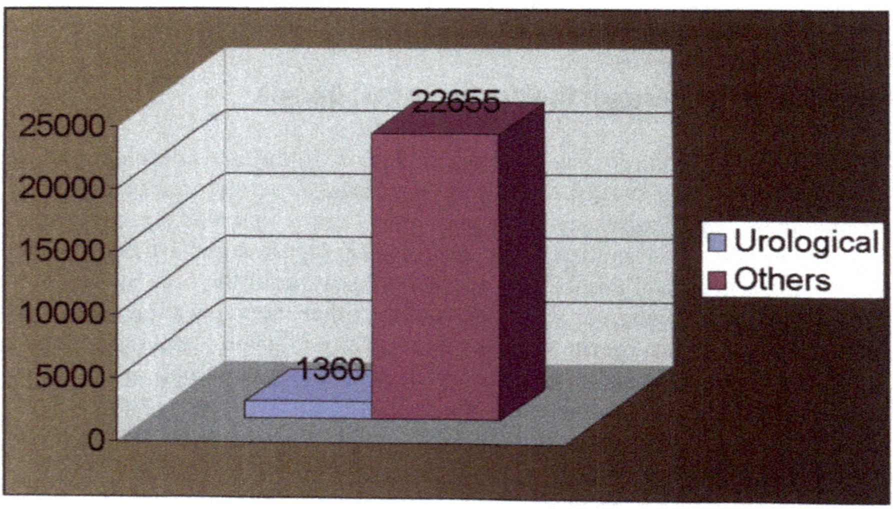

Fig. 2. A comparison between laparoscopic urological and total laparoscopic articles published

while an average laparoscopic urologist is mostly looking for the chance to perform such a procedure, in general surgery and gynecology, there is generally a long waiting list for a variety of procedures, such as cholecystectomy, fundoplication, appendectomy, herniorrhaphy, and tubectomy.

There was one more reason for the comparatively smaller number of laparoscopic urological procedures. While the role of laparoscopy in gynecology and general surgery soon was established, its role for most urological procedures is still being debated. Consequently, only a few retroperitoneoscopic procedures in urology have actually become established.

Retroperitoneoscopic Urological Procedures of Limited Value

Many retroperitoneoscopic urological procedures, such as renal biopsy, varicocelectomy, colposuspension, renal cyst decortication, nephropexy and pelvic lymphadenectomy, which were frequently being performed earlier, have now been either discontinued or are performed far less frequently. This is because either there are not many indications for these procedures or their long-term results are not satisfactory or other less invasive therapeutic procedures are available.

Retroperitoneoscopic Urological Procedures of Proven Value

Simple Nephrectomy

The first published report of simple nephrectomy by the retroperitoneal laparoscopic approach was by Gaur et al., although Clayman et al. had performed it earlier [9]. Since then retroperitoneoscopic nephrectomy has been established as the minimally invasive procedure of choice for treating patients with symptomatic, benign nonfunctioning kidneys [10-12]. Its efficiency, efficacy and safety was demonstrated in a recent series of 185 retroperitoneal laparoscopic simple nephrectomies by Hemel et al., who had an operative time of 100 min, an open conversion rate of 10.3% and a major complication rate of 3.78% [13]. With more experience in this field even a tubercular nonfunctioning kidney would not have to be considered a contraindication [14,15].

Adrenalectomy

Uchida et al. reported the first retroperitoneoscopic adrenalectomy and since then it has been performed both by the posterior and the lateral approach [11,12,16]. However, most agree that the upper limit of the size of the adrenal tumor for retroperitoneoscopic removal should not be more than 5 or 6 cm due to the high incidence of malignancy in larger adrenal tumors [17,18]. Waltz et al. have suggested that a total adrenal resection is not necessary and partial adrenalectomy with an adequate tumor-free adrenal margin is enough for most adrenal tumors [18].

Sasagawa et al. and Suzuki et al. have suggested the use of a stapler and an ultrasonic knife, respectively, for performing retroperitoneoscopic partial adrenalectomy [19,20]. Fernandez-Cruz et al. have compared the results of retroperitoneoscopic and transperitoneal laparoscopic adrenalectomy and found no difference in operative time, analgesic requirement, hospital stay and return to normal activity [21]. However, according to these authors the retroperitoneal approach should be preferred if one expects Intraperitoneal adhesions. Baba et al. compared the results of the transperitoneal laparoscopic, the lateral retroperitoneoscopic and the posterior retroperitoneoscopic approaches in 51 procedures and found that the posterior approach was most effective for retroperitoneoscopic adrenalectomy in regard to the simplicity of vascular control [22]. Terachi et al. feel that, although retroperitoneoscopic adrenalectomy has a lower morbidity rate than the transperitoneal procedure, more skill is required to overcome the drawback of the narrow working space and fewer anatomical landmarks [23]. The efficiency, efficacy and safety of the posterior retroperitoneoscopic approach was shown in a recent series of 142 adrenalectomies by Waltz et al., who had an operative time of 101 min (range 35-185 min), success rate of 95% and no major complications [24]. Gill et al. and Suzuki et al. feel that a lateral retroperitoneoscopic approach is an equally effective, simple and safe procedure [25,26].

Evolving Retroperitoneoscopoic Urological Procedures

Reconstructive Procedures

Retroperitoneoscopic ablative surgery is being performed at many centers throughout the world, but because of inherent problems in laparoscopic suturing and problems of manipulation due to space restrictions, reconstructive surgery has not yet been widely accepted. Consequently, nondismembered pyeloplasty procedures for ureteropelvic junction obstruction such as exopyelotomy and Fenger-plasty were initially performed [27,28]. Nevertheless, they were soon followed by retroperitoneoscopic dismembered pyeloplasty, which was first reported by Eden and associates [29-31]. The efficiency and efficacy of the procedure is reflected in a recent series of 50 by Eden et al. with a mean operative time of 164 min, open conversion rate of 4% and success rate of 95% [32].

Radical Nephrectomy

Retroperitoneal laparoscopic radical nephrectomy is gaining in popularity as an effective minimally invasive method for treatment of T1-T2N0M0 renal tumors since it was first reported by Kinukawa et al. in 1995 [33]. Clayman and associates in a 9-year follow-up study have shown that the results of laparoscopic radical nephrectomy for T1-T2 renal tumors up to 10 cm were quite comparable with the open radical nephrectomy series and that there were no port site recurrences in any patient [34]. The results of retroperitoneal laparoscopic radical nephrectomy recently published by Gill et al. have not only shown identical results but these authors have also shown that T1-T2N0M0 tumors even as large as 12 cm can be safely removed by the retroperitoneal approach [35].

Radical Nephroureterectomy

The most difficult part of the retroperitoneal laparoscopic radical nephroureterectomy procedure is the dissection of the juxtavesical ureter and excision of the bladder cuff. Gill et al. used a novel endoscopic approach for this purpose and have recently compared the results of retroperitoneoscopic radical nephroureterectomy and the open surgical procedure [36,37]. They found that laparoscopy was superior in regard to duration of surgery, blood loss, specimen weight, resumption of oral intake, narcotic analgesia requirements, hospital stay, return to normal activities and convalescence. To simplify the procedure, Salomon et al. make a small iliac incision for distal ureterectomy and excision of the cuff of bladder and Igarshi et al. use a gasless hand-assisted retroperitoneoscopic technique [38,39].

Partial Nephrectomy

Gill et al. reported the first retroperitoneal laparoscopic partial nephrectomy using a double loop apparatus and argon beam coagulator for obtaining hemostasis [40]. Since then ultrasound, radiofrequency, microwave, cable-tie, fibrin glue, biological glue, hydrojet and electrosurgical snare have all been used for achieving hemostasis during this procedure [41-46]. Retroperitoneal laparoscopic renal cryoablation, a much simpler nephron-sparing procedure, seems to be a safe and effective alternative to partial nephrectomy, but the long-term results are still outstanding [47].

Ureterolithotomy

The real indication for laparoscopic ureterolithotomy is a salvage procedure as an alternative to an open procedure in patients in whom URS and ESWL have failed. However, according to Gaur the retroperitoneoscopic approach may be used as a primary procedure, if the surgeon feels that the chances of failure with the existing minimally invasive procedures could be high due to size of the stone, degree of its impaction or a coexisting ureteral anomaly [48].

After going through various reports on laparoscopic ureterolithotomies, it is a bit surprising to note that the transperitoneal approach is still being routinely used at some centers. If open ureterolithotomy is not performed by this route, there is not much justification in its routine use for the laparoscopic procedure.

Pyelolithotomy

Since Gaur et al. reported the first retroperitoneal laparoscopic pyelolithotomy in 1994, only a few papers have appeared in the medical literature as there are not many indications for the procedure [49-51]. However, due to its being less invasive to the renal parenchyma and having a better chance of total stone clearance, it can be given priority over percutaneous nephrolithotripsy in a select group of patients with large renal stones [52]. With improvement in technique and instrumentation, retroperitoneal laparoscopic pyelolithotomy might eventually become an acceptable minimally invasive alternative for patients with staghorn stones.

Live Donor Nephrectomy

Retroperitoneoscopic live donor nephrectomy has been performed in the past but, mainly due to the problem of limited space, it has not become popular [53]. Gasless retroperitoneoscopy-assisted live donor nephrectomy using specially designed retractors, a simpler procedure, is slowly gaining in popularity [54,55]. A hand-assisted standard retroperitoneoscopic live donor nephrectomy has also recently been reported [56].

Radical Prostatectomy

Since Schuessler et al. first reported laparoscopic radical prostatectomy in 1992 and Guillonneau et al. popularized the technique, it is regularly being performed at many centers by the transperitoneal laparoscopic approach [57,58]. However, Bollens et al. were the first to perform it retroperitoneoscopically and have since reported 42 procedures with a reasonable mean operative time of 317 min [59].

Future Perspectives in Retroperitoneoscopy

Improvement in Human Skill

There is a great scope for improving one's skill in performing retroperitoneoscopic reconstructive procedures such as pyeloplasty, partial nephrectomy, uretero-ureterostomy, ureteral re-implantation and others. All these procedures require a high degree of proficiency in suturing and knot tying, which can be quite difficult due to the limited space available in the retroperitoneum but can be mastered with perseverance and diligence. However, until one acquires a reasonable amount of proficiency in knot tying, there is no harm in using the simpler clip ligation technique for some of the reconstructive procedures [60,61].

In an attempt to make retroperitoneoscopic suturing and knotting a bit easier, Frede et al. studied and analyzed the geometry of laparoscopic suturing and knotting techniques [62]. They have suggested that, if an isosceles triangle is formed between the instruments, it increases the suturing and knotting efficiency. However, the crux of the matter is that with dedication, perseverance and patience, one should be able to achieve the same degree of dexterity in laparoscopic free-hand suturing as in open surgery. Mechanical suturing aids are commercially available but in their present form are not very suitable for retroperitoneoscopic reconstructive surgery.

Due to the inherent problems in laparoscopy and a steep learning curve, the suggestion made by Breda et al. that there should be a two-tier system for future advancement of urological laparoscopy and for providing maximal patient benefits applies more to retroperitoneoscopy [63]. This is a good suggestion and the author fully agrees that the more complicated laparoscopic procedures should be performed only at tier-one referral centers while tier-two centers, in addition to carrying out straightforward procedures, should also concentrate on making urological laparoscopic procedures simpler, so that more and more urologists could be inducted into laparoscopy.

Improvement in Technology

Intraoperative Imaging

The use of ultrasonography during laparoscopy can improve the efficiency and efficacy of laparoscopic urological surgery. Linear-array transducers with frequencies of 7.5-10 MHz can be very useful during decortication of a renal cortical cyst, marsupialization of a lymphocele, renal stone surgery and cryotherapy of renal tumors [64]. It provides vital information during laparoscopic cryoablation of renal tumors about the extent and depth of the ice ball, which is crucial in preventing inadvertent damage to the neighboring structures and assuring total ablation of the tumor.

Even computer-generated assistance has been used during retroperitoneoscopy to simplify the operative procedure. Chaffanjon et al. have used it for performing retroperitoneoscopic staging pelvic lymphadenectomy in difficult cases with good results [65,66].

Hemostasis

The control of hemorrhage is of utmost importance for performing complex retroperitoneoscopic procedures. Hydrodissectors and pneumodissectors are useful evolving adjuncts for reducing blood loss during retroperitoneoscopic surgery [45,67]. Bipolar diathermy, argon beam, ultrasound, microwave and radiofrequency have been found to be quite effective in controlling bleeding from the renal parenchyma. However, Clayman et al. have shown that their new electrosurgical snare device is equally effective in achieving hemostasis and is less traumatic to the renal parenchyma [46]. Fibrin glue and the biological glue consisting of gelatin, resorcinol and formaldehyde are also quite effective in controlling renal parenchymal bleeding [43,44]. A recent report of the use of radiofrequency for retroperitoneoscopic ablation of multiple renal tumors under ultrasound control might open new vistas for patients with multiple bilateral renal tumors as in von Hippel-Lindau disease [68]. However, all these are evolving techniques and have to be established before they can be widely used in clinical practice.

Video Imaging

Kourambas and Preminger feel that the introduction of technological advances, such as HDTV, three-dimensional laparoscopy, and further miniaturization of high-resolution digital video cameras, will allow significantly enhanced opportunities for laparoscopic surgical proficiency and further broadening of laparoscopic applications in urology [69].

Although a blind, closed percutaneous primary access for retroperitoneoscopy is being used at some centers, for obvious reasons it is not as easy as in the transperitoneal approach. Micali et al. have used the optical trocar for this purpose for their pediatric patients, but it was not found to be of much use at our institute [70]. Maybe with improved quality of the optical trocars, this would be adopted as a reliable, less invasive closed access technique for retroperitoneoscopy. With the development of this closed access technique, it might be possible to perform a needlescopic retroperitoneoscopy in the near future.

Improvement in Robotics and Telementoring

With the development of robotics and the de Vinci telemanipulation system, telepresence radical nephrectomy has now been performed between countries as far as half way round the world [71]. More recently, even laparoscopic radical prostatectomy was performed by this technique [72-74]. Telerobotic laparoscopic surgery, though expensive, has some advantages over the standard technique as there is stereovision and it provides programs for dexterity enhancement and tremor filtering. As the Internet becomes universally available, the cost of higher bandwidth telecommunication lines will decrease and it will be possible to have telepresence systems installed even in remote countries at an affordable price to enable patients in the less developed part of the world to have laparoscopic surgery performed by an expert from another country.

Because of the steep learning curve for most urological laparoscopic procedures, there are lengthy operative sessions and an unacceptably high complication rate for less experienced laparoscopic surgeons. According to Kavoussi and associates urological laparoscopy can be made easier and safer through telesurgical mentoring, whereby less experienced surgeons with basic laparoscopic skills could receive guidance and training in advanced techniques from a world expert without having to travel [75]. This would certainly have a great impact on future laparoscopic training programs.

Conclusions

With perfection of tissue approximation techniques, tissue retrieval methods, tissue ablation techniques, hemostasis techniques, intraoperative imaging techniques, virtual reality, three-dimentional video imaging, miniaturized robotics and telerobotics, it will soon be possible to universally perform almost all reconstructive and ablative urological procedures by the laparoscopic approach [76,77]. The use of needlescopes and microlaparoscopic instruments will go a long way in further reducing the invasiveness of the retroperitoneal laparoscopic procedure. Although these microlaparoscopic procedures are being performed at some centers by the transperitoneal laparoscopic approach, none has been performed by the retroperitoneal approach [78]. This is because of the problem of needlescopic access to the retroperitoneal space, and it is hoped that soon this barrier will also be overcome.

References

1. Bartel M (1969) Die Retroperitoneoskopie. Eine endoscopische Methode zur Inspektion unt bioptischen Untersuchung des retroperitonealen Raumes. Zentralbl Chir 94: 377.
2. Wittmoser R (1973) Die Retroperitoeoskopie als neue Methode der lumbalen Sympathicotomie. Fortschr Endosc 4:219-223
3. Sommerkamp H (1974) Lumboscopie: ein neues diagnostich-therapeutisches Prinzip der Urologie. Acta Urol 5: 183
4. Wickham JEA (1979) The surgical treatment of renal lithiasis. In: Wickham JEA (ed) Urinary calculus disease. Churchill Livingstone, New York, pp 145-198
5. Bay-Nielsen H, Schultz A (1982) Endoscopic retroperitoneal removal of stones from the upper half of the ureter. Scand J Urol Nephrol 16: 227-228
6. Clayman RV, Preminger GM, Franklin JF, Curry T, Peters PC (1985) Percutaneous ureterolithotomy. J Urol 133: 671-673
7. Clayman RV, Kavoussi LR, Soper NJ, Dierks NJ, Meretyk S, Darcy MD, Roemer FD, Pingleton ED, Thomson PG, Long SR (1991) Laparoscopic nephrectomy: initial case report. J Urol 146: 278-281
8. Gaur DD (1992) Laparoscopic operative retroperitoneoscopy: use of a new device. J Urol 148: 1137- 1139
9. Gaur DD, Agarwal DK, Purohit KC (1993) Retroperitoneal laparoscopic nephrectomy: initial case report. J Urol 149: 103-105
10. Barreto H, Doublet JD, Peraldi MN, Gattegno B, Thibault P (1995) Kidney surgery using lumbar endoscopy: initial experiences. Prog Urol 5(3):384-389
11. Gaur DD (1995) Retroperitoneal surgery of the kidney, ureter and adrenal gland. Endosc Surg Allied Technol 3(1):3-8
12. Mandressi A, Buizza C, Antonelli D, Chisena S, Servadio G (1995) Retroperitoneoscopy. Ann Urol (Paris) 29(2):91-96.
13. Hemal AK, Gupta NP, Wadhwa SN, Goel A, Kumar R (2001) Retroperitoneoscopic nephrectomy and nephroureterectomy for benign nonfunctioning kidneys: a single-center experience. Urology 57(4):644-649
14. Gaur DD (2000) Simple nephrectomy: retroperitoneal approach. J Endourol 14(10): 787-790
15. Hemal AK, Gupta NP, Kumar R (2000) Comparison of retroperitoneoscopic nephrectomy with open surgery for tuberculous nonfunctioning kidneys. 14: J Urol 164(1):32-35
16. Uchida M, Imaide Y, Yoneda K et al (1994) Endoscopic adrenalectomy by retroperitoneal approach for primary aldosteronism. Hinyokika Kiyo 40(1):43-46
17. Heintz A, Junginger T (1998) Technique and results of the retroperitoneoscopic adrenalectomy via a lumbar approach. Langenbecks Arch Surg 383(3-4):286-288
18. Walz MK, Peitgen K, Saller B, Mann K, Eigler FW (1998) Subtotal retroperitoneoscopic adrenal gland resection—an alternative to adrenalectomy? Langenbecks Arch Chir [Suppl Kongressbd] 115:1038-1040
19. Sasagawa I, Suzuki H, Tateno T, Izumi T, Shoji N, Nakada (1998) Retroperitoneoscopic partial adrenalectomy using an endoscopic stapling device in patients with adrenal tumor. Urol Int 61(2):101-103
20. Suzuki K, Sugiyama T, Saisu K, Ushiyama T, Fujita K (1998) Retroperitoneoscopic partial adrenalectomy for aldosterone-producing adenoma using an ultrasonically activated scalpel. Br J Urol 82(1):138-139
21. Fernandez-Cruz L, Saenz A, Taura P, Benarroch G, Astudillo E, Sabater L (1999) Retroperitoneal approach in laparoscopic adrenalectomy: is it advantageous? Surg Endosc 13(1):86-90

22. Baba S, Miyajima A, Uchida A, Asanuma H, Miyakawa A, Murai M (1997) A posterior lumbar approach for retroperitoneoscopic adrenalectomy: assessment of surgical efficacy. Urology 50(1):19-24
23. Terachi T, Yoshida O, Matsuda T et al (2000) Complications of laparoscopic and retroperitoneoscopic adrenalectomies in 370 cases in Japan: a multi-institutional study. Biomed Pharmacother 54 [Suppl 1]: 211-214
24. Walz MK, Metz KA, Hellinger A, Pfeiffer T, Peitgen K (1997) Surgery of primary unilateral adrenal gland tumors—results of 154 patients. Zentralbl Chir 122(6):481-486
25. Sung GT, Hsu TH, Gill IS (2001) Retroperitoneoscopic adrenalectomy: lateral approach. J Endourol 15(5):505-511
26. Suzuki K (2001) Laparoscopic adrenalectomy: retroperitoneal approach. Urol Clin North Am 28(1): 85-95
27. Gaur DD, Purohit KC, Jain M, Kashyapi BD, Joshi AS (1997) If endopyelotomy works, why not 'exopyelotomy'? MITAT 5/6: 463-466
28. Janetschek G, Peschel R, Bartsch G (1996) Laparoscopic and retroperitoneoscopic kidney pyeloplasty. Urologe A 35(3): 202-207
29. Eden CG, Sultana SR, Murray KH, Carruthers RK (1997) Extraperitoneal laparoscopic dismembered fibrin-glued pyeloplasty: medium-term results. Br J Urol 80(3): 382-389
30. Yeung CK, Tam YH, Sihoe JD, Lee KH, Liu KW (2001) Retroperitoneoscopic dismembered pyeloplasty for pelvi-ureteric junction obstruction in infants and children. BJU Int 87(6): 509-513
31. Ben Slama MR, Salomon L, Hoznek A et al (2000) Extraperitoneal laparoscopic repair of ureteropelvic junction obstruction: initial experience in 15 cases. Urology 56(1):45-48
32. Eden CG, Cahill D, Allen JD (2001) Laparoscopic dismembered pyeloplasty: 50 consecutive cases. BJU Int 88: 526-531
33. Kinukawa T, Hattori R, Ono Y et al (1995) Laparoscopic radical nephrectomy. analysis of 10 cases and preliminary report of retroperitoneal approach. Nippon Hinyokika Gakkai Zasshi 86(11): 1625-1630
34. Dunn MD, Portis AJ, Shalhav AL et al (2000) Laparoscopic versus open radical nephrectomy: a 9-year experience. J Urol 164: 1153-1159
35. Gill IS, Schweizer D, Hobart MG, Sung GT, Klein EA, Novick AC (2000) Retroperitoneal laparoscopic radical nephrectomy: the Cleveland clinic experience. J Urol 163: 1665-1670
36. Gill IS, Soble JJ, Miller SD, Sung GT (1999) A novel technique for management of the en bloc bladder cuff and distal ureter during laparoscopic nephroureterectomy. J Urol 161(2):430-434
37. Gill IS, Sung GT, Hobart M et al (2001) Laparoscopic radical nephroureterectomy for upper tract transitional cell carcinoma: the Cleveland Clinic experience. J Urol 164(5): 1513-1522
38. Salomon L, Hoznek A, Cicco A et al (1999) Retroperitoneoscopic nephroureterectomy for renal pelvic tumors with a single iliac incision. J Urol 161(2):541-544
39. Igarashi T, Tobe T, Mikami K et al (2000) Gasless, hand-assisted retroperitoneoscopic nephroureterectomy for urothelial cancer of the upper urinary tract. Urology 56(5):851-853
40. Gill IS, Delworth MG, Munch LC (1994) Laparoscopic retroperitoneal partial nephrectomy. J Urol 152(5 Pt 1):1539-1542
41. Gettman MT, Bishoff JT, Su LM et al (2001) Hemostatic laparoscopic partial nephrectomy: initial experience with the radiofrequency coagulation-assisted technique. Urology 58(1): 8-11
42. Yoshimura K, Okubo K, Ichioka K, Terada N, Matsuta Y, Arai Y (2001) Laparoscopic partial nephrectomy with a microwave tissue coagulator for small renal tumor. J Urol 165(6 Pt 1): 1893-1896
43. Cadeddu JA, Corwin TS, Traxer O, Collick C, Saboorian HH, Pearle MS (2001) Hemostatic laparoscopic partial nephrectomy: cable-tie compression. Urology 57(3) 562-566

44. Hoznek A, Salomon L, Antiphon P et al (1999) Partial nephrectomy with retroperitoneal laparoscopy. J Urol 162(6):1922-1926
45. Shekarriz H, Shekarriz B, Upadhyay J et al (2000) Hydro-jet assisted laparoscopic partial nephrectomy: initial experience in a porcine model. J Urol 163(3): 1005-1008
46. Elashry OM, Wolf JS Jr, Rayala HJ, McDougall EM, Clayman RV (1997) Recent advances in laparoscopic partial nephrectomy: comparative study of electrosurgical snare electrode and ultrasound dissection. J Endourol 11(1):15-22
47. Chen RN, Novick AC, Gill IS (2000) Laparoscopic cryoablation of renal masses. Urol Clin North Am 27(4):813-820
48. Gaur DD (1997) Retroperitoneal laparoscopic ureteral surgery. In: Gaur DD (ed) Retroperitoneal laparoscopic urology. Oxford University Press, New Delhi, pp 106-132
49. Gaur DD, Agarwal DK, Purohit KC, Darshane AS (1994) Retroperitoneal laparoscopic pyelolithotomy. J Urol 151: 927-929
50. Sinha R, Sharma N (1997) Retroperitoneal laparoscopic management of urolithiasis. J Laparoendosc Adv Surg Tech A 7: 95-98
51. Ghoneimi A, Valla JS, Teyaert H, Aigrain Y (1998) Laparoscopic renal surgery via a retroperitoneal approach in children. J Urol 160: 1138-1140
52. Gaur DD, Punjani HM, Madhusudhana HR, Rathi SS (2001) Retroperitoneal laparoscopic pyelolithotomy: how does it compare with percutaneous nephrolithotomy for larger stones? Min Invas Ther Allied Technol 10(2): 105-1090
53. Gaur DD (1997) Retroperitoneal laparoscopic nephrectomy. In: Gaur DD (ed) Retroperitoneal laparoscopic urology. Oxford University Press, New Delhi, pp 153-173
54. Suzuki K, Ushiyama T, Ishikawa A, Mugiya S, Fujita K (1997) Retroperitoneoscopy assisted live donor nephrectomy: the initial 2 cases. J Urol 158(4):1353-1356
55. Yang SC, Ko WJ, Byun YJ, Rha KH (2001) Retroperitoneoscopy assisted live donor nephrectomy: the Yonsei experience. J Urol 165(4):1099-1102
56. Gaur DD, Garg RK, Trivedi SP, Trivedi S, Prabhudesai MR (2002) Retroperitoneal laparoscopic hand assisted live donor nephrectomy: our initial experience. Min Invas Ther Allied Technol (in press)
57. Schuessler WW, Kavoussi LR, Clayman RV et al (1992) Laparoscopic radical prostatectomy: initial case report. J Urol 147: 246A
58. Guillonneau B, Rozet F, Barret E, Cathelineau X, Vallancien G (2001) Laparoscopic radical prostatectomy: assessment after 240 procedures. Urol Clin North Am 28(1):189-202
59. Bollens R, Vanden Bossche M, Roumeguere T et al (2001) Extraperitoneal laparoscopic radical prostatectomy: results after 50 cases. Eur Urol 40(1):65-69
60. Gaur DD (1997) Retroperitoneal laparoscopic suturing. In: Gaur DD (ed) Retroperitoneal laparoscopic urology. Oxford University Press, New Delhi, pp 68-86
61. Holman E, Salah MA, Toth C (1995) Endoscopic clip-knot suturing technique: preliminary report of application in retroperitoneal ureterolithotomies. J Laparoendosc Surg 5(3):177-180
62. Frede T, Stock C, Renner C et al (1999) Geometry of laparoscopic suturing and knotting techniques. J Endourol 13(3):191-198
63. Breda G, Nakada SY, Rassweiler JJ (2001) Future developments and perspectives in laparoscopy. Eur Urol 40(1): 84-91
64. Matin SF, Gill IS (2001) Laparoscopic ultrasonography. J Endourol 15(1): 87-92
65. Chaffanjon P, Bainville E, Cinquin P, Sarrazin R (1995) Place of computer-assisted surgery in the evaluation of lymphatics metastases in pelvic cancers. Exploration by retroperitoneoscopy. Bull Cancer 82 [Suppl 5]:569-572
66. Bainville E, Chaffanjon P, Cinquin P (1995) Computer generated visual assistance during retroperitoneoscopy. Comput Biol Med 25(2):165-171
67. Seifman BD, Wolf JS Jr (2000) Technical advances in laparoscopy: hand assistance, retractors, and the pneumodissector. J Endourol 14(10): 921-928
68. Pautler SE, Pavlovich CP, Mikityansky I et al (2001) Retroperitoneoscopic-guided radiofrequency ablation of renal tumors. Can J Urol 8(4): 1330-1333

69. Kourambas J, Preminger GM (2001) Advances in camera, video, and imaging technologies in laparoscopy. Urol Clin North Am 28(1) :5-14
70. Micali S, Caione P, Virgili G et al (2001) Retroperitoneal laparoscopic access in children using a direct vision technique. J Urol 165(4):1229-1232
71. Lee BR, Png DJ, Liew L (2000) Laparoscopic telesurgery between the United States and Singapore. Ann Acad Med Singapore 29(5): 665-668
72. Rassweiler J, Frede T, Seemann O, Stock C, Sentker L (2001) Telesurgical laparoscopic radical prostatectomy. initial experience. Eur Urol 40(1):75-83
73. Binder J, Kramer W (2001) Robotically assisted laparoscopic radical prostatectomy. BJU Int 87: 408-410
74. Abbou CC, Hoznek A, Salomon L et al (2001) Laparoscopic radical prostatectomy with a remote controlled robot. J Urol 165(6 Pt 1): 1964-1966
75. Link RE, Schulam PG, Kavoussi LR (2001) Telesurgery. Remote monitoring and assistance during laparoscopy. Urol Clin North Am 28(1): 177-188
76. Matsuda T, Kawakita M, Terachi T (2000) Future of urologic laparoscopy. World J Surg 24(10): 1172-1175
77. Hedican SP (2000) Laparoscopy in urology. Surg Clin North Am 80(5): 1465-85
78. Gill IS (2001) Needlescopic urology: current status. Urol Clin North Am 28(1): 71-83

Chapter 3

Retroperitoneal Anatomy

Guido Virgili, Flavio Forte

Introduction

The retroperitoneum is a part of the abdominal cavity located between the posterior parietal peritoneum and the posterior abdominal wall. The upper part extends to the hepatic peritoneal reflection, the lower part to the extraperitoneal pelvic region.

The retroperitoneal space contains fatty areolar tissue, in which the abdominal aorta and its branches, the inferior vena cava and its roots, lymph nodes, nervous plexuses, the kidneys and adrenal glands, the renal pelvis, and the lumbar portion of the ureters are located. Furthermore, a portion of the pancreas and the second and third portion of the duodenum are also found there. Embryologically, these are intraperitoneal organs; subsequently they lost the posterior serosa, which joined with the posterior parietal peritoneum to become retroperitoneal organs and their anterior surface joined with the posterior parietal peritoneum. The retroperitoneal soft tissue is connected with the abdominal serous spaces through the mesenteric roots and the insertions of the ligaments.

Posterior Wall

The posterior wall of the retroperitoneum delimits the posterior wall of the abdominal cavity; there it consists of the bodies of lumbar vertebrae and, on the side, of the ileo-psoas and quadratus lumborum muscles (Fig. 1). The deep layer of the lumbodorsal aponeurosis and the transverse processes of the lumbar vertebrae represent a border between the retroperitoneal posterior wall and the lumbodorsal region.

Limits

Superiorly the retroperitoneal space extends to the 12th rib and down to the pelvic rim; on the side it reaches the quadratus lumborum muscle and the pelvic rim.

Muscular Layer

Quadratus Lumborum Muscle. The quadratus lumborum muscle is a square-shaped lamina placed between the 12th rib and the pelvic rim. Posteriorly, it connects

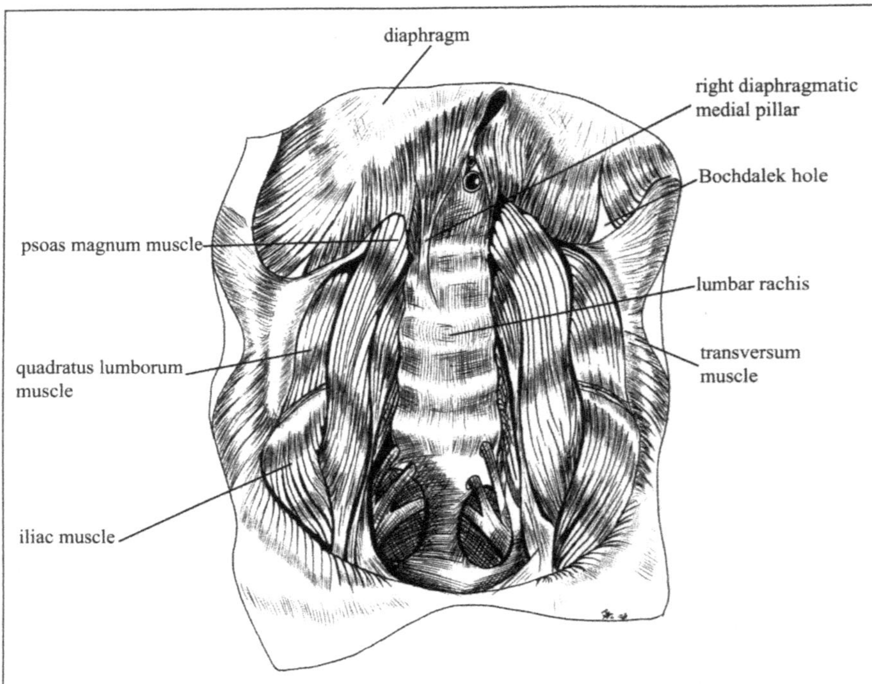

Fig. 1. Frontal view of the retroperitoneal posterior wall

with the deep layer of the lumbodorsal fascia; before that it is covered by a fascia which fixes the boundaries of the abdominal retroperitoneal space. Medially its insertions on the transverse processes of lumbar vertebrae are covered by psoas muscle. On the sides the border of the quadratus lumborum muscle projects from the sacrolumbar muscular mass and joins with the aponeurosis of transverse muscle and the posterior border of the internal oblique muscle. On the upper part the superior lumbar space of Grynfeltt is circumscribed between the borders of quadratus lumborum and internal oblique muscles, the 12th rib, and the inferolateral border of the serratus posteroinferior muscle.

Ileopsoas Muscle. The *psoas magnum muscle* and by the *iliac muscle* make up the ileopsoas muscle. The psoas magnum muscle is a long cylindric muscle originating from the transverse processes of lumbar vertebrae via its dorsal bundles, and from the lateral surfaces of the bodies of D12 - L4 and the intervertebral disks via its ventral bundles. The muscles insert on the vertebrae by fibrous arches through the lumbar vessels and pass the sympathetic branches. The lumbar nerves proceed from the intervertebral spaces; their anterior branches are anastomosed under the muscular fascia, forming the lumbar plexus. The psoas magnum muscle reaches its maximum diameter at the promontorium level; then it slopes down towards the pelvis, forming a groove for the femoral nerve with the iliac muscle. The terminal tendon passes through the *lacuna musculorum* up to the small trocanter of the femur. The *iliac muscle*, flat and triangle shaped, lies on the iliac fossa, extending towards the coxo-femural articulation. Its bundles join with the psoas magnum muscle.

Fascial Layer

The muscular layer is separated from the retroperitoneal connective tissue by a fascia which assumes different names according to the muscles that it covers. It is thin: the upper part is strengthened by the lateral lumbocostal tendinous arch of the diaphragm, which originates from L2 and the 12th rib. Sideways, it extends to the transverse fascia; medially, it passes on the psoas muscle. The lumbar portion of the psoas fascia is strengthened by the medial lumbocostal tendinous arch of the diaphragm; medially, the fascia is fixed to the vertebral column. The inferior part of the psoas fascia is known as the iliac fascia: it covers the iliac muscle, the iliac portion of the psoas magnum, and forms the sheath for the external iliac vessels. It is fixed at the terminal line of the pelvis. The iliac fascia passes behind the inguinal ligament; at this point it is strengthened and its medial portion reaches the ileopectineal eminence, forming the ileopectineal fascia which separates the *lacuna vasorum* from the *lacuna musculorum*.

Anterior Wall

The posterior parietal layer of the peritoneum constitutes the retroperitoneal anterior wall, which is separated by the retroperitoneal muscles by adipose connective tissue containing vessels and nerves.

Retroperitoneal Vessels

The Abdominal Aorta

The abdominal aorta reaches the retroperitoneum through the diaphragmatic hiatus of the aorta; it passes along the anterior surfaces of the bodies of the lumbar vertebrae, lying on the anterior longitudinal ligament. At the L4 level it is divided into the two common iliac arteries and ends with the medial sacral artery (Fig. 2).

The parietal branches of the aorta are distributed along the abdominal walls and are anastomosed with the intercostal arteries, the internal thoracic artery, the deep circumflex iliac arteries, and the inferior epigastric artery. The aorta proceeds from the body of pancreas, the third portion of the duodenum, and the mesenteric root. On the right side is the inferior vena cava; between the two great vessels lies the right medial pillar of diaphragm, the right celiac ganglion, and the caudal lobe of the liver (Table 1).

Table 1. Aortic branches

Abdominal Aorta

Parietal branches	Visceral branches
Inferior Diaphragmatic Arteries	Celiac trunk
Lumbar arteries	Superior mesenteric a.
	Inferior mesenteric a.
	Middle suprarenal aa.
	Renal aa.
	Gonadal aa.

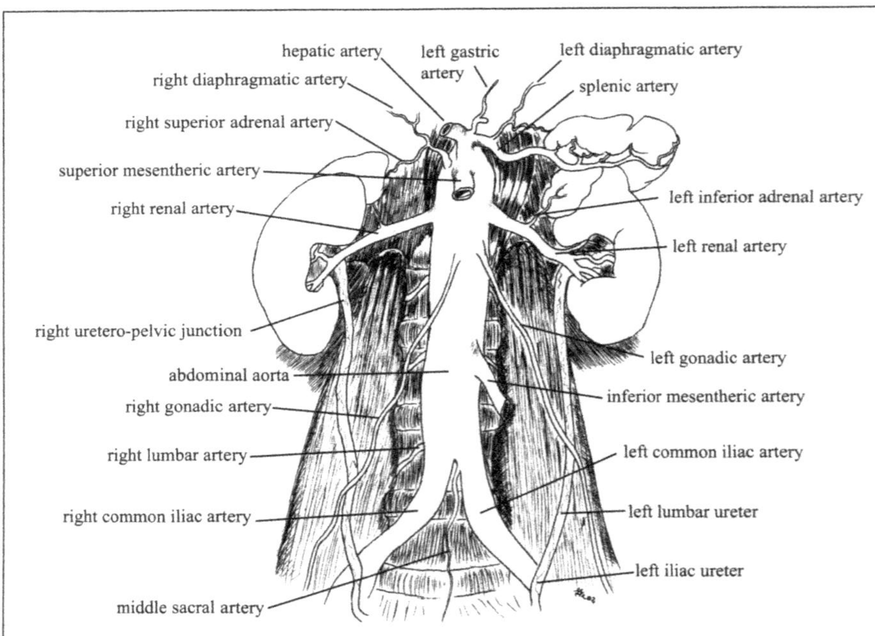

Fig. 2. The abdominal aorta and the retroperitoneal arteries

The Inferior Vena Cava

The inferior vena cava lies along the right side of the vertebral column; it starts at the confluence of the common iliac veins, at the L4 level. It passes behind the head of pancreas and crosses the diaphragm through the caval diaphragmatic cavity (Fig. 3). Interposed between the inferior vena cava and the abdominal wall are the right sympathetic trunk, the lumbar vessels, the right renal vein, and the right adrenal gland. Its tributary vessels are the inferior diaphragmatic veins, the lumbar veins (as parietal branches), the right gonadal vein, the middle adrenal veins, the renal veins, and the hepatic veins (as visceral branches).

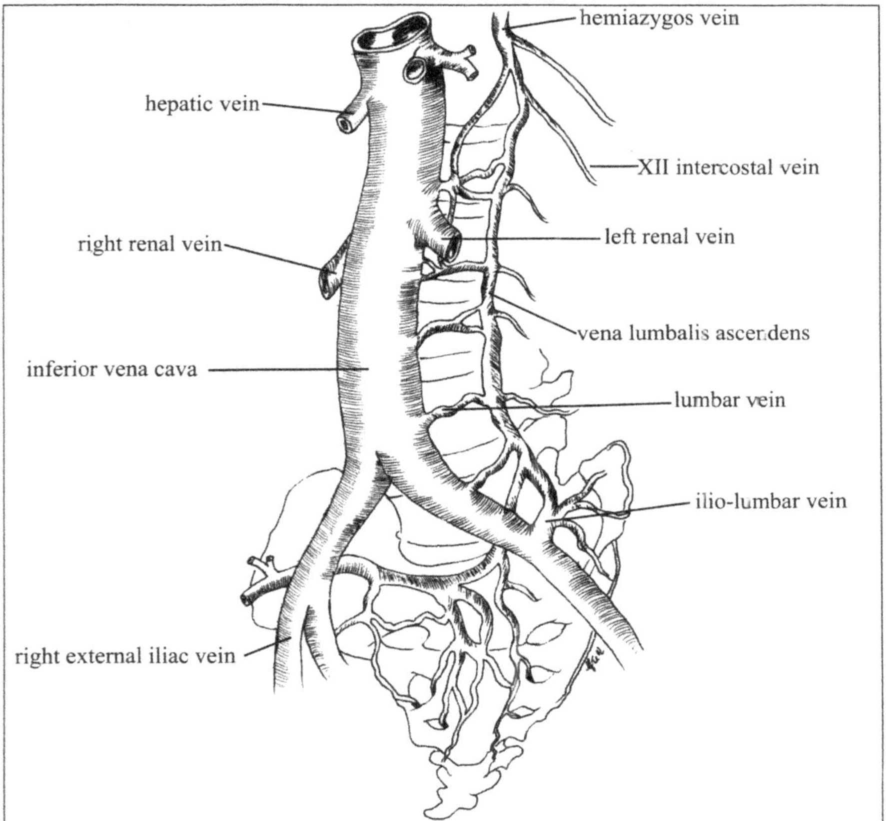

Fig. 3. The inferior vena cava and the retroperitoneal veins

Other Vessels

The common iliac artery proceeds inferolaterally towards the sacroiliac joint, where it divides into the internal and external iliac arteries. The right common iliac vein is behind the corresponding artery, while the left one is medially situated at the left common iliac artery and passes behind the right artery to reach the inferior vena cava. Its tributaries are the iliolumbar veins and the branches of the sacral venous plexus. The middle sacral vein reaches the left common iliac vein. The common iliac vessels pass along the medial border of the psoas magnum muscle: the muscular fascia forms a sheath which contains the vessels and the internal iliac lymph nodes. Behind the common iliac vessels lie the lumbosacral nervous trunk, the obturator nerve, and the sympathetic trunk; the sympathetic branches of the abdominal aortic plexus lie in front of the vessels. In females the ovarian vessels and their sympathetic nervous plexuses are present. The ureters pass over the vessels.

The external iliac artery passes laterally to the sacroiliac joint, under the inguinal ligament; the vein is situated behind and below the artery. Before the inguinal ligament the vas deferens in males and the roundish ligament in females cross the vessels. The external iliac lymph nodes lie on the vessels, extending into the vascular sheath.

The gonadal vessels, the lumbar vessels, the iliolumbar artery, and the deep circumflex iliac arteries pass to the side of the spinal trunk. The gonadal arteries are accompanied by the gonadal veins, which drain the testes in males and the ovaries in females, and also the ureteral, peritoneal, and retroperitoneal vessels.

Usually five lumbar arteries derive from the aorta; they pass under the psoas arches at the level of the lumbar vertebrae. The lumbar veins extend to the inferior vena cava; the left lumbar veins pass behind the aorta to reach the vena cava. Sideways the lumbar veins are connected by anastomoses which are located behind the psoas muscle and in front of the transverse processes of the lumbar vertebrae, forming the ascending lumbar vein, which extends from the iliolumbar vein to the azygos and hemiazygos veins.

The iliolumbar artery, deriving from the internal iliac artery, extends upward, behind the psoas muscle, where it gives off a lumbar branch, a spinal branch, and an iliac trunk.

Nervous Structures

The sympathetic lumbar trunks lie on the side of the spinal trunk; the right one is covered by the inferior vena cava and the left one by the aorta. From these trunks several branches are derived that form the celiac plexus; this is located in front of the aorta at the level of D11 - D12, L1 - L2 (Fig. 4). The celiac plexus covers the aorta, the celiac trunk, and the superior mesenteric artery; to the side it gives off branches for the adrenal glands and the kidneys and inferior branches for the pancreas, too. It is covered by the peritoneum, at the level of the posterior wall of the omental bursa. The celiac plexus is formed by several ganglia. The right one, semilunar shaped, lies on the diaphragmatic right medial pillar; its left portion takes the celiac trunks of the posterior vagal nerve, while the right portion receives the splanchnic nerves, forming the nervous ansa of Wrisberg. The left celiac ganglion lies on the diaphragmatic left medial pillar: it gives off branches for the left adrenal vein and receives the left splanchnic nerve. The aortoabdominal plexus lies below the celiac plexus, in front of the aorta: it continues along the internal iliac arteries as the hypogastric plexus. Between the muscular bundles of the psoas muscle the lumbar plexus is found.

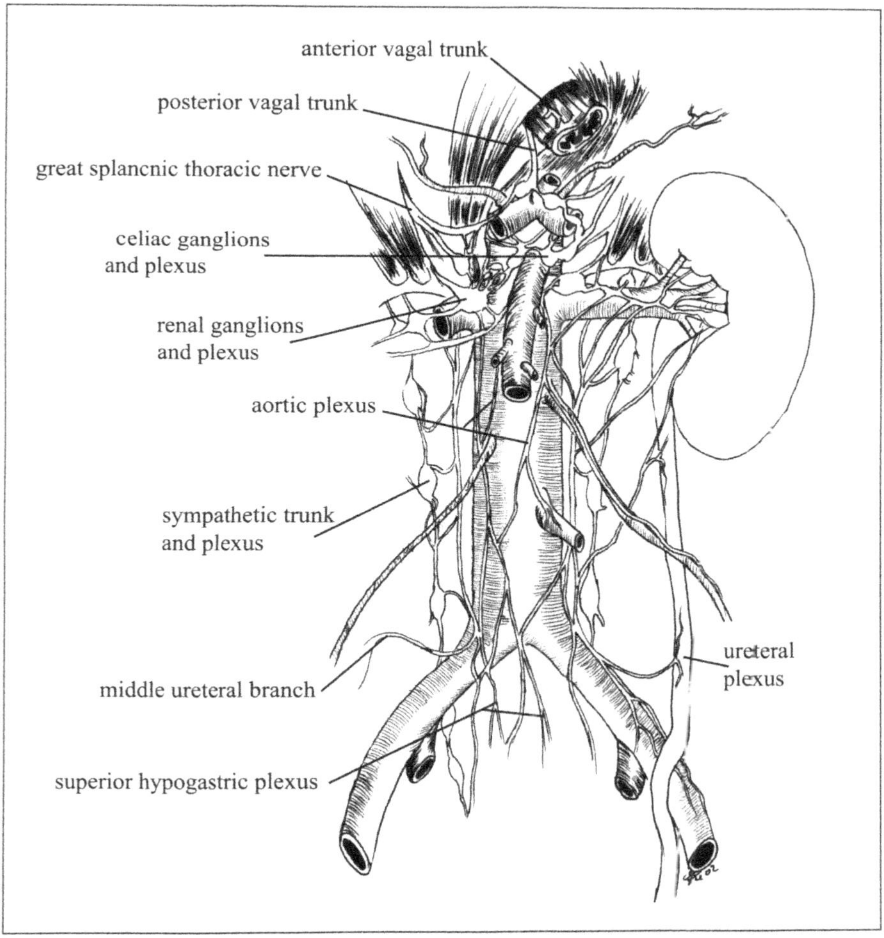

Fig. 4. The retroperitoneal nervous structures

Lymph Nodes

The retroperitoneal lymph nodes are divided into four groups: left para-aortic, right para-aortic, preaortic, and retroaortic lymph nodes (Fig. 5). The para-aortic lymph nodes are the most important in the lymphatic drainage of the kidney. The left kidney drains into four to five para-aortic lymph nodes located at the left side of the aorta, near the renal vein. The left para-aortic lymph nodes form a chain along the left aortic border: the upper lymph node lies at the level of the left diaphragmatic pillar and gives off some lymphatic branches which reach the thoracic duct. The right para-aortic lymph nodes lie around the inferior vena cava: the prevenous ones are below the renal veins and the retrovenous ones lie on the roots of the psoas muscle and the right diaphragmatic pillar.

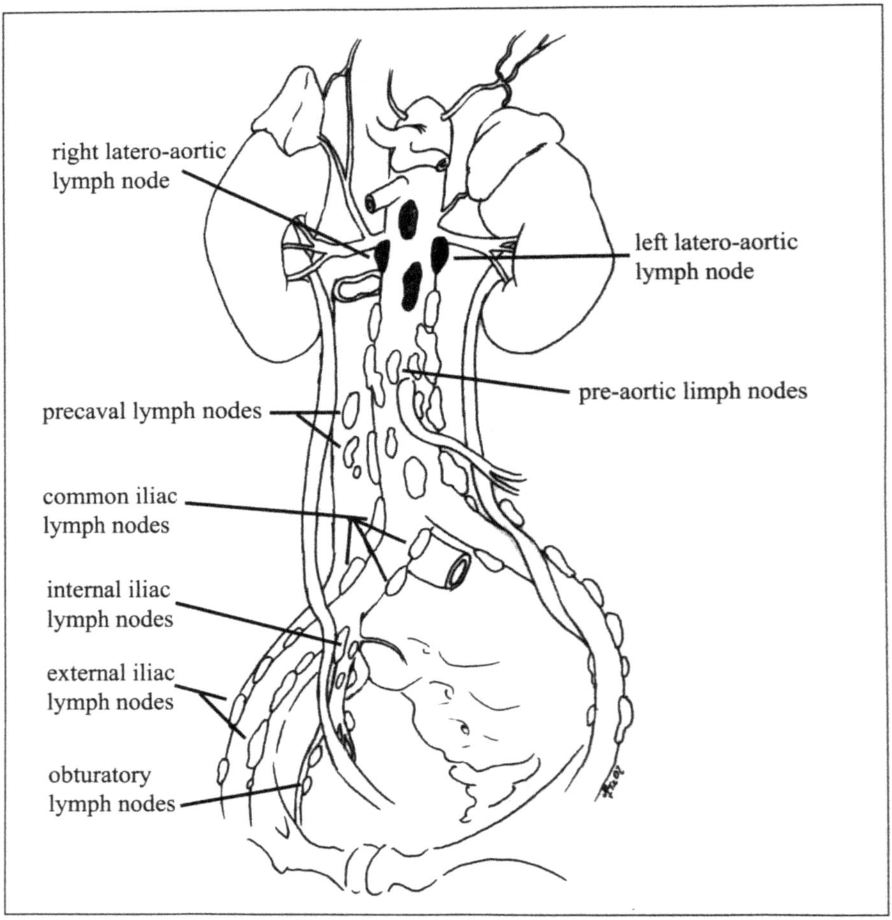

Fig. 5. The retroperitoneal lymph nodes

Renal Loggia

The renal loggia is formed by an anterior fibrous layer known as the prerenal fascia, and a posterior one known as Zuckerkandl retrorenal fascia. The prerenal fascia ex-

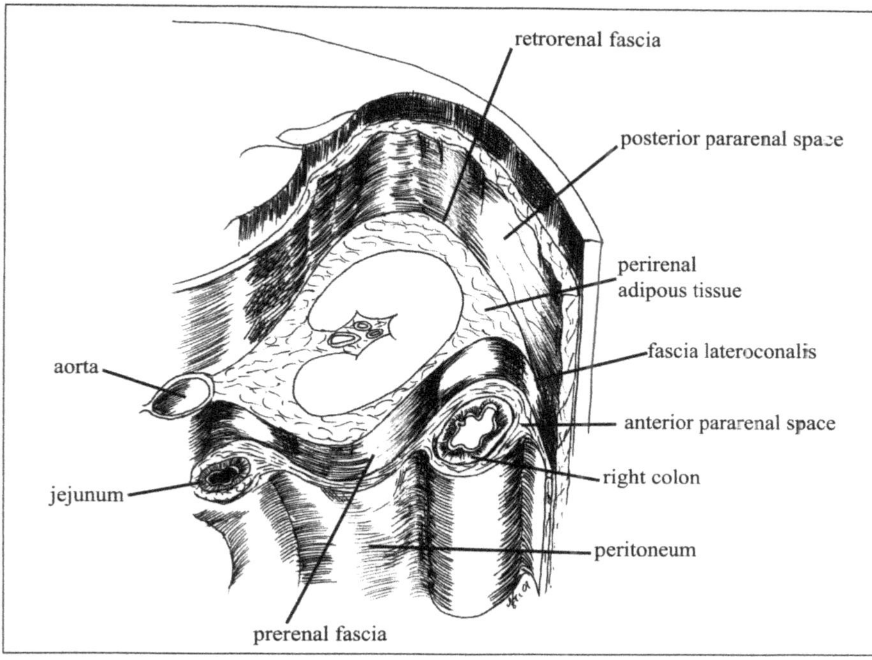

Fig. 6. The renal loggia

tends from the lateral border of the kidney to the anterior surface of the aorta and the inferior vena cava, where it joins the contralateral one (Fig. 6). The prerenal fascia is thickened by the Toldt lamina at the level of the right and left colon. The Zuckerkandl fascia lies behind the kidneys: it is separated from the transverse fascia via Gerota's adipose layer or pararenal adipose body. The Zuckerkandl fascia ends at the level of the lumbar vertebrae. The prerenal and Zuckerkandl fascia are fixed to the diaphragm at the adrenal glands, whereas inferiorly, under the kidneys, they usually end in the retroperitoneal tissue. To the sides, behind the right and left colon, the prerenal and Zuckerkandl fascias are joined with n the so-called fascia lateroconalis, which divides the posterior pararenal space from the anterior one. The fascia lateroconalis joins the Toldt line and, sideways, closes the anterior pararenal space.

The renal loggia contains Gerota's capsule, the adrenal gland, and the kidney with its vascular pedicle and the renal pelvis. Gerota's capsule is an adipose layer, its posterior wall being thicker, which envelops the kidney and the adrenal gland; it is covered by the prerenal and Zuckerkandl fasciae.

The Adrenal Gland

The adrenal glands cover the upper poles of both kidneys. The right one is triangle shaped, with its anterior surface facing the liver and the inferior one the upper

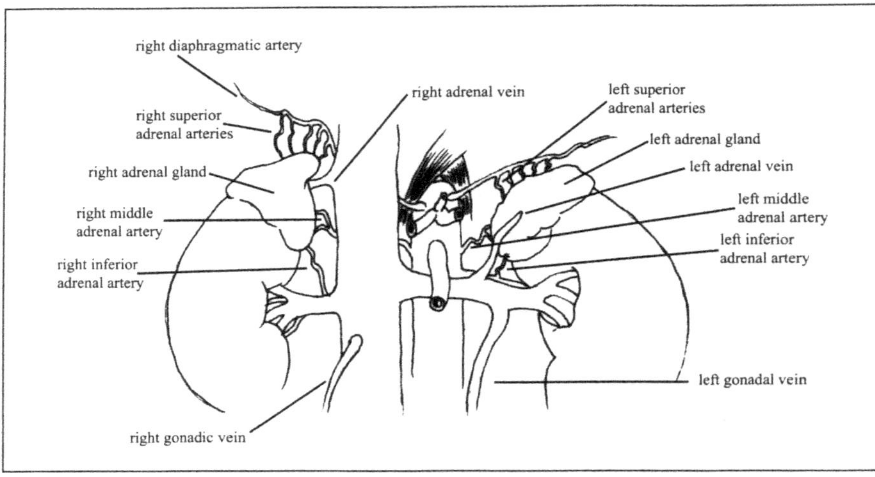

Fig. 7. Vascularization of the adrenal glands

pole of the kidney and, usually, directly on the renal vascular pedicle. The posterior surface lies on the diaphragm. The left adrenal gland is smaller than the right; it faces the stomach anteriorly, the spleen sideways, the upper pole of the kidney and the diaphragm posteriorly, and the pancreas and splenic vessels inferiorly.

The Adrenal Vessels

The adrenal arteries are usually divided into three groups: the superior adrenal arteries, which arise from the inferior diaphragmatic artery; the middle adrenal artery, which arises usually from the aorta (sometimes from the renal artery or the celiac trunk); and the inferior adrenal artery, arising from the renal artery (Fig. 7). The right adrenal vein is short and drains directly into the inferior vein, whereas the left one is longer and drains into the left renal vein.

Lymphatic Vessels And Nerves

Two trunks that lie on the adrenal vein are responsible for lymphatic drainage. The adrenal gland is innervated by the great splanchnic nerve and the great splanchnic ganglion.

The Kidney

The kidneys are bean shaped; the left one extends from D11 to L2 - L3, the right one from the 12th rib to L3 (Fig. 8). The renal axis is oblique and so the upper poles are closer to the sagittal or middle line, represented by the vertebral column and the aorta and inferior vena cava. The right kidney faces the posterior surface of the right lobe

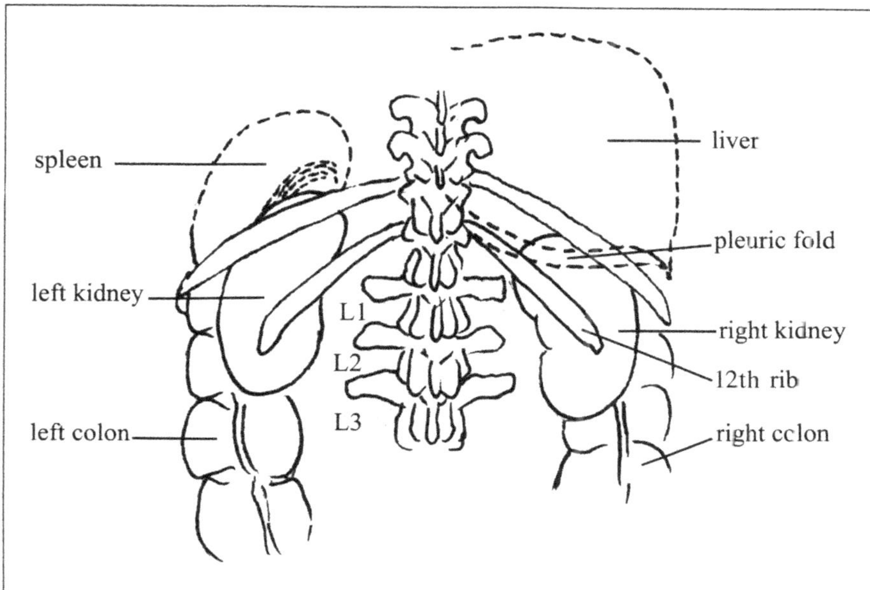

Fig. 8. Topographic relationships of the kidneys

of the liver. The posterolateral border of the liver extends to cover the right kidney posteriorly: this is important if a percutaneous approach to the upper pole of the right kidney is required. Moreover, the right hepatic triangular ligament, which joins the liver to the diaphragm, passes between the right renal hilum and the inferior vena cava: it must be resected in surgical renocaval neoplastic thrombosis procedures. The inferior portion of the right kidney is covered by the right colon, whereas the duodenum covers its hilum and the renal pelvis. The spleen is found medial to the left kidney, whereas its anterior surface faces the stomach and pancreas.
The upper half of the left kidney and the upper third of the right one are in the thorax; behind the upper pole of both kidneys is the pleural fold, which lies on the periosteum of the 12th rib, thus limiting the percutaneous approach to the kidney at an inferior level.

As the upper half of the left kidney and the upper third of the right one are considered to be in the thorax, the middle inferior portion of both kidneys is found at the lumbar level and, with its posterior surface, lies on the quadratus lumborum muscle, in front of the 12th intercostal nerve and the iliohypogastric and ilioinguinal nerves. Sideways this part of the renal posterior surface exceeds the lateral border of the quadratus lumborum muscle and faces the muscles of the abdominal lateral wall, at the level of the Grynfellt square and the Petit triangle.

In the middle part of the medial border of both kidneys is the hilum, which contains first the renal vein, in the middle the renal artery, and then the renal pelvis. The renal pelvis is subdivided into two to three major calyces, from which arise seven to eight minor calyces. From a surgical point of view the pelvis is de-

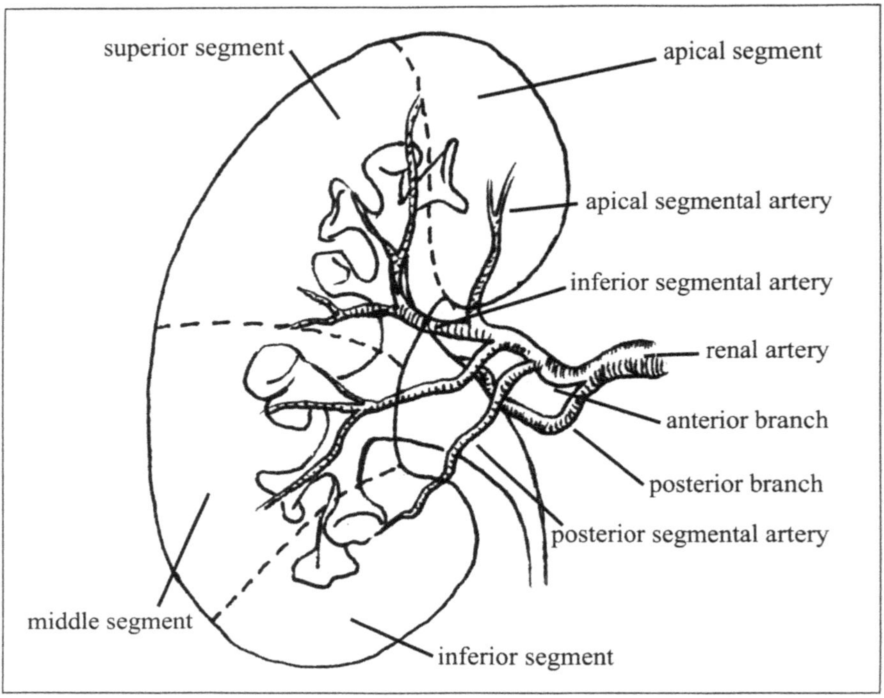

Fig. 9. Vascularization of the right kidney

fined as intrarenal or extrarenal; an intrarenal pelvis originates from a later division of the ureteral bud, which gives shorter calyces.

Renal Vessels

The renal artery arises from the aorta (Fig. 9). The double renal artery is most commonly found on the right side: sometimes small supranumerary vessels reach the renal poles arising from the aorta. Most of the accessory arteries which go to the lower pole extend directly into the cortex. The arteries for the upper pole are small and arise from the main renal artery: in some cases accessory arteries may be found arising from the gonadal or superior mesenteric arteries. From the renal artery derive anterior and posterior branches. Five main segmental arteries arise from these two trunks: the apical or suprahilar artery, the superior artery, the middle artery, the inferior artery, and the posterior artery. During a percutaneous approach to the collector system of the kidney, any bleeding usually stems from injury to one of the anterior or posterior segmental arteries. The arteries for the renal adipose capsule are represented by a plexus constituted by three trunks: a superior capsular artery, arising from the middle and superior adrenal arteries; the middle capsular artery, arising from the renal artery; and the inferior capsular artery, deriving from the ureteral and gonadal arteries. The venous drainage of the kidney is represented by the renal vein, into which the inferior diaphragmatic vein, the gonadal vein, and one to three lumbar veins drain. The renal vein drains directly into the inferior vena cava.

Renal Innervation

The renal innervation derives from the renal plexus, which lies on the anterior surface of the renal artery. It receives branches from the celiac plexus, from the splanchnic nerves, which extend directly to the kidney or up to the aortorenal ganglia, from the second sympathetic lumbar ganglion, from the posterior renal ganglion, and from the superior hypogastric ganglion. Renal lymphatic drainage and lymph nodes are described in the section "Lymph Nodes".

The Ureter

Three morphofunctional regions can be distinguished in the ureter: the uretero-pelvic junction, the intermediate tract, and the vesicoureteric junction (Fig. 2).

The ureters are about 28-34 cm long; the left one, longer than the right, ends in the intermediate layer of the retroperitoneal fascia, joining the renal fascia, and is strongly adhered to the peritoneum. In males the ureters pass along the middle part of the psoas muscle and the left colic artery and cross over the genitofemoral nerve. After crossing the common iliac artery, the ureter follows the path of the hypogastric artery, passing medially to the sciatic spine and crossing the vas deferens, then reaching the bladder. In females, after the sciatic spine, the ureter passes behind the ovary, strongly connected with the ovarian suspending ligament, forming the posterior border of the ovarian fossa; it then enters the parametrium and passes along the uterosacral, cardinal, and uterovesical ligaments. The uterine artery crosses the ureter near the point at which the latter is surrounded by the vaginal and perivesical venous plexuses; the ureter passes the lateral vaginal fornix for almost 1 cm and sideways to the cervix for 1-4 cm and then reaches the bladder.

Ureteral Vessels

The ureteral vessels arise from the renal artery (30%), the aorta (15.4%), the gonadal arteries (7.7%), the superior and inferior vesical arteries (12.8% and 12.9%, respectively), and the internal iliac arteries (8.5%). The superior ureteral veins usually drain into the lower branch or main trunk of the renal vein or, alternatively, into the gonadal vein. The lower ureteral vein drains into the perivesical plexus and, in females, into the vaginal and ovarian plexuses.

Ureteral Lymph Nodes

The upper ureteral lymphatic vessels drain into the aortic lymph nodes located around the origin of the gonadal artery: the middle ureteral lymphatic vessels follow the arteries and extend to the common iliac lymph nodes, whereas the lower ureteral ones extend to the common, the internal, and the external lymph nodes and the interaortocaval lymph nodes.

Ureteral Nerves

The ureter is innervated by the superior ureteral nerve through the renal and aortic plexuses, by the middle ureteral nerve through the superior hypogastric plexus, and by the inferior ureteral nerve through the pelvic plexus.

Chapter 4

Retroperitoneal Access

SALVATORE MICALI, PAOLO CAIONE

Introduction

The first attempts to explore the retroperitonem were made almost 80 years ago, when gas was insufflated into the retroperitoneum for gas contrast studies to delineate renal and adrenal tumors [1]. Endoscopes were not used until the 1970s. Early animal experiments proved the feasibility and safety of pneumoretroperitoneum, and Roberts placed a fetoscope into Gerota's fascia under radiologic guidance and with CO_2 insufflation was able to visualize the kidney [2]. Retroperitoneoscopic urological surgery using CO_2 insufflation to create a pneumoretroperitoneum was first reported by Wickham's pioneering efforts in performing an extraperitoneal laparoscopic ureteral lithotomy in 1978 [3]. Ten years later no further improvements in retroperitoneoscopy had been accomplished; in fact, Clayman et al. performed the first nephrectomy using a retropeitoneal approach, but the difficulty in creating a pneumoretroperitoneum that permitted a satsifactory work space prompted them to pursue the transperitoneal approach in subsequent cases [4].

The laparoscopic approach has been applied to a wide variety of procedures in the field of urology. Since 1992 urologists have adopted laparoscopy from other specialities; most of the procedures described have been based on the traditional transperitoneal approach. Well-defined organ systems and a relative paucity of introperitoneal fat allow for rapid identification of landmarks. Instilled gas expands the space in a predictable manner to allow for optimal visualization. In contrast, in traditional open urologic surgery, most urogenital organs are approached through a retroperitoneal access. However, it is technically difficult to develop a consistent working space in the retroperitoneum, which is occupied by areolar and fat tissues. This may explain why most of the initial urologic laparoscopic procedures were performed transperitoneally [5]. Concern also exists regarding the risk of postoperative adhesions with a transperitoneal approach compared with extraperitoneal surgery. Adhesions have been associated with postoperative pain, bowel obstruction, and difficulty in performing subsequent surgical procedures. Moreover, laparoscopic procedures have a risk of injury to intraperitoneal structures [6].

The posterior peritoneum is attached to the body wall by delicate and dense fibrous bands, which can restrict the ability of simple insufflation to create this working space. Gaur was the first to describe preliminary balloon distension of the retroperitoneal space [7]. This is the underlying concept of the increased interest in retroperitoneoscopy and pelvic extraperitoneoscopy. During the past 7–8 years, increasing experience at various centers has led to the refinement of laparoscopic techniques that take advantage of the strengths of the retroperitoneal approach while overcoming its perceived disadvantages [8-12].

Techniques To Create a Retroperitoneal Space

Patient Preparation

Preoperative preparation for establishing pneumoretroperitoneum is similar to the open or laparoscopic procedure except for minor variations dictated by the type of surgery. The patient should be informed about possible vascular and bowel injuries that may necessitate open intervention. For major extirpative surgeries, two units of autologous blood are donated. The immediate preoperative placement of a urethral catheter is routinely advised. A rigid ureteral catheter, open tip, could be inserted to facilitate identification of the ureter during the procedures and furthermore a contrast study can be done.

Patient Positioning

The patient is placed in the lateral decubitus position with the table flexed and the kidney rest extended close to the skin. Additionally, a rolled towel can be placed between the operating table and the patient, to maximize the space between the 12th rib and the iliac crest; then the patient is secured on the operating table with roll tape. Some authors suggest, in indications such as adrenalectomy, the prone position for a retroperitoneal posterior approach. The advantages and disadvantages are not clear yet, except for better vascular control of the adrenal and kidney pedicles. Unfortunately, this technique is not as popular as the flank access and the worldwide experience has been limited [13, 14].

Access to the Retroperitoneum

Several techniques were developed in the last decade to establish a correct and safe access to the retroperitoneum.

Closed Technique with the Veress Needle

Following retrograde placement of a ureteral occlusion balloon catheter, the patient is placed prone on a table with fluoroscopy capability. The collecting system of the affected kidney is opacified by injecting contrast dye through the ureteral catheter. At the inferior lumbar triangle, bounded by the latissimus dorsi, external oblique muscle, and iliac crest, a small skin incision is made and the Veress needle is introduced perpendicularly for a distance of 3–4 cm. The needle is gradually advanced under fluoroscopic control until the tip lies just above the horizontal plane of the kidney. Anatomically, the tip of the needle should now reside within Gerota's fascia and just below the lower pole of the kidney. Insufflation with CO_2 is begun with the pressure set at 15 mmHg and, initially, at least 2 l/min of insufflation in the retroperitoneum is necessary. Insufflation pressure may have to be increased up to 25 mmHg to achieve adequate pneumoretroperitoneum.

Alternatively, the patient may be placed in the lateral decubitus position and similar steps followed. The Veress needle may be introduced at the lumbar triangle without floroscopic guidance. This technique was the first attempt to create a retroperitoneal space, but retroperitoneal fat is dense and a minimal dissection is required to create an adequate working space; in such cases an additional device such as a balloon should be used to create a reasonable working space [15].

Balloon Technique

A 1.5- to 2-cm skin incision is created below the tip of the last rib and the flank muscle fibers are bluntly separated. Entry is gained into the retroperitoneum by gently piercing the anterior thoracolumbar fascia. Finger dissection of the retroperitoneum is performed in a cephalad direction, remaining anterior to the psoas muscle and posterior to the Gerota's fascia to create a space for placement of the balloon dilator.

The most common dissecting balloon device is fashioned from a middle finger of a sterile number 8 surgical glove and tied to the end of a 14 Fr red rubber catheter. The balloon device is inserted in the retroperitoneum and gradually distended with normal saline, according to the individual patient's body (1.0–1.2 l in thin adults and 1.2–1.8 l in slightly obese adults). The balloon is kept inflated for 5 min to facilitate hemostasis. Alternatively, balloon devices are made following Gaur's idea, using condoms, whole surgical gloves, party balloons, a Foley catheter, saline distension balloons, and nephroscope balloon devices [16-18]. Unfortunately, homemade balloon devices are associated with a high rupture risk with loose fragments [19]. For safe use, employing a trocar-mounted industrial-made balloon distension device with a balloon rupture guarantee is recommended. Balloon dilation in the pararenal fat, between the psoas muscle posteriorly and Gerota's fascia anteriorly, effectively displaces the kidney anteromedially and expedites direct access to the posterior aspect of the renal hilum and adjacent great vessel [20]. This facilitates retroperitoneal nephrectomy; dilation of other retroperitoneal areas can be employed for other retroperitoneoscopic indications. Following balloon deflation and removal, a trocar is placed as the primary port and pneumoretroperitoneum is created to 15 mmHg with CO_2. Finally, accessory trocars can be placed under direct vision of the primary trocar.

Blunt Finger Dissection

A 15- to 18-mm incision is made in the lumbar (Petit's) triangle between the 12th rib and the iliac crest, bounded by the lateral edges of the latissimus dorsum and external oblique muscles. A tunnel is created down to the retroperitoneal space by blunt dissection. This tunnel is dilated until an index finger can be inserted to push the retroperitoneum forward, thus creating a retroperitoneal cavity. Finger dissection continues in the space between the lumbar aponeurosis and Gerota's fascia and secondary trocars are inserted under laparoscopic guidance. Additional working space is created by gas insufflation dissection aided by a swinging movement of the laparoscope, which allows blunt dissection of the loose perirenal tissue [21, 22].

Direct Vision Technique

The initial retroperitoneal access site is the lumbar triangle (Petit's triangle) (Fig. 1). With the patient secured in the standard flank position, and the operating table flexed, the space between the 12th rib and the iliac crest is maximized (Fig. 2). This allows the surgeon to find Petit's triangle. A 12-mm incision is made within this area and a laparoscopic visual trocar, Visiport (Auto Suture, US Surgical Corporation, Norwalk, Conn.), is advanced directly into the retroperitoneum under direct vision using the Visiport. This device incises each tissues layer under direct vision, thus giving the surgeon complete visual control so as to avoid injuring blood vessels, nerves, etc., as he enters the retroperitoneum. Penetration of Scarpa's fascia, the flank muscle, and lumbodorsal fascia can be felt and seen subsequently in some patients. The lumbodorsal fascia was clearly seen in all cases and most obviously was felt to "give" once the fascia was cut [Fig. 3]. After the lumbodorsal fascia is traversed the retroperitoneum is encountered and the characteristic fat is seen. Insufflation with CO_2 at 15 mmHg is then instituted. The laparoscope is then used to bluntly dissect the retroperitoneal space and mobilize the lateral peritoneal from the anterior abdominal wall. Care must be taken when dissecting to prevent

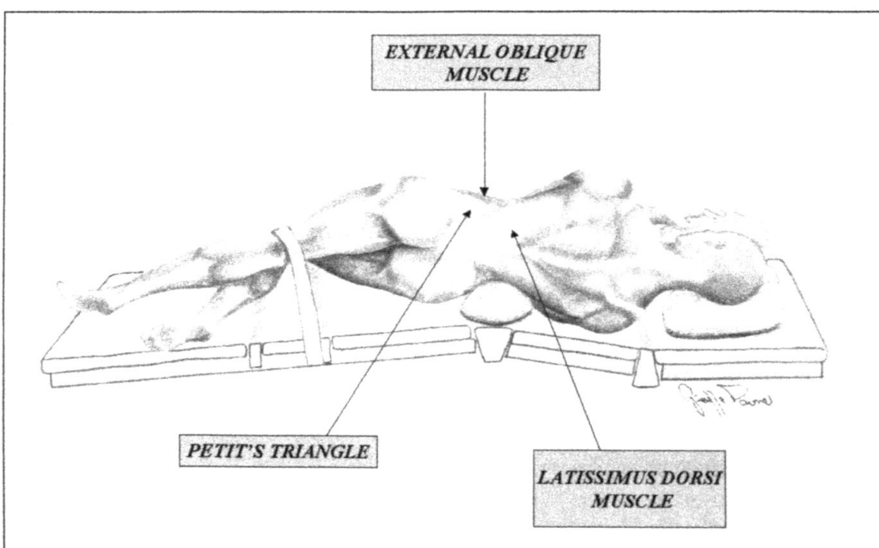

Fig. 1. Location of Petit's triangle in relation to patient position

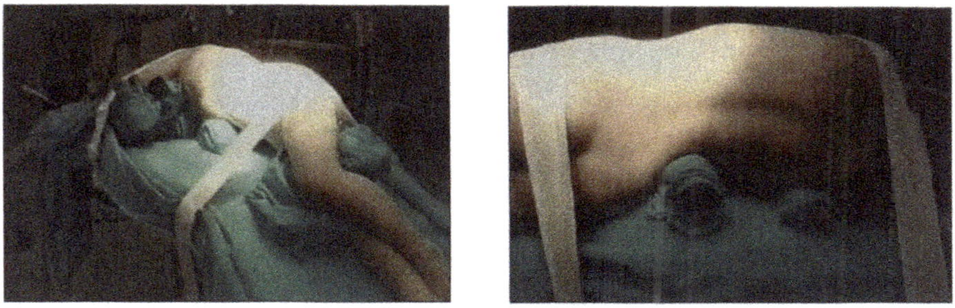

Fig. 2. Patient positioning for retroperitoneal access

peritoneal tearing. In a series of 31 retroperitoneal laparoscopic procedures, direct vision access was achieved within 3 min (range, 1-5 min) [23].

The direct visual retroperitoneal access technique is simple and safe and does not require extensive laparoscopic experience. Moreover, this tecnique is rapid and reliable for retroperitoneal access and creation of a retroperitoneal space in the pediatric population. Recently, a 5-mm, direct visual access device has become available, which represents a very good advantage for a pediatric popolation.

Conclusions

The performance of retroperitoneal and pelvic extraperitoneal laparoscopy is increasing. A questionnaire survey of 24 urologic centers worldwide revealed that, in 1993, only 28% of laparoscopic procedures were performed retroperitoneoscopically (72% were performed by transperitoneal laparoscopy). In comparison, in 1996, the retroperitoneal/extraperitoneal approach was performed in 51% of urologic laparoscopic interventions (49% of procedures were perfored transperitoneally) [24]. Compared with transperitoneal laparoscopy, retroperitoneoscopy has distinct drawbacks and advantages. Its primary drawback is the smaller working space in the retroperitoneum; this results in crowding of trocars, restricted maneuverability of the instruments, and problems with orientation. During the learning curve phase, retroperitoneoscopy may be technically somewhat more demanding than transperitoneal laparoscopy: despite the fact that survey respondents are highly experienced laparoscopists, 48% feel more comfortable while performing transperitoneal laparoscopy as compared to 30% who prefer retroperitoneoscopy. However, retroperitoneoscopy offers inherent advantages. By allowing direct access to the retroperitoneum, it obviates the need to enter the peritoneal cavity and mobilize the colon, thus minimizing, although not entirely eliminating, the chances of intraperitoneal organ injury. The posterior approach should be better evaluated, advantages and disadvantages need to be studied carefully, since this approach could be considered as an alternative to the flank position. With the increasing acceptance of laparoscopy in urologic surgery, the scope and application of retroperitoneoscopy will develop further. More experience

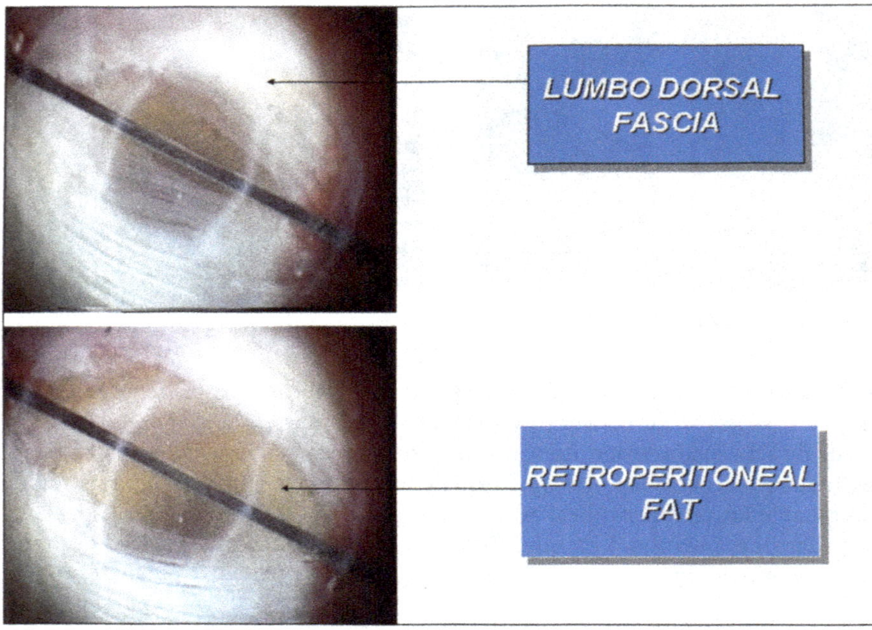

Fig. 3. Internal view of retroperitoneal space and lumbodorsal fascia in a patient in whom incision was made by the Visiport device

with technique and instrumentations will make the retroperitoneum a more "familiar" space for the urologic surgeon.

Retroperitoneoscopy is an important adjunct to the laparoscopic armamentarium in urology. For the experienced laparoscopist, facility in both transperitoneal and retroperitoneal techniques is essential for providing patients with the optimal minimally invasive approach.

References

1. Robertson LH, Andersen EE, Glenn JF (1965) Retroperitoneal contrast study: simplified bilateral perirenal carbon dioxide insufflation. J Urol 93: 414
2. Robert JA (1976) Retroperitoneal endoscopy. J Med Primatol 5: 124
3. Wickham JEA (1979) The surgical treatment of renal lithiasis. In: Wickham JEA (ed) Urinary calculus disease. Churchill Livingstone, New York, pp 145-198
4. Clayman RV, Kavoussi LR, Soper NJ et al (1992) Laparoscopic nephrectomy: review of the initial 10 cases. J Endourol 6: 127
5. Clayman RV, Kavoussi LR, Soper NJ, Dierks SM, Meretyk S, Darcy MD, Roemer FD, Pingleton ED, Thomson PG, Long SR (1991) Laparoscopic nephrectomy: initial case report. J Urol 146: 278-282
6. Capelouto CC, Kavoussi LR (1993) Complications of laparoscopic surgery. Urology 42: 2
7. Gaur DD (1992) Laparoscopic operative retroperitoneoscopy: use of a new device. J Urol 148: 1137
8. Rassweiler JJ, Henkel TO, Stock C, et al (1994) Retroperitonel laparoscopic nephrec-

tomy and other procedures in the upper retroperitoneum using a balloon dissection technique. Eur Urol 25: 229-236

9. McDougall EM, Clayman RV (1996) Laparoscopic nephrectomy for benign disease: comparison of the transperitoneal and retroperitoneal aproach. J Endourol 10: 45-49
10. Gill IS (1998) Reteroperitoneal laparoscopic nephrectomy. Urol Clin North Am 25: 343-360
11. Rassweiler JJ, Seemann O, Frede T et al (1998) Retroperitoneoscopy: experience with 200 cases. J Urol 160: 1265-1269
12. Adams JB, Micali S, Moore RG, Babayan RK, Kavoussi LR (1996) Complications of extraperitoneal balloon dilation. J Endourol 10:(4), 375-378
13. Baba S (2000) Laparoscopic adrenalectomy: posterior approach. Biomed Pharmacother 54(1): 161-163
14. Siperstein AE, Beber E, Engle KL, Duh QY, Clark OH (2000) Laparoscopic posterior adrenalectomy: technical considerations. Arch Surg 135(8): 967-971
15. Chiu AW, Chen K, Wang J, Huang WJS, Chang LS (1995) Direct needle insufflation for pneumoretroperitoneum: anatomic confirmation and clinical experience. Urology 46(3): 432-437
16. Chan YK, Pope AJ, Webb DR (1996) Extraperitoneal laparoscopy: anatomical dissections with experimental balloon dilators. BJU Int 77: 296-301
17. Keeley FX, Tolley DA (1999) Retroperitoneal laparoscopy. BJU Int 84: 212-215
18. Ono Y, Katoh N, Kinukawa T, Matsuura O, Ohshima S (1996) Laparoscopic nephrectomy via the retroperitoneal approach. J Urol 156: 1101-1104
19. Adams JB, Micali S, Moore RG, Babayan RK, Kavoussi LR (1996) Complications of extraperitoneal balloon dilation. J Endourol 10(4): 375-378
20. Gill IS (1998) Retroperitoneal laparoscopic nephrectomy. Urol Clin North Am 25(2): 343-360
21. El-Ghoneimi A, Valla' HS, Aigrain Y (1998) Laparoscopic renal surgery via a retroperitoneal approach in children. J Urol 160: 1138-1141
22. Rassweiler JJ, Seemann O, Frede T, Henkel TO, Alken P (1998) Retroperitoneoscopy: Experience with 200 cases. J Urol 160: 1265-1269
23. Micali S, Caione P, Virgili G, Capozza N, Scarfini M, Micali F (2001) Retroperitoneal laparoscopic access in children using direct vision technique. J Urol 165: 1229-1232
24. Gill IS, Clayman RV, Albala DM et al (1998) Retroperitoneal and pelvic extraperitoneal laparoscopy: an international perspective. Urology 52(4): 566-571

Chapter 5

Laparoscopic Instrumentation

Pierluigi Bove, Ennio Matarazzo

Introduction

Despite the time-consuming and costly nature of laparoscopy, the decreased morbidity and brief convalescence associated with this procedure are evident and well documented. This and the most recent developments in "high-tech" instruments have allowed many advances to be made in laparoscopic surgery. Laparoscopy depends on new technology results for several reasons: lack of the three-dimensional view as in open surgery; reduction in depth perception; and alterations in video images due to magnification and color resolution. The movements of the instrument are limited by fixation at the trocar entry site, and tactile sensation is blunted because the instruments must pass through trocars and their valves. In order to overcome the aforementioned limitations, manufacturers have been continually improving research on laparoscopy so as to offer a wide variety of high-quality equipment and instruments. A good knowledge of this specialized equipment and proper training are essential to perform laparoscopy in the easiest and safest way.

For surgeons who want to use minimally invasive surgery, it is crucial to become familiar with the basic instrumentation needed for laparoscopy and retroperitoneoscopy, and to know the basic techniques used in performing these kinds of procedures. Laparoscopic equipment can be divided into the following categories of instruments: (a) those for approaching the operative site; (b) for visualizing the surgical field, and (c) for performing operative procedures.

Approaching the Operative Site

During laparoscopic procedures, the operative field is determined by creating a working space inside the patient's abdomen or the extraperitoneal space. This can be performed by establishing a pneumoperitoneum: CO_2 is insufflated into a preexistent space (e.g., the peritoneal cavity) or in a surgically created cavity (e.g., Retzius' space and retroperitoneal space).

Insufflation Needle

The insufflation needle is the first instrument used to obtain the pneumoperitoneum. The needle most commonly used for insufflation of the peritoneal cavity is

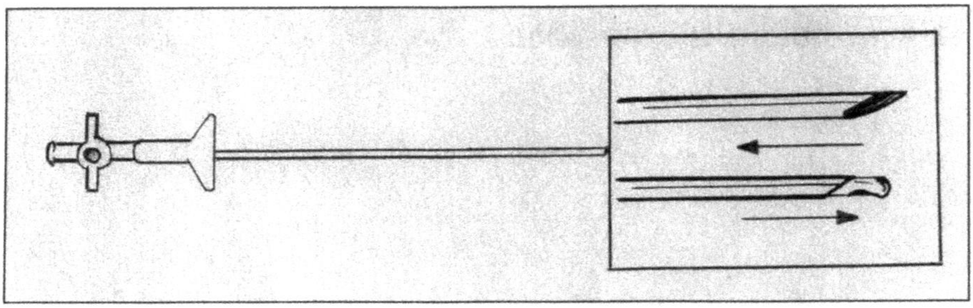

Fig. 1. Veress needle. *Inset*: the tip has an inner blunt core that retracts when encountering resistance from tissue but pops forward once the needle is in the peritoneal cavity (i.e., no resistance)

the Veress needle. Standard needle diameter is 14 gauge (6 Fr or 2 mm) and needle lengths are 12 and 15 cm. The needle consists of an inner blunt tip (safety mechanism) and a sharp outer beveled sheath. The inner blunt tip is spring-loaded so that it retracts when it meets resistance, thus exposing the sharp outer beveled sheath. As the needle is advanced, the sharp sheath penetrates the muscular fascia and then the peritoneum; once this resistance is overcome, the blunt tip springs forward, protecting the underlying abdominal structures from inadvertent injury. This movement is indicated by a click and a red marker in the hub of the needle. The hub of the needle contains a Luer lock connector for attachment to the insufflation tubing (Fig. 1).

Insufflation System

The insufflation system provides adequate working space to initiate and maintain the pneumoperitoneum; it consists of a gas and an insufflator. The most useful gas used is carbon dioxide (CO_2).When absorbed, CO_2 rapidly dissolves in blood, with only little risk of embolism. It is not combustible; therefore, electrosurgical instruments can be used safely. The insufflator controls the flow of pressurized gas into the patient's abdomen. The insufflator's front panel shows the rate of flow (liters per minute), intra-abdominal pressure (mmHg), and total volume (liters) of gas used for insufflation (Fig. 2).

The gas flow rate can also be predetermined: insufflation begins with a flowrate of 1 l/min, reaching a maximum rate of 16 l/min and an abdominal working pressure of around 15-20 mmHg, which is suitable for most laparoscopic procedures in adults. A microprocessor arrests the gas insufflation once the preset intra-abdominal pressure has been reached. In case of gas loss (and subsequent pressure decrease), insufflation is restored immediately. We suggest always positioning the insufflator directly in front of the surgeon so as to better control any variation in abdominal pressure. Abdominal pressures over 25 mmHg expose the patient to an increased risk of CO_2 absorption, decreased venous return from the inferior vena cava, and impaired ventilation as a result of increased pressure on the diaphragm, which ultimately increases the risk of systemic acidosis.

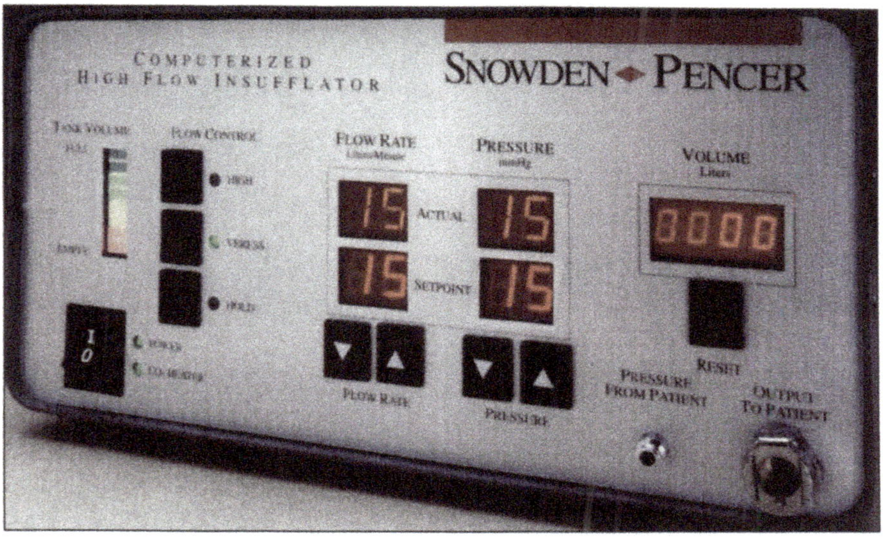

Fig. 2. Insufflator's front panel

Gasless Laparoscopy

The concept of gasless laparoscoy was introduced to avoid complications linked to gaseous laparoscopy (hypercarbia [1]). Many systems are available for creating a gasless work space: through a small incision, twin-blade retractors are positioned to lift the anterior abdominal wall [2, 3], such as with the Laprolift System (Origin Med-systems, Inc., Menlo Park, Calif.); the retractors are suspended by a mechanical arm attached to the operating table and it is possible to have different configurations for various regions of the abdominal cavity. As an option, when an extraperitoneal approach is chosen, the access can be facilitated by the use of a balloon in the targeted extraperitoneal space [4]. Recently, many transparent balloon systems have been developed that can be attached directly onto trocars (PBD, Origin Med-systems, Inc.), allowing a safer dissection under direct visualization (Fig. 3 A, B). Whereas the open balloon technique is valuable for gaining access to the retroperitoneum and pelvic extraperiptoneum, the complications associated with this technique (such as CO_2 leakage, blind access, and balloon rupture [5], make it less than ideal. For this reason , we prefer to use alternative retroperitoneal access methods. One of these is blunt finger dissection (see Chap. 4 "Retroperitoneal Access," this volume). Recently, a new, closed technique for creating the retroperitoneal space using an optical trocar has been described: the laparoscope is used to mobilize the lateral peritoneum from the anterior abdominal wall.

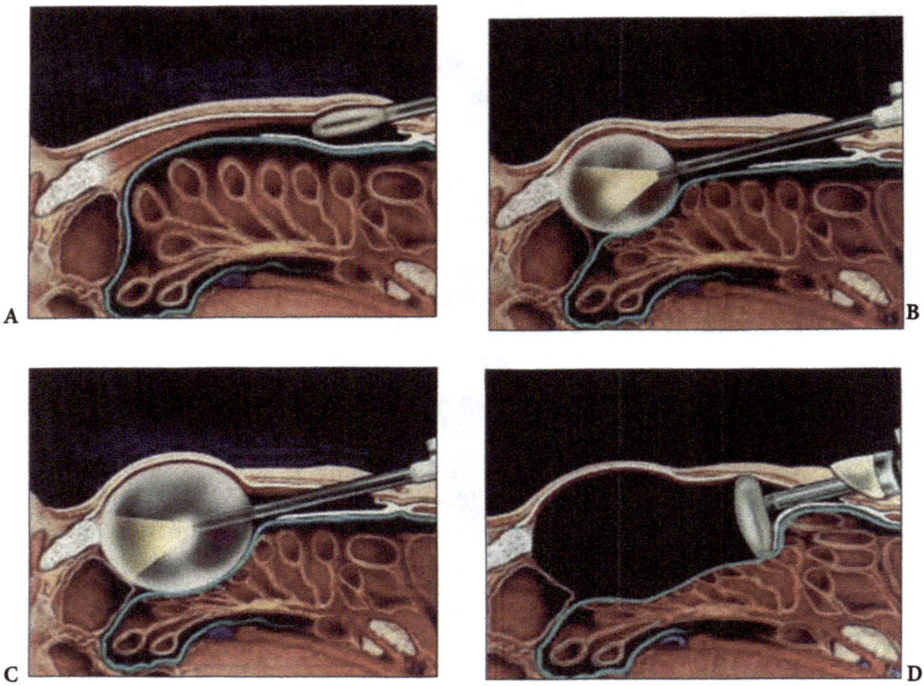

Fig. 3 A-D. Balloon system. It provides a rapid access to and maintenance of the extraperitoneal space under direct visualization (**A, B**). Inflation is continued until adequate space is created (**C**); balloon system is removed before extraperitoneal space insufflation (**D**)

Trocars

Once a space, whether gaseous or gasless, has been created, the trocars can be positioned. These devices allow the surgeon to introduce surgical instruments into the abdominal or retroperitoneal cavities. Trocars are available in disposable and reusable forms. The reusable types are metallic trocars: they are heavier than the disposable ones and their tips tend to dull with use, requiring periodic sharpening. The disposable trocars are made of plastic material; they are lighter than their metallic counterparts and easier to handle. Each trocar has four components (Fig. 4 A): the trocar sheath, removable obturator, a safety mechanism, and a valve mechanism.

Trocar Sheath

Both reusable and disposable trocars are available in various working diameters (range from 3 to 15 mm) and lengths (range from 5 to 15 mm). Suitable trocar selection depends on the type of laparoscopic procedure and the individual characteristics of the patient. For example, there is a direct correlation between the size of the patient and the size of the trocar (i.e., pediatric patients require a small trocar). The working length of a standard 5-mm trocar is 7 cm, and that of a 10-mm

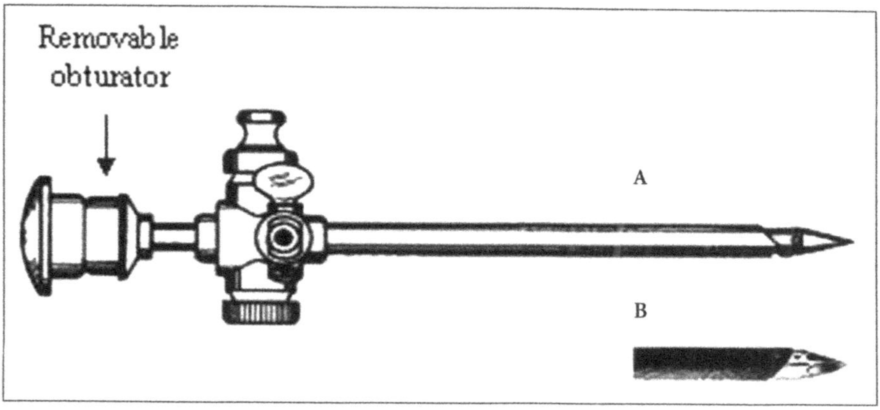

Fig. 4. Trocar. The tip of the obturator can be conical (**A**) or pyramidal (**B**)

trocar is 11 cm. Trocars that are 5 mm in diameter are adequate for the passage of most working instruments, such as graspers, scissors, forceps, and smaller laparoscopes. The 10- to 12-mm trocars are suitable for standard size instruments (10-mm laparoscope) and for instruments such as clip appliers, laparoscopic stapplers, tissue morcellators, and intralaparoscopic ultrasonography instruments.

Recently, the concept of microlaparoscopy was introduced. This means using laparoscopic instruments whose outer sheath is less than 2 mm in diameter. Microlaparoscopy has been proposed as the new standard procedure for abdominal entry and for performing some diagnostic and therapeutic techniques. These "mini" instruments are already the preferred choice when performing laparoscopic procedures in younger patients, but it is important that they are used properly. For instance, because they are extremely delicate, they do not seem to be useful for retroperitoneoscopic procedures.

To prevent inadvertent removal of the sheath from its port site, which involves leakage of the pneumoperitoneum, the risk of subcutaneous emphysema, and loss of time, several design changes in either reusable (i.e., nondisposable) or disposable trocars have been made. There are many methods of trocar fixation:

A simple and efficient way of anchoring the sheath is to use nonabsorbable sutures to secure the trocar sleeve to the skin.

Nondisposable trocars have been projected with a roughened shaft to offer a greater resistance towards abdominal wall tissues.

Disposable trocars have been crafted with a separate plastic covering to be applied on the trocar sheath, so that they can be screwed together into the abdominal wall. These trocars have the disadvantage of considerably enlarging the skin incision, leaving an ugly scar.

Malecot-type disposable trocars have a retention device in the tip. As soon as the tip of the obturator pierces the peritoneum, the wings of the Malecot expand, locking the sheath into the abdomen. In addition, an outer sliding ring can be locked onto the trocar sheath at skin level, to prevent unintentional trocar retraction or advancement.

With blunt tip trocars internal sealing is provided by an inflatable balloon and a collar-compressed sponge forms the external seal. Together, this enables pneumoperitoneum to be established and maintained without the need for sutures.

Removable Obturator

The removable obturator has a conical or pyramidal pointed tip to puncture the abdominal wall (Fig. 4 A,B). A conical tipped obturator is more difficult to insert, but involves less risk of injury to the underlying viscera or vessels. A pyramidal tip obturator is more traumatic and represents a higher risk of injury. However, insertion is easier. It is preferable to use a pyramidal, pointed tip for the primary trocar placement. Secondary trocars, which are placed under direct endoscopic vision, should possibly have conical tips; they can be reused and are not equipped with a safety shield.

Safety Mechanism

Similar to a Veress needle mechanism, the outer atraumatic shield of the obturator retracts as the assembled trocar is pushed against the abdominal wall, thus exposing the sharp tip of the obturator (Fig. 5 A). As soon as the trocar has pierced the peritoneum, the shield springs forward, covering the sharp tip of the obturator (Fig. 5 B) and protecting the underlying abdominal organs from injury. The position (locked vs. unlocked) of the safety shield at any given time is indicated by a spring-loaded red marker on the handle.

A 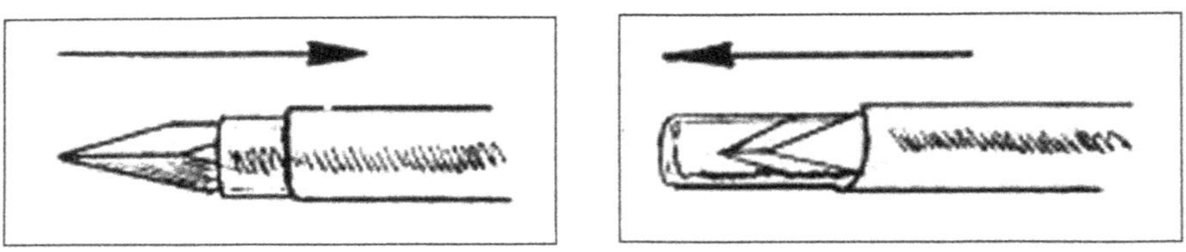 B

Fig. 5 A, B. Trocar safety mechanism

Valve Mechanism

Most trocars have two valve mechanisms located in the handle. The first of them is an external side arm with a stopcock that can be attached to the CO_2 insufflation tube in order to maintain the pneumoperitoneum. The second valve mechanism consists of a flap valve that is incorporated into the body of the trocar; it prevents gas from escaping from the pneumoperitoneum when no instrument is inside it. In the disposable trocars, this mechanism is usually provided by a flap valve that can be manually opened by a lever on the handle (Fig. 6). The closed, at rest, flap valve

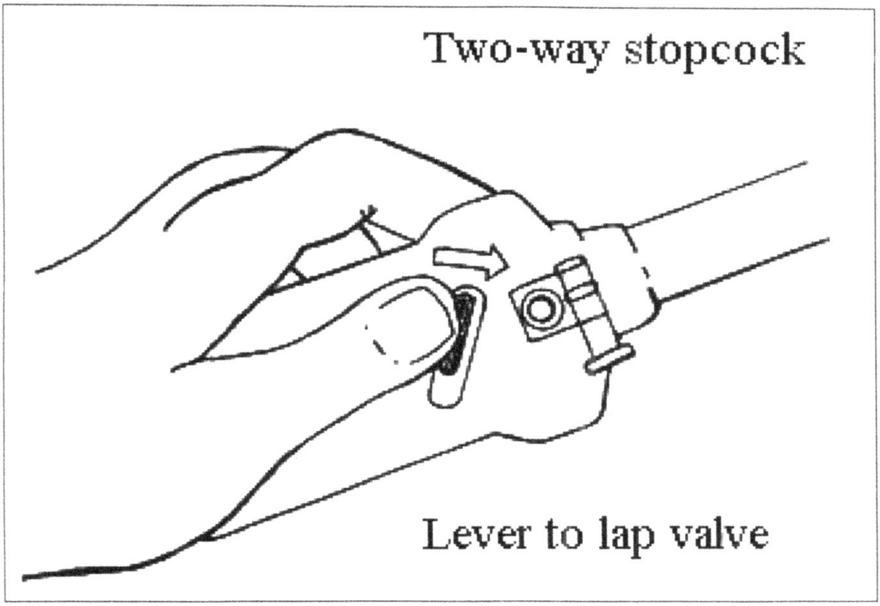

Fig. 6. Valve mechanism

opens automatically if any pressure from the tip of an instrument is applied. In the reusable trocar, the valve has a trumpet-shaped design. It must be opened manually, by pressing the protruding metal knob to pass instruments into the trocar sheath.

When the valve is in its open position, a series of additional seals prevent gas from escaping around an inserted instrument. The valve must be held in its open position when removing certain instruments (e.g., hook electrode) or tissues. Recently, a removable valve for specimen retrieval was designed (GeniCon L.C.). Specially designed reducer caps or reducer-sheaths are available to down-size the larger trocars. This facilitates the use of smaller instruments, for example, through a 10-mm trocar, without gas escaping from the abdomen. The convertible trocars such as the Versaport RPF Trocar (USSC) obviate the need for adapters or converters when using instruments of various sizes, by reducing the number of steps required to switch instruments. These trocars can accommodate from 5- to 12-mm instruments.

Special Trocars

There are many types of special trocars:

A. Optical trocars were created so as to be able to safely place the first trocar. With these systems the surgeon can place them under direct vision, while dissecting through the layers of the abdominal wall directly into the peritoneum [6]. Optical trocars are available in two different sheath sizes: the Visiport trocar with a 12-mm diameter (Visiport RPF Optical Trocar. United States

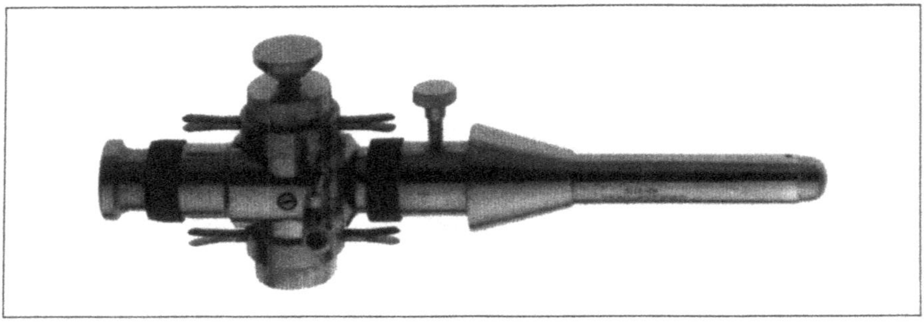

Fig. 7. Hasson cannula

Surgical Corp.[USSC]. Norwalk. Conn.) or the Optiview trocar with a 5-mm diameter (Ethicon Endosurgical, Inc.).

B. New disposable trocars without a safety mechanism and with no sidearm stopcock have been introduced. They can be used as secondary trocars and must be positioned under direct vision. These trocars are less expensive and handier to use.

C. The Hasson cannula is a specially designed trocar that can be used when "open" trocar placement is required (in patients with a high risk of injury, e.g., with abdominal adhesions or in obese patients) during the first trocar positioning. The cannula consists of a blunt-tipped obturator and an adjustable outer conical sleeve which allow an airtight sealing of the incision. A mini-laparotomy access (2-cm incision) is made in the abdominal wall and a suture is positioned on both sides of the fascial incision. The peritoneum is incised after it is identified; then, the surgeon may introduce one of his fingers inside the abdominal cavity to ensure the absence of bowel or omental adhesions. The obturator is then inserted into the incision and the outer conical sleeve is pushed into the fascial opening. Finally, the cannula is secured to the fascia on each side of the sheath by the previously fixed sutures (Fig.7). A Hasson cannula with a retention feature Malecot-type (Auto Suture) is also now available.

D. Flexible trocars (Storz) may be used when curved instruments must be passed. Often used for thoracoscopy, their application in laparoscopy is rare.

Visualizing the Surgical Field

Once the access has been created, the optical system allows the surgeon to visualize the surgical field. The basic system consists of a laparoscope for direct visualization, a camera and video system for the remote visualization and documentation, and a light source.

Laparoscope

The laparascope consists of a rigid optical system through which light and an image are transmitted by a camera, from the operative field directly to a television

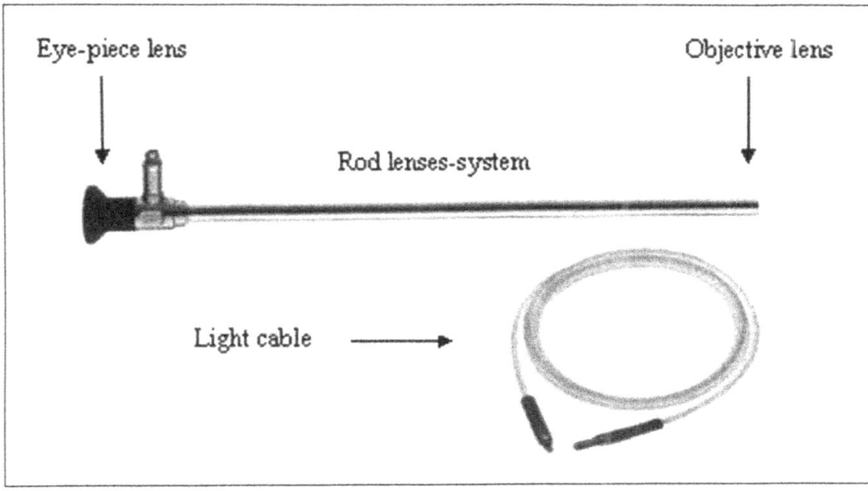

Fig. 8. Laparoscope

monitor. The laparoscope consists of a rigid rod-lens imaging system (objective lens, rod lens system with or without an eyepiece lens) and a light cable (Fig. 8).

The objective lens is located on the tip of the laparoscope. It gathers the light that has been reflected by the tissue and focuses the inverted image on the end of the rod lens system. The rod lens system consists of a series of long glass lenses, separated by short air spaces which transmit the image and reverse it at the eyepiece; the image is then magnified and transferred to the camera and then to the television monitor. The light is transmitted by a fiberoptic cable both in the laparoscope and in the light cord. Nowadays, a variety of laparoscopes are available and they typically come in a number of different sizes (ranging from 2.7 to 12 mm) and different angles of view (e.g., 0°, 30°, 45°, 50°, or 70° lenses). Operative laparoscopes equipped with a built-in working channel for passing instruments directly into the surgical field are rarely used in urologic surgery.

Recently, attempts have been undertaken to solve the problem of lens fogging, one of the problems most commonly encountered during laparoscopic procedures, with various lens cleaning systems. The Murdoch Laparoscopic Lens Cleaner (Cook Urological, Inc. Spencer, Ind.) passes through an 11-mm access port, permitting saline flushing of the laparoscope's lens without having to remove it from the port. More refined are the Hydro Laparoscopes (Circon ACMI, Stanford, Conn.) which offer a distal lens-washing and a tissue irrigation device along with a distal lens warming function.

Camera and Video System

The camera, in terms of optimizing the optics, is as critical as the laparoscope. It allows the endoscopic image to be magnified, providing an excellent visualization

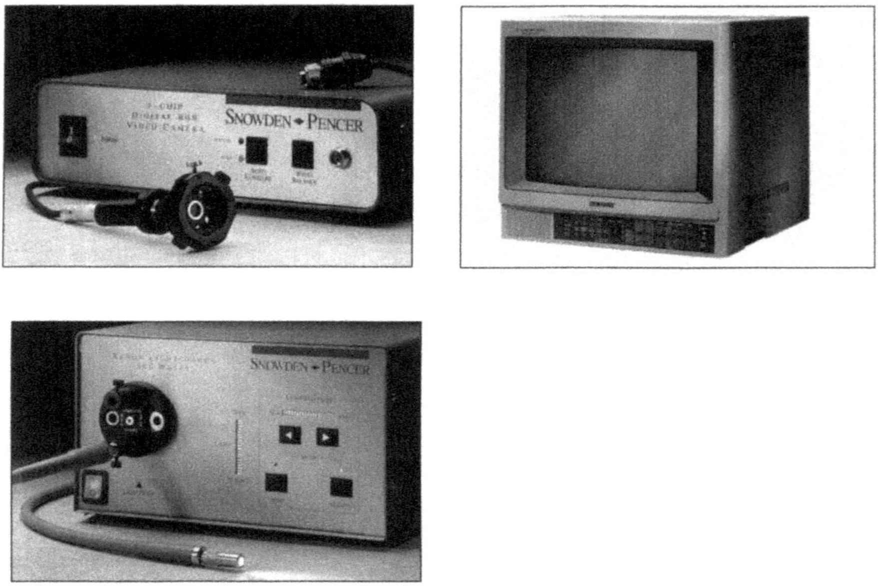

Fig. 9. Camera (A), video system (B) and light source (C)

of many fine anatomic details. The camera locks the eyepiece of the endoscope and receives optical information. The image is transmitted through a cable to the camera box and then it is reconstructed and sent to the video monitor where optical information is finally displayed, providing a view of the surgical field to all operating room personnel (Fig. 9 A, B).

Before introducing the laparoscope through the trocar, it is important to check that the focus and white balance have been adjusted. The laparoscope should be pointed at a white object (e.g., gauze sponge) so that the strands of the gauze sponge become sharp and clear on the monitor. Then, the corresponding button on the camera box should be pressed to white balance the camera image. Constant improvements in camera design are producing better images with increasingly smaller units. At present, the three-chip cameras (Stryker Endoscopy; Circon ACMI; Richard Wolf Medical Instruments Corp.; Olympus America, Inc., Melville, N.Y.) combine a high resolution with a low minimum illumination requirement, while the digital signal processing provides a distortion-free image.

Differently from open surgery, where the surgeon has stereoscopic vision, conventional laparoscopic camera systems limit the surgeon to a two-dimensional view. A three-dimensional (3D) image would be analogous to open surgery and extremely helpful when performing complicated reconstructive laparoscopic procedures. An example can be provided by the 3D Video-laparoscope System (Richard Wolf Medical Instruments Corp.).

Light Source

There are many different light sources which produce a high-intensity light (Fig. 9 C). These light sources can use a xenon, mercury, or halogen vapor bulb to produce illumination. A fiberoptic cable, different for every kind of laparoscope and light source, transports the light from the light source to the laparoscope. Remember to handle the light cord with care because damage to the delicate optical fibers can result in a lower illumination of the operative field.

Each piece of imaging equipment must be checked before initiating every procedure.

Performing Operative Procedures

Laparoscopic procedures require tissue manipulation in a fashion similar to an open surgical procedure. Therefore, many laparoscopic instruments parallel the design of standard open surgical equipment [7, 8]. Laparoscopic instruments can be classified into instruments for dissection, instruments for suturing, retractors, irrigation, and aspiration systems, and instruments for tissue removal. Finally, a wide assortment of miscellaneous instruments is available to facilitate each kind of laparoscopic procedure.

Instruments for Dissection

These instruments are generally held in the surgeon's dominant hand. This category of instruments includes graspers, dissectors and scissors.

Graspers

Graspers are available in various sizes (diameter ranging from 3 to 12 mm) and designs. Variations in design include electrosurgical capability, type of handle, and type of tip.

Several variations in the design of the handle allow the locking of the jaw on the tip of the instrument: spring-loaded locking handles (Fig. 10 A) can be opened by squeezing the handle. It is useful to tightly grasp and retract structures for a pro-

A
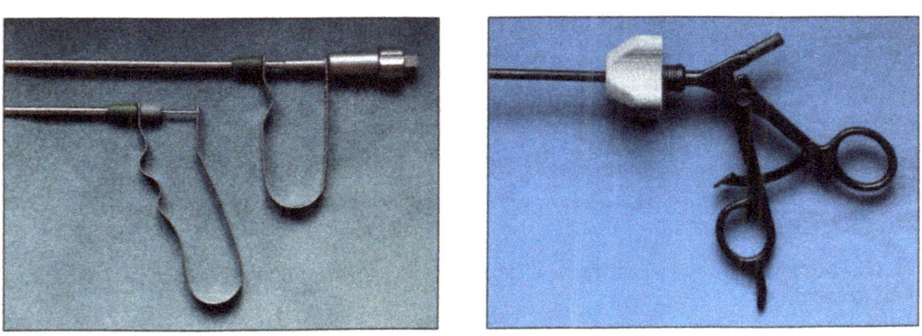
B

Fig. 10. Spring-loaded (A) and bar type locking handles (B)

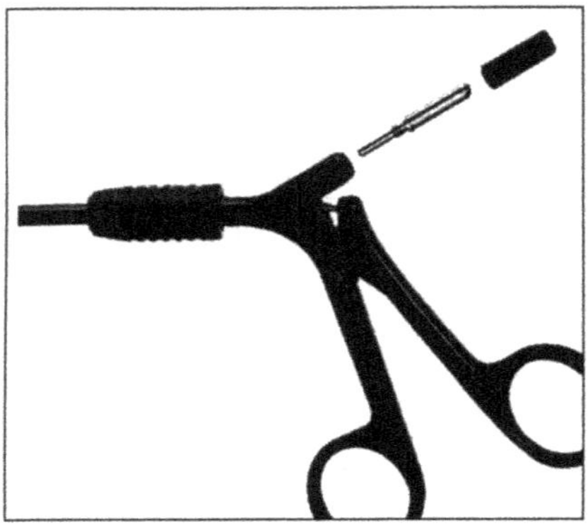

Fig. 11. Electrosurgical capability enhances the value of an instrument, allowing one either to grasp or coagulate tissue

longed time, thus obviating the need to exert constant pressure on the handle. A second mechanism used to lock the tip in closed position is the bar-type handle (Fig. 10 B). It allows the surgeon to place various degrees of tension on grasped tissue. An electrosurgical capability (Fig. 11) enhances the value of an instrument, allowing tissue to be both grasped and coagulated.

Grasping instruments can be divided, as regards the different kind of tips, into different categories, these ranging from instruments equipped with coarse, toothed, or clawed jaws (traumatic) (Fig. 12) to fine instruments for grasping bowel, vessels, or any kind of delicate structures (atraumatic) (Fig. 13). A rotational mechanism, close to the handle, allows the surgeon to rotate the tip of the instrument by means of a single-handed control (e.g., finger).

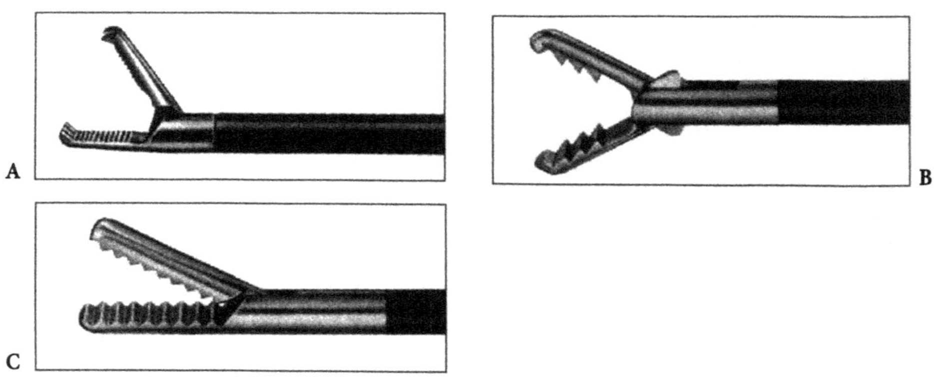

Fig. 12. Traumatic graspers: claw extraction forceps (**A**), spoon cup grasper (**B**), gator toothed grasper (**C**)

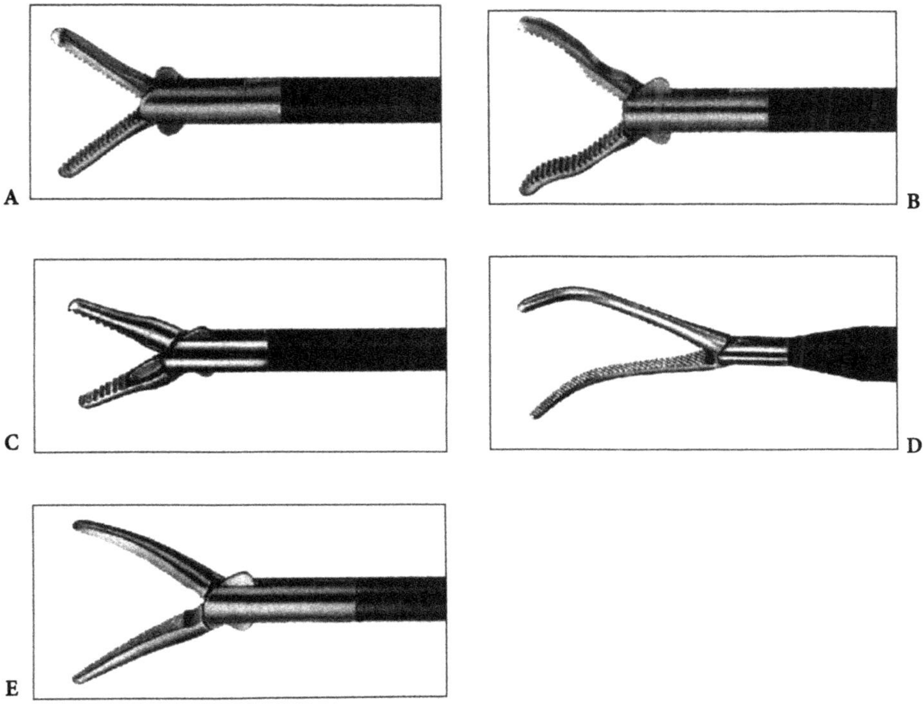

Fig. 13 A-E. Atraumatic graspers (A-C) can be used for precise spread dissection of delicate structures: i.e. 60° angle dissector (D) and Maryland dissector (E)

Dissectors

Various dissectors, with slightly curved jaws, have proven to be useful for tissue dissection. The most commonly used dissectors are the Maryland and the atraumatic-curved types (Fig. 13 D,E). These dissectors are generally held in the surgeon's dominant hand and are equipped with a rotational mechanism.

New methods for soft tissue dissection have been developed. With the Harmonic Scalpel and the LaparoSonic Coagulating Shears (Ethicon Endo-Surgery, Inc.) ultrasonic energy delivered through a vibrating blade is used to denature tissue proteins and to form a coagulum. If compared with electrocautery, it produces less tissue injury and minimal eschar formation, tissue dessication, and smoke formation. Another innovative method for tissue dissection is the use of a high-pressure fluid system. With Hydro-dissection Probes (Circon Surgitek, Santa Barbara Calif.), the fluid stream can be accurately directed to cleave tissue planes.

Scissors

Scissor tips are available in a variety of configurations: serrated tips for fascia cutting, curved tips for dissection, and hooked tips for suture cutting (Fig. 14). Many scissors are provided with an electrosurgical connection, which allows simultaneous monopolar coagulation. Unfortunately, these scissors tend to dull within

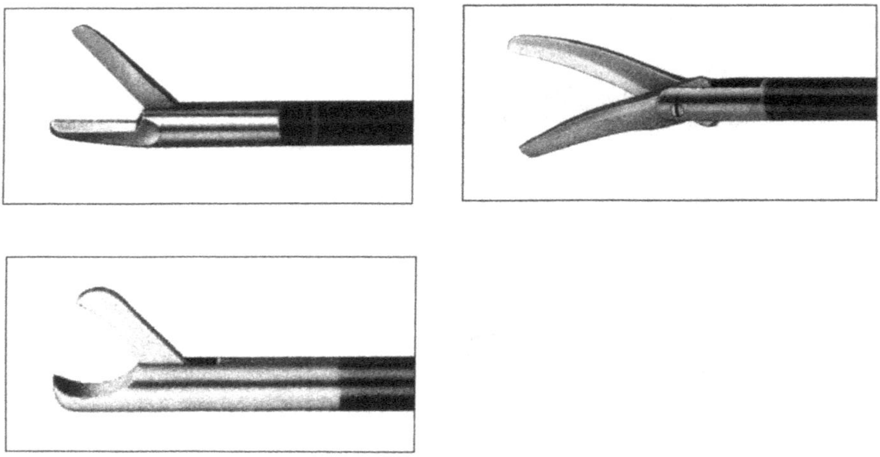

Fig. 14. Scissor tips: serrated (A), curved (B) and hooked (C)

a short time because they are also used for electrocoagulation. Disposable instruments are preferable, even if reusable scissors may be less expensive. A good compromise is to use instruments with exchangeable blades and reusable handles (Fig. 15).

Needle electrodes, with different tip angles, are useful to produce a vary fine incision.

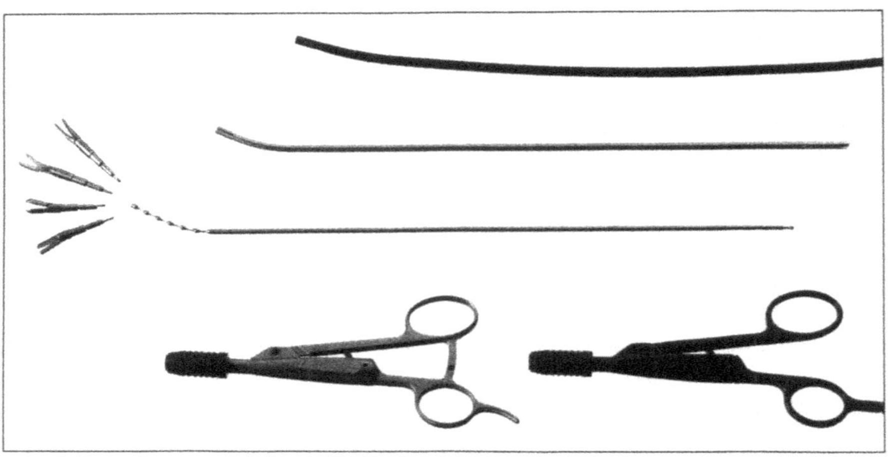

Fig. 15. Instruments with exchangeable blades and reusable handles

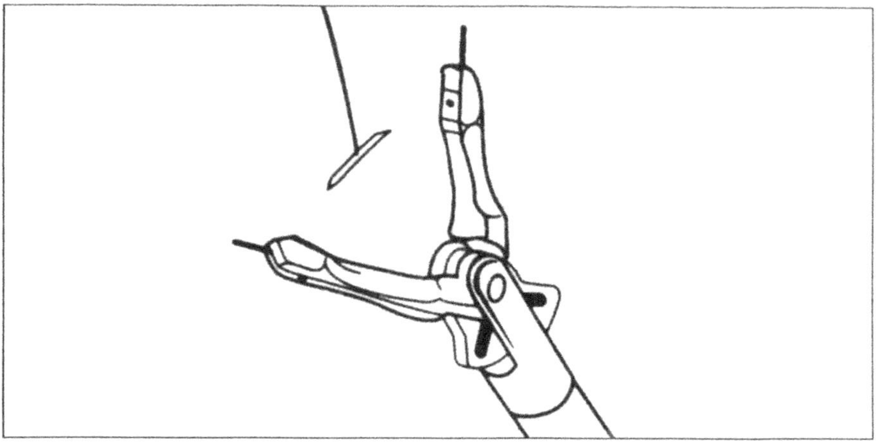

Fig. 16. The Endo Stich device

Instruments for Suturing

Several types of needle holders are available. The handle should have a locking mechanism to prevent inadvertent needle rotation while suturing. Two basic types of needle holder tips exist: a hinged-jaw and sliding sheath design. The hinged-jaw needle holders usually have one fixed jaw to guarantee an easier positioning of the needle. The sliding sheath needle holders consist of a cylindrical tube with a distal notch for needle positioning.

Recent advances in suturing instruments have truly simplified laparoscopic reconstructive surgery. The Endo Stich device (U.S. Surgical, Norwalk, Conn.) can pass a tapered, double-pointed needle between its jaws. This greatly facilitates suturing, obviating intracorporeal needle grasping and reloading (Fig. 16). However, in those situations where knotting is difficult, the Lapra-ty instrument (Ethicon, Inc., Somerville, N.J.) can be used to secure the suture with a reabsorbable (polyglicolic acid) clip.

The knot pusher is used to slide an extracorporeally formed "throw" through the laparoscope sheath down onto tissue within the surgical field.

A 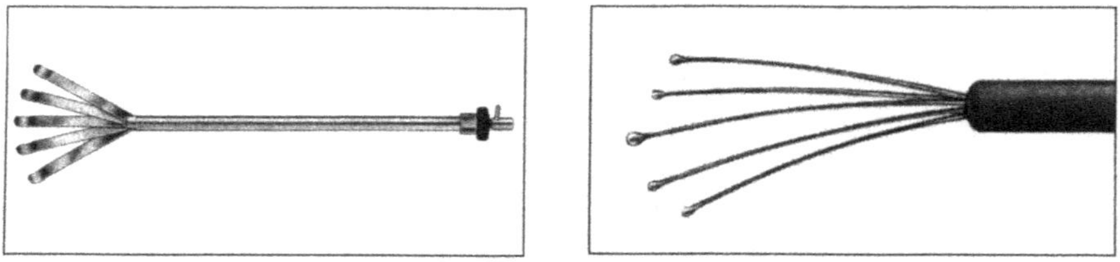 B

Fig. 17. Basic retractor (**A**), and retractor with finger-like projections (**B**)

Retractors

Retractors are indispensable in major laparoscopic surgery, providing for a better visualization of the surgical field. Various models are available in diameters of 5 and 10 mm. Previously, some special retractors were exposed when conducting gasless laparoscopy.

The basic retractor consists of a solid metal bar with a rounded, atraumatic tip. Most sophisticated retractors have a fan-like array of finger-like projections (Fig. 17). This fan is opened by a rotating mechanism (Auto Suture). Some models have an angled tip (Snowden Pencer).

Irrigation and Aspiration Systems

The irrigation and aspiration unit is a critical device for clearly identifying potential sites of bleeding. Normal saline solution at a temperature of 37°C is used for irrigation; heparin (5000 U/l) may be added to prevent the formation of blood clots. With a one way stopcock or trumpet valve, it is possible to control a pressurized mechanism of irrigation. For this purpose, a compressor working with room air is available. Irrigators, powered by the compressor, can also produce a vacuum for the purpose of suction.

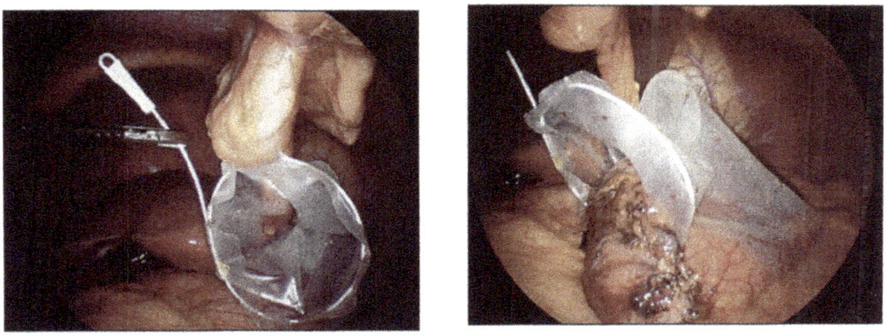

A B

Fig. 18 A, B. Lap-sack. It is designed to temporarily contain tissue or stones and facilitate their emoval from the patient without wound contamination during laparoscopic surgery

Instruments for Tissue Removal

The possibility of removing entire tissue specimens depends directly on the specimen's dimensions. While smaller tissue specimens (e.g., lymph node) may be removed through the major laparoscopic sheath, larger tissues or organs (e.g., kidney), may need to be entrapped in a sack and morcellated before retrieval (Fig. 18). The Lap-sack (Cook Urological Inc.) is made of either a durable double layer of impenetrable nylon and plastic or a single layer of thick-walled plastic.

The morcellators presently available (Karl Storz Endoscopy-America, Inc.; Cook Urological Inc.) consist of motor-driven cutting tubes that can be inserted directly into the entrapment sack.

Miscellaneous Instruments

Diagnostic Ultrasound

Ultrasound probes 5 and 10 mm in size have been used to locate vessels, renal cysts, or uretheral stones during laparoscopic procedures.

Clip Appliers

Disposable clip appliers preloaded with titanium clips of various size have proven to be the most suitable. Because the tip of the applier can be angled and the shaft rotated, the surgeon can place the instrument at a favorable angle to the structure to be occluded. With some new instruments, the clipped structure can be simultaneously resected (Ethicon). Reusable clip appliers are also available, but they have to be removed through the trocar sheath after every single clip application.

Today the Endo-GIA Tissue Stapler is used for a simple and safe renal vein transection. However, its application is limited because it cannot be angled.

Tripolar Cutting Forceps

The Seitzinger Tripolar Cutting Forceps (Circon Surgitek) is a new device that grasp, coagulates, and transects using bipolar electrocautery. The tissue is simultaneously grasped and coagulated by the current before the transection is completed by the guillotine blade.

Argon Beam Coagulator

The argon beam coagulator is very useful for controlling hemorrhage from renal, hepatic, or splenic parenchyma. The argon beam coagulator electrifies a jet of argon gas as it passes through a nozzle located at the tip of the device. Delivery of current in this fashion is diffused across a broad area, the probe not having any direct contact with the tissue. Penetration of the electrical current is ≤ 2 mm; as such, deeper tissue injury does not occur with this device.

Room Setup

The positioning of surgeon, assistants, and surgical nurse and the laparoscopic equipment should be carefully planned before initiating every laparoscopic procedure. Although some changes in the surgical room setup may occur, some basic rules can be defined (Fig. 19): (a) Two video-systems are required to grant the operating room staff optimal visualization of the operative field. (b) Insufflator and light source always should be placed right in front of the primary surgeon or his assistant, in order to constantly check data and functioning. Special trays are currently available to hold, transport, and store the main instruments and the wires belonging to them: this avoids having any vacant electrical or optical wires and gas tubes in the room, thus helping to avoid any accidents involving staff and patients. The position of irrigation-aspiration devices, laser or electrocautery units, anesthesia equipment and instruments trays in the operating room should facilitate comfortable movements of the surgeons and an easy and fast access to all instruments and devices for the nurses.

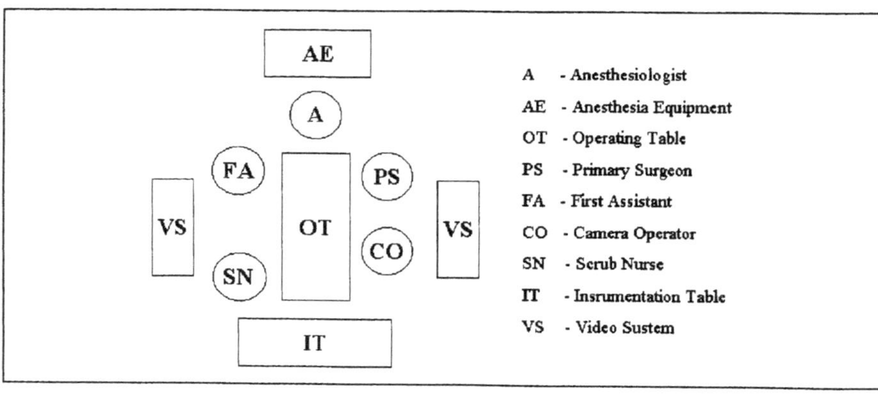

Fig. 19. Room setup

References

1. Luks FI, Peers KH, Deprest JA, et al (1995) Gasless laparoscopy in infants: the rabbit model. J Pediatr Surg 30: 1206-1208
2. Paolucci V, Gutt CN, Schaeff B, et al (1995) Gasless laparoscopy in abdominal surgery. Surg Endosc 9: 497-500
3. Smith RS, Fry WR, Tsoi EK, et al (1993) Gasless laparoscopy and conventional instruments: the next phase of minimally invasive surgery. Arch Surg 128: 1102-1107
4. Gaur DD (1992) Laparoscopic operative retroperitoneoscopy: use of a new device. J Urol 148: 1137-1139
5. Adams JB, Micali S, Moore RG, Babayan RK, Kavoussi LR (1996) Complications of extraperitoneal balloon dilatation. J Endourol 10: 375-378
6. Melzer A, Weiss U, Roth K, et al (1993) Visually controlled trocar insertion by means of the optical scalpel. Endosc Surg Allied Technol 1(4): 239-242
7. Semm K (1987) Instruments and equipment for endoscopic abdominal surgery. In: Semm K, Friedrich ER (eds) Operative manual for endoscopic abdominal surgery. Year Book Medical Publishers, Chicago, pp 46-124
8. Talamini MA, Gadacz TR (1991) Laparoscopic equipment and instrumentation. In: Zucker KA (ed) Surgical laparoscopy. Quality Medical Publishing, St. Louis, pp 23-27

Chapter 6

Preparation of the Patient

Marco Bitelli, Salvatore Micali

Introduction

A prepared patient and skilled surgeon are prerequisites for successful laparoscopic procedures. Laparoscopic surgical candidates must be fully informed and medically suitable. Surgeons should be cognizant of the physiologic changes characteristic of specific laparoscopic surgery and proficient in laparoscopic techniques. The open surgery expertise does not fully prepare a surgeon for the specific demands of operating in the confines of a limited working space and laparoscopic instrumentation [1,2].

To perform laparoscopic surgery safely, the surgical, anesthetic, and nursing staff must be experienced with laparoscopic techniques and familiar with specialized instrumentation. An open line of communication between personnel before, during, and after the surgery is mandatory.

Patient evaluation begins by assessing the general risks associated with anesthesia and surgery.

Laparoscopic procedures require tolerance to general anesthesia, fluid shifts, and cardiopulmonary system stress, as in open surgery.

Anesthetic risks are related to absorption of insufflating CO_2, head-down positioning, and transmitted pneumoperitoneal pressure. Patients with impaired pulmonary function and/or significant cardiovascular dysfunction may not tolerate hypercarbia and/or respiratory compromise from peritoneal CO_2 insufflation; both Trendelenburg position and increased abdominal pressure decrease pulmonary vital capacity.

Contraindications to Laparoscopic Surgery

Contraindications can be classified as infectious, anatomic, and systemic.
Infectious diseases such as peritonitis, abdominal wall infections, and sepsis should be an indication for open surgery. Anatomic conditions "against" laparoscopic surgery are multiple prior laparotomies, large interabdominal mass organomegaly, ascites, umbilical hernia, and, most of all, severe obesity, which should be treated only by the most experienced laparoscopists.

Patients with severe cardiac or pulmonary disease are not candidates for laparoscopic surgery because of the possible side effects of CO_2 absorption [3].

For laparoscopic surgeons there are eight absolute contraindications to laparoscopy:

1. Abdominal wall infections
2. Generalized peritonitis
3. Bowel obstructions
4. Uncorrected coagulopathy
5. Massive hemoperitoneum
6. Intra-abdominal advanced neoplasms
7. Severe obesity
8. Ventral hernia

In fact, the establishment of pneumoperitoneum in the patient with abdominal wall infection or generalized peritonitis presents the risk of dissemination of the infectious processes. Then, a bowel obstruction with associated bowel distension clearly increases the risks of visceral injury during Veress needle or primary trocar insertion. Finally, any laparoscopic procedure is fraught with hazard when an uncorrectable coagulopathy is encountered.

Relatives contraindications to laparoscopy are:

1. Cardiovascular disease: High intra-abdominal pressure could cause severe problems during the procedure in patients with cardiovascular disease.
2. Diaphragmatic hernia: Possibility of pneumothorax due to expansion of pneumoperitoneum.
3. Previous abdominal surgical procedures or intraperitoneal infections: Risks of intra-abdominal organ damage increase by the presence of adhesions following abdominal surgical procedures. Pleissner [4] found a 7% of incidence of adhesions in 1,658 laparoscopic procedures.
4. Ascites: In these patients abdominal wall is very weak and the possibility of bowel injury during Veress needle positioning is very high.
5. Obesity not severe
6. Coagulopathy
7. Hepato/splenomegaly

Ethical and Legal Aspects: Informed Consent

The current idea of informed consent comes from the concept that one can choose what should be done on one's own body.

Informed consent by means of a thorough discussion of the risks, benefits, alternatives to and potential complications of laparoscopic surgery is the initial step in preparing patients for laparoscopic procedures. This should result in a clear understanding by the patient of the potential need for open surgery. The patient must consent to having an open surgical procedure if laparoscopy results in an emergency situation such as hemorrage or bowel injury.

The patient should be informed long before the operation, giving him/her the possibility to ask questions, talk with the family and, possibly, ask the advice of another surgeon.

If the patient is under age, a guardian is requested to be present during the conversation.

First of all the patient has to be informed clearly about his/her disease. The surgeon then should explain, as best as he/she can, the laparoscopic procedure without using specific medical terms that could be misunderstood by the patient. The patient must also receive informations regarding the surgical team and their past laparoscopic experiences. This point is very important at the beginning of a surgeon's laparoscopic experience.

Informed consent must include knowledge of all risks of laparoscopic procedures, generic (bound infection, hematoma), specific (vascular or bowel injury), and fatal with the relative recurrence rate of each complication based on international scientific data [5] and not on personal data.

Laparoscopic techniques represent "minimal access" surgery not "minimally invasive" surgery: the potential risks of an open surgical approach also apply to laparoscopic techniques.

General Preparation of the Patient

Depending on the nature of the procedure and an assessment of the patient's individual risks for bowel injury, mechanical or full bowel preparation should be given the day before the procedure.

For simple and diagnostic procedures, the bowel preparation consists of a full liquid diet for 48 h before the procedure. For longer procedures some institutions routinely order an outpatient bowel preparation for maximal decompression of the bowels. By giving a complete outpatient bowel preparation, a primary repair can also be undertaken if a bowel injury occurs. The bowel preparation popularized by Clarke et al. [6] consists of a mechanical bowel preparation followed by three oral doses of both erythromycin and neomycin base on the day prior to surgery: in addition, broad-spectrum intravenous antibiotics are given when the patient is called to the operating room.

All patients undergoing elective renal and major retroperitoneal procedures should be given the opportunity to donate autologous blood preoperatively. Ideally, 2 units of autologous packed red blood cells should be available prior to laparoscopic nephrectomy.

Patients are advised to discontinue aspirin, anticoagulants, and other platelet-affecting medications at least 5 days before laparoscopy.

Routine laboratory studies are obtained before laparoscopic procedures; for older patients a chest radiograph and electrocardiogram are also required.

To prevent visceral injuries, placement of a nasogastric tube (major surgical procedures) and Foley catheter is recommended prior to establishing the pneumoperitoneum and is removed at the end of the laparoscopic procedure. The surgical area should be cleansed and sterile drapes placed. Skin preparation should accommodate the need for conversion to an open procedure, although this is rare. Surgical preparation for transperitoneal procedures extends from the nipple line to thighs and laterally to the posterior axillary line; limiting skin preparation to the subcostal margin is adequate for pelvic procedures.

For retroperitoneal laparoscopic procedures bowel preparation and placement of a ureteral catheter is strictly recommended.

Prolonged laparoscopic procedures induce hypothermia due to cold CO_2 insufflation; therefore the patient should be covered with a warm blanket during the procedure.

Patient Positioning

Appropriate patient positioning helps optimize surgical exposure and, we can say, is equivalent to placing retractors during open surgery.

An operative table that enables intraoperative Trendelenburg and a lateral side-to-side position is a necessity: the table should also allow attachments for devices for dorsolithotomy positioning and fluoroscopy for radiological procedures.

Transperitoneal access is preferred for approaching the adrenal glands, intrabdominal organs, and pelvic genitourinary organs; it is considered the standard approach for laparoscopic varicocelectomy. Standard position begins with the patient supine. After the pneumoperitoneum is established, the patient may require repositioning into the lateral decubitus position for trocar placement.

A retroperitoneal approach to the adrenal glands and upper and middle ureters requires that the patient be placed in lateral decubitus or prone position. The Gaur balloon expansion device is used to create a retroperitoneal work space; advantages are avoidance of hazards associated with pneumoperitoneum, a direct approach to renal ileum, optimal visualization of renal collecting; and the exposure of a short right adrenal vein is improved with a retroperitoneal approach.

For pelvic procedures patients are placed in either supine or low lithotomy position; access to the perineum and vaginal cavity allows transvaginal elevation of the bladder neck while placing suspension sutures during incontinence procedures. Further, Trendelenburg and lateral positioning may aid surgical exposure by displacing the bowel.

Very important is patient positioning before a retroperitoneal laparoscopic procedure: a correct positioning reduces injuries during trocar introduction. Patients should be positioned supine with a pillow under the operating side: this allows the lateral rotation of 15-20°.

Conclusions

Patient selection, complete informed consent, preparation, and positioning are prerequisites for successful laparoscopic procedures and are as important as the actual procedures.

If general anesthesia is necessary and techniques must be modified to carry out laparoscopic procedures, difficulties can be avoided with adequate preoperative preparation.

Laparoscopic surgery requires an integrated approach, including physicians and personnel, with the surgeon acting as the team leader.

As with all urologic procedures the safety and success of laparoscopic procedures rely on proper patient selection and specific surgical training.

References

1. Kerbl K, Clayman RV et al (1993) Staging pelvic lymphadenectomy for prostate cancer: a comparison of laparoscopic and open techniques. J Urol 150:396-399
2. Hawasli A., Lloyd LR (1991) Laparoscopic cholecystectomy. The learning curve: report of 50 patients. Am Surg 57: 542-544
3. Roger KL, Stoller ML (1996) Patient preparation and operating room setup. In: Smith's textbook of endourology. Quality Medical Publication, St. Louis, pp 697-709
4. Pleissner J, Berndt H, Gutz HI (1978) Laparoscopy following abdominal operations. Endoscopy 10:187-191
5. Donovan JF (1992) Legal issues in Laparoscopy. Contemp Urol 4:74-81
6. Clarke JS et al (1977) Preoperative oral antibiotics reduce septic complications of colon operations :results of prospective, randomised, double blind clinical study. Ann Surg 186:251-259

Chapter 7

Aspects of Anesthesiology in Adults

M. Dauri, F. Coniglione, N. Heffawi

Introduction

Laparoscopic techniques often constitute a valid alternative to traditional surgery. In urology, the indications for such procedures vary among the different authors. Nonetheless, thanks to technological innovations and progress in anesthesiology, the number of patients that are able to undergo these procedures is increasing constantly.

Surgical procedures such as radical nephrectomy, pyeloureteral junction plastic reconstruction, adrenalectomy, and spermatic cord ligature can now be easily performed with minimally invasive techniques, which provide low surgical stress, rapid re-canalization, and, consequently, fast functional recovery.

It is then important for anesthesia to be similarly adequate in granting fast recovery and a reduced incidence of side effects that may affect the postoperative course and hence prolong the in-hospital stay.

Pathophysiology

In order to perform an extraperitoneal approach, it is necessary to create a space between the peritoneum and the adjacent structures. Different means can be used to acheive this aim; as a matter of fact, the various methods can be divided into "gas" and "gasless" procedures according to whether the creation of this virtual cavity is performed by loosely injecting a substance or by confining it inside a ballon which prevents its uncontrolled spreading [1].

Methods using free gas injection, however, are more commonly employed since they allow better surgical vision of the field, are cheaper, and provide more room to operate. CO_2 is the most commonly used gas because of its availability, low cost, relative sterility, and easy elimination.

It is not possible to use N_2O for surgical procedures due to its flammability, and helium is not soluble in blood and consequently might raise the percentage of embolic accidents [2].

Physiological changes during the formation of the retroperitoneal space are essentially due to CO_2 insufflation, hence its absorption and effects on respiratory and circulatory functions. Pain is another relevant factor both during and after the operation.

As far as ventilation dynamics are concerned, the effects are minimal: in fact, gas insufflation does not substantially affect ventilatory pressures since the volume of gas used to create the operating space is not relevant and does not affect diaphragmatic mobility.

On the other hand, CO_2 partial pressure in the blood increases. Such an increase is due to the widening of the surface exposed to the gas, the pressure of the gas inside the space, and the the velocity of elimination.

The elimination of the gas is initially a function of its systemic absorption, which depends on the coefficient of solubility. Once the gas is absorbed, ventilation plays an important role, since CO_2 is basically eliminated by breathing.

The effect of the absorption of CO_2 can be easily highlighted by arterial blood sampling during the first 60 min of surgery, during which time a constant increase in $PaCO_2$ values can be observed, without a similar increase in end-tidal CO_2 values ($EtCO_2$), probably due to a change in the V/Q ratio [3].

Such a phenomenon can also be explained by the fact that the retroperitoneal space is not a defined one; even a small amount of the gas causes a continuous micro-dissection through soft tissues. Thus, the contact surface exposed to CO_2 keeps becoming wider, consequently increasing absorption of the gas until an equilibrium between the peritoneal, interstitial, and serum concentrations is established (plateau $EtCO_2$).

Patient positioning on the surgical table may also affect the CO_2 alveolar—arterial gradient; hence, especially when using prone positioning, end-tidal CO_2 evaluation must be accompanied by arterial blood sampling, at least during the first 60 min of surgery [3].

Evaluation of Respiratory Function During Retroperitoneoscopy

Table 1 shows the standard values during retroperitoneoscopy. From a hemodynamic point of view, a retroperitoneoscopic approach is decidedly less destabilizing than an intraperitoneal one [4].

During the formation of pneumoperitoneaum, the caval compartment is subjected to an increase in the pressure gradient from the inferior to the superior compartment (measured at diaphragmatic level): such an increase is caused by insufflation pressure

Table 1. Standard values

Airway peak pressure	Slightly increased
Intrathoracic pressure	No change
Compliance	Slightly increased
Pa02	No change
PaC02	Increased
CFR	Slightly decreased

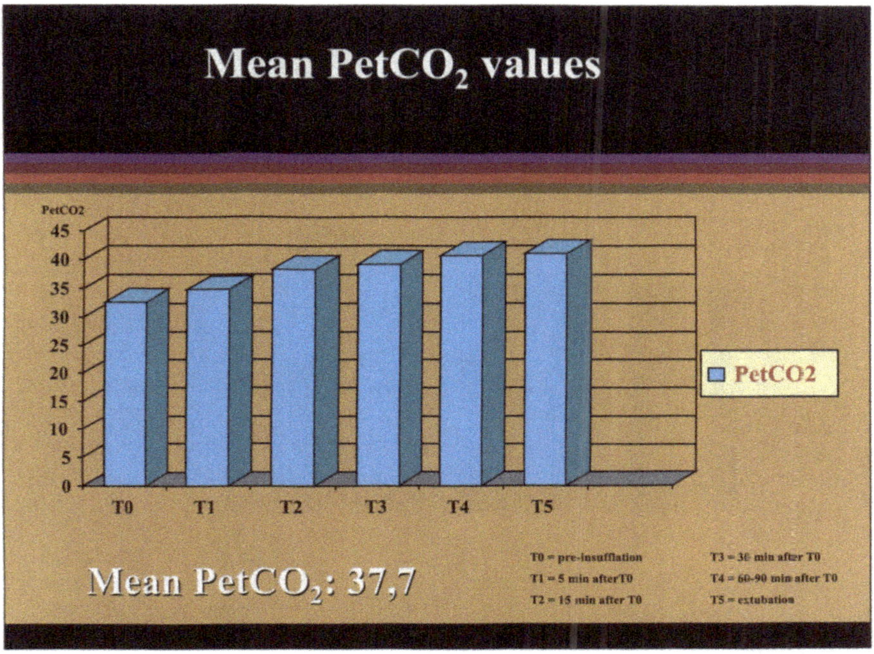

Fig. 1. PetCo$_2$ variations during the different phases of anesthesia (S. Micali, personal case reports)

and the resulting effect influences resistance in Starling's cardiac system.

The Trendelenburg position accentuates such a gradient, and this change in resistance might affect cardiac output by altering the pre-load. This alteration has not been observed during retroperitoneoscopic surgery. According to Starling, variations in the final resistive load, if present, can mainly be attributed to the blood shifting as a result of the tilting position [4].

Systemic and renal hemodynamic variations have been investigated by several experimental studies; the impact of pneumoperitoneum has always appeared to be less severe than in other laparoscopic procedures [5, 6] (Figs. 1–3).

Anesthesia

The anesthesia protocol should always be chosen according to the ASA classification of the patient, surgical requirements, and, not less important, personal proficiency of the anesthetist (ASA and SIAARTI recommendations). As a matter of fact, the possible choices are general anesthesia or central neuraxial blocks.

However, no matter what the choice, adequate monitoring is fundamental. Cardiac electrical activity in cardiopathic patients is best monitored by an ECG machine that is able to measure S-T segment length.

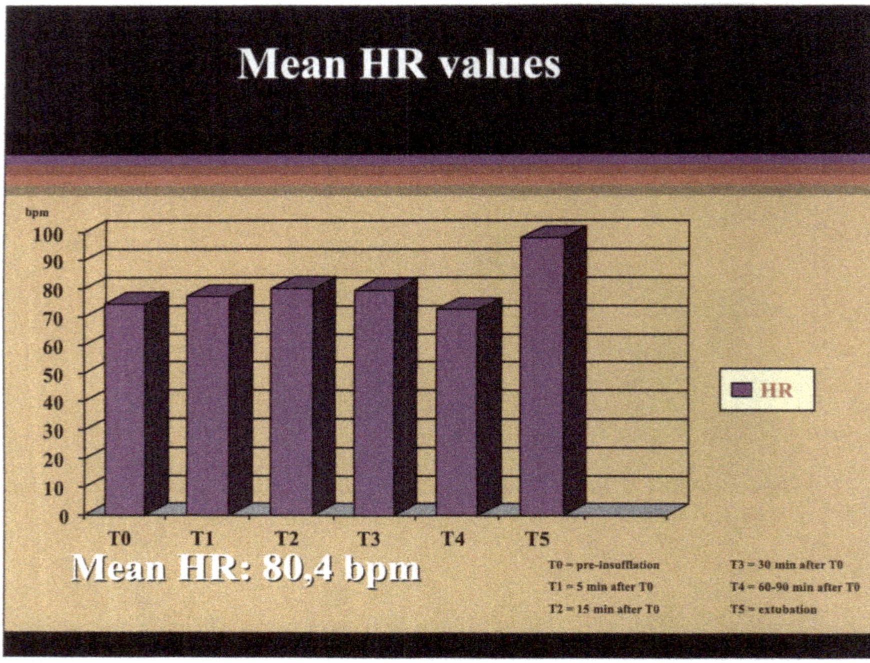

Fig. 2. Heart rate variations during the different phases of anesthesia (S. Micali, personal case reports)

General anesthesia, normally preferred by many anesthetists, can be administered either as purely inhalation anesthesia, balanced anesthesia, or totally intravenous anesthesia (TIVA).

Leaving purely inhalatory anesthesia aside, since it is nowadays scarcely used, it is worth noting that balanced anesthesia can now be performed using new low-solubility halogenated agents, such as sevoflurane, which allow a fast emergence from anesthesia and whose kinetics are only slightly or not affected by the action of other gases, such as CO_2, a well-know condition during laparoscopic surgery.

At present, N_2O use is no longer considered controversial by several authors, at least as far as intraperitoneal laparoscopic procedures are concerned [7].

However, it must still be considered that the diffusion of gas inside the intestinal loops for longer periods of time causes a certain degree of stretching, which might hinder surgical maneuvers; this is even more relevant in retroperitoneosopic surgery where operative space is normally limited.

N_2O solubility is very low: consequently in the event of a gaseous embolism, the hypothesis of a summation in volume between circulating gas and inhaled N_2O becomes a real threat [8]. The use of this gas might be completely avoided by administering the patient a pharmacologic mix intravenously (TIVA).

As far as central neuraxial anesthesia is concerned, epidural anesthesia deserves particular consideration; it is, in fact, well known that this kind of anesthsia only dis-

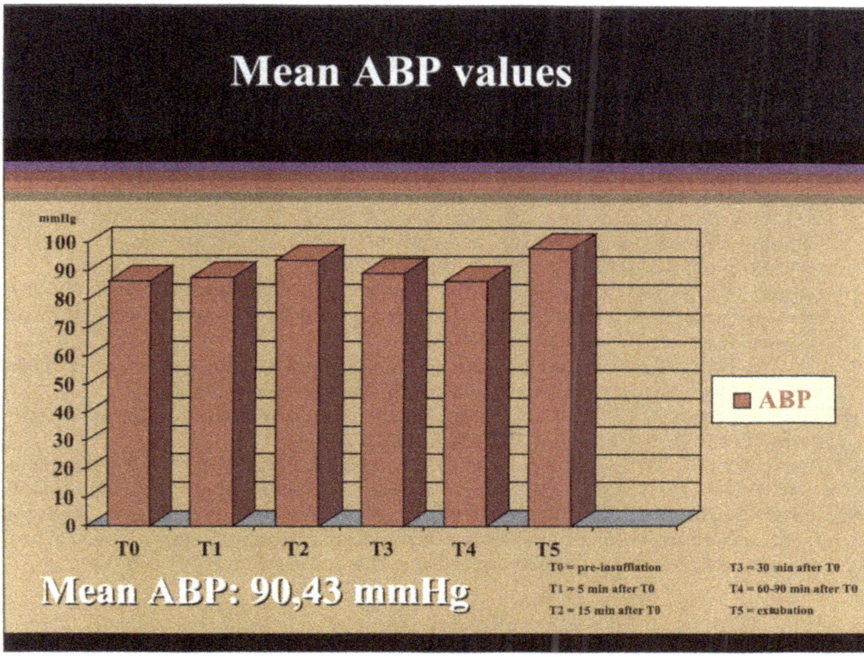

Fig. 3. Variations in arterial blood pressure during the different phases of anesthesia (S. Micali, personal case reports)

turbs hemodynamic homeostasis to a minor degree, as demonstrated by the reports of several authors of retroperitoneal surgery in ASA I-II coronary artery disease patients [9]. It is also useful to remember that this method has been proven to increase renal perfusion, thus improving the overall condition of the patient.

The advantages of epidural anesthesia are also evident in short surgical operations and, most of all, when dealing with bronchopneumopathic patients, in whom it is possible, by taking opportune precautions, to avoid mechanical ventilation. This procedure, even if well performed, alters the ventilation/perfusion ratio, increasing the shunt and eventually leading to a decrease in expiratory CO_2 levels [10].

Finally, another option is represented by combined anesthesia, which consists in ensuring analgesia by means of a central neuraxial block while providing narcosis by administering a purely hypnotic drug. The choice of whether to provide myoresolution mainly depends on the surgical needs or, as mentioned above, on the opportunity of applying mechanical ventilation [10].

References

1. Gill IS, Schweizer D, Hobart MG, Sung GT, Klein EA, Novick AC (2000) Retroperitoneal laparoscopic radical nephrectomy: the Cleveland Clinic experience. J Urol 163: 1665-1670

2. Wolf JS Jr, Carrier S, Stoller S (1994) Gas embolism: helium is more lethal than carbon dioxide. J Laparendosc Surg 4:173
3. Sasagawa I, Suzuki H, Izumi T, Shoji N, et al (1999) Influence of carbon dioxide on respiratory function during posterior retroperitonoscopic adrenalectomy in prone position. Eur Urol 36:413-417
4. Giebler RM, Behrends M, Steffens T, Walz MK, Peitgen K, Peters J (2000) Intraperitoneal and retoperitoneal carbon dioxide insufflation evoke different effects on caval vein pressure gradients in humans. Anesthesiology 92:1568-580
5. Chiu AW, Chang LS, Birkett DH, Babayan RK (1995) The impact of pneumoperitoneum, pneumoretroperitoneum, and gasless laparoscopy on the systemic and renal hemodynamics. J Am Coll Surg 181(5):397-406
6. Giebler RM, Kabatnik M, Stegen BH, Scherer RU, Thomas M, Peters J (1997) Retroperitoneal and intraperitoneal CO2 insufflation have markedly different cardiovascular effects. J Surg Res 68: 153-160
7. Taylor E, Feinstein R, White PF, Sopor N (1992) Anesthesia for laparoscopic cholecystectomy; is nitrous oxide contraindicated? Anesthesiology 76:541
8. Blaser A, Rosset P (1999) Fatal carbon dioxide embolism as an unreported complication of retroperitoneoscopy. Surg Endosc 13:713-714
9. Rosenbaum GJ, Arroyo PJ, Silvina M (1994) Retroperitoneal approach used exclusively with epidural anesthesia for infrarenal aortic disease. Am J Surg 168: 136-139
10. Kolker AR, Hirsch CJ, Gingold BS, Stamatos JM, Wallack MK (1997) Use of epidural anesthesia and spontaneous ventilation during transabdominal colon and rectal procedures in selected high-risk patient groups. Dis Colon Rectum 40 : 339-343

Chapter 8

Anaesthesiological Aspects in Children

Antonio Villani, Patrizia Bozza

Introduction

Laparoscopic surgery has gained widespread popularity over the last decade. Compared with open surgery, this technique is associated with less access trauma, a significant reduction in postoperative pain, reduction in postoperative respiratory impairment, shorter hospital stay and convalescence, as well as better cosmetic results.

Because of these evident advantages, laparoscopic techniques have more recently been extended to paediatric patients.

A variety of laparoscopic surgical procedures have been developed, not only for intraperitoneal but also for extraperitoneal organs. Initially, a transperitoneal laparoscopic approach was used to perform retroperitoneal surgery. Today, surgery on the kidney, adrenal gland or ureter is also carried out with the patient in the lateral decubitus position with exposure of the retroperitoneal space.

During these laparoscopic procedures, significant respiratory and cardiovascular modifications may occur, which are related to the patient's underlying health status, patient positioning and insufflation of gas into body cavities. Knowledge of these cardiorespiratory changes is very important for the anaesthesiologist, because it is essential in planning the different phases of anaesthetic care.

Therefore, in this chapter, the respiratory and cardiovascular changes produced by retroperitoneoscopy will be considered before discussing the pre-, intra- and postoperative anaesthetic care of patients undergoing retroperitoneal laparoscopic surgery.

Respiratory Changes

Although various gases may be used for insufflation, carbon dioxide (CO_2) is the most commonly employed since it does not sustain combustion and, as it is highly soluble, any residual gas is rapidly absorbed, thus decreasing the duration of postoperative abdominal discomfort.

Nevertheless, the absorption of CO_2 from the extraperitoneal cavities plays a major role in alterations in the respiratory function during extraperitoneal laparoscopy.

In fact, the hypercarbia observed during extraperitoneal laparoscopic insufflation is due primarily to the absorption of CO_2, even if several factors, such as alterations in cardiac output and ventilation—perfusion matching, might contribute to increasing the level of $PaCO_2$ [1, 2].

Much controversy exists concerning the extent of CO_2 absorption during extraperitoneal laparoscopy. Many experimental studies performed on animals and human adults have shown that CO_2 absorption during the retroperitoneal or extraperitoneal approach is similar to that observed during transperitoneal laparoscopy [3]. Nevertheless, Bannenberg et al. in their experimental animal study demonstrated that with the extraperitoneal approach, a less marked increase in $ETCO_2$, arterial CO_2 pressure and respiratory acidosis occurs than with the intraperitoneal approach [4]. Wolf and Mullet, on the other hand, suggested that there is a greater CO_2 absorption with retroperitoneal or extraperitoneal insufflation than with transperitoneal laparoscopy [5, 6].

These conflicting results could be explained by some differences in the protocols used to evaluate the effects of intraperitoneal versus extraperitoneal insufflation, and also by differences between animal species concerning absorptive surface, anatomy and compartment compliance.

In fact, absorption of a gas from a cavity depends on its diffusibility, on the size of the absorptive area as well as on the perfusion of the walls of that cavity.

The peritoneal membrane is a wide absorptive area, and during intraperitoneal insufflation, a marked systemic absorption of CO_2 may occur. During retroperitoneal laparoscopy, CO_2 insufflation is performed exclusively in the retroperitoneal space, which, for CO_2 absorption, is much smaller than the peritoneal area. Moreover, the peritoneum is more perfused than the retroperitoneal fatty tissue, and, therefore, the absorption rate of CO_2 during pneumoperitoneum would be more pronounced than during retro- or extrapneumoperitoneum. However, during transperitoneal laparoscopy, increased intra-abdominal pressure may cause a reduction in peritoneal perfusion and, consequently, a decrease in CO_2 absorption from the peritoneum. On the other hand, retroperitoneal CO_2 insufflation may induce an extensive dissection, exposing a large area of the tissue surface and resulting in increased capacity for gas absorption. Furthermore, minute undetected peritoneotomies may certainly occur during retroperitoneoscopy, leading to combined pneumoperitoneum and pneumoretroperitoneum.

From a practical point of view, it should be noted that the insufflation pressure and duration, as well as the development of subcutaneous emphysema, represent the most important determinants of CO_2 absorption [7, 8].

A prolonged operative time (more than 60 min) may increase the absorption of CO_2 during insufflation, so that the CO_2, which is not excreted by ventilation, is accumulated in the skeletal muscle and in the bones. Therefore, after completion of the laparoscopic procedure, CO_2 is gradually released from the tissues, increasing the CO_2 levels observed after extubation in the recovery room [7].

Another important factor regarding CO_2 absorption is the operative site. In fact, peak CO_2 elimination averaged 53% during pelvic laparoscopy compared to 80% during renal laparoscopy. The role of the operative site, which is independent of the laparoscopic approach, could be attributed to the more extensive dissection created during renal laparoscopy than during pelvic laparoscopy, resulting in a greater area for gas absorption [9].

Although few data are available as yet, the respiratory alterations observed in children during laparoscopic surgery are considered to be similar to those seen in adults [1, 10]. Nevertheless, in infants under 4 months of age, CO_2 absorption may be more efficient due to the peculiar anatomical and physiological features of neonates and infants (reduced thickness of tissues between the gas-containing cavity and the capillaries and more absorptive surface in proportion to weight). Moreover, after CO_2 insufflation and deflation, a faster reaction time of the PET-CO_2 change has been observed in younger than in the older children [11].

Diemunsch, in an experimental study on pigs, observed that retroperitoneoscopy was not associated with any adverse effects on ventilation despite an insufflation pressure of 10 mmHg, which allowed a satisfactory working area to be created. The author concluded that the retroperitoneoscopy technique could be carried out in children with fewer respiratory repercussions than those seen during laparoscopy at any equivalent level of pressure [12].

Cardiovascular Effects

The cardiovascular changes induced by an extraperitoneal surgical approach have not yet been completely defined, probably due to their complex pathophysiology, with interaction of many mechanical, chemical and neurohumoral mechanisms.

Moreover, results reported so far differ considerably, depending on the kind of patients studied, and are apparently affected by CO_2 pressure, blood volume expansion or positioning.

However, several studies have suggested that the retropneumoperitoneum has a different impact on the circulatory system compared to that of the pneumoperitoneum [13, 14]. The increase in cardiac output, pulmonary artery, central venous and iliac venous pressures seems to be significantly greater with intraperitoneal than with retroperitoneal CO_2 insufflation [15]. The haemodynamic effects are probably due to the intra-abdominal pressure, since it has been demonstrated — by transoesophageal measurements of the stroke volume and cardiac output — that during laparoscopy, a high intra-abdominal pressure (15 mmHg) induces an increase in heart rate and mean arterial blood pressure associated with a decrease in stroke volume (26%) and cardiac output (28%). In contrast, low intra-abdominal pressure (7 mmHg) induces an increase in heart rate, mean arterial blood pressure, stroke volume and cardiac output [16].

Bearing in mind the results of the experimental work of Guyton and Adkins on the relationship between abdominal pressure and inferior caval venous return, the haemodynamic response to CO_2 insufflation may be due to the inferior-to-superior caval pressure gradient, which for comparable insufflation pressures is greater during pneumoperitoneum than during retropneumoperitoneum [14, 17].

Marathe, studying the potential contribution of altered left ventricular contractility to haemodynamic modifications in pigs during CO_2 pneumoperitoneum with an intra-abdominal pressure from 5 to 25 mmHg, concluded that the haemodynamic modifications are secondary to impaired left ventricular preload and not to marked changes in contractility or left ventricular afterload [18].

Other mechanisms have also been hypothesized to explain the cardiovascular changes observed during laparoscopic surgery.

Hypercarbia may produce an increase in systemic vascular resistance or even myocardial depression; likewise, the moderate increase in heart rate observed during retropneumoperitoneum may represent a sympathetic response to the increase in $PaCO_2$ [19].

In an experimental animal study, it has been observed that during pneumoperitoneum the absorption of CO_2 initiates a pathophysiological process that stimulates vasopressin release. Therefore, vasopressin may possibly play a pivotal role in the haemodynamic response to a CO_2-induced laparoscopy [20].

On the other hand, Mikami suggested that haemodynamic parameters should be carefully monitored at the beginning of the laparoscopic procedure, since he found that epinephrine and norepinephrine levels increase significantly 5 min after CO_2 insufflation [21].

Although limited data are as yet available, the cardiovascular alterations in children undergoing extraperitoneal laparoscopy appear to be qualitatively similar to those of healthy adults [22].

The results of a study performed on 126 children aged between 11 months and 13 years showed that an intra-abdominal CO_2 pressure of 10 mmHg has no effect on haemodynamic stability. A considerable decrease in aortic blood flow and stroke volume, and a marked increase in systemic vascular resistance with no significant changes in mean arterial pressure, was observed by continuous oesophageal echo-Doppler monitoring during laparoscopy in infants. Nevertheless, in spite of this, cardiovascular changes had no clinically deleterious effects, as these haemodynamic alterations were completely reversed after CO_2 deflation [11].

In some children, non-specific decreases in heart rate and in blood pressure can be observed. These alterations can be elicited by a surgical complication, hypovolaemia, head elevated position or deep anaesthesia [19].

Complications

Although the majority of patients recover quickly from laparoscopic surgery, recognition of the most common complications helps the anaesthesiologist to plan appropriately.

The most frequent risk in extraperitoneal laparoscopy concerns CO_2-related morbidities, such as subcutaneous emphysema, pneumomediastinum and pneumothorax. These complications appear to be greater during extraperitoneal insufflation than during intraperitoneal insufflation.

In a study carried out by Ng et al., immediate postoperative chest radiography revealed subcutaneous emphysema in 12.5% and 45% of the patients submitted, respectively, to transperitoneal or retroperitoneal laparoscopy. Irrespective of the laparoscopic approach, patients with subcutaneous emphysema had higher CO_2 elimination during the initial 2.5 h of insufflation than those not presenting evidence of this complication [23].

It has been reported that changes in gas exchange and haemodynamics are associated with marked subcutaneous emphysema. In fact, whereas the vast majority of extraperitoneal CO_2 is easily released through existing trocar holes, CO_2 distributed subcutaneously is not readily vented and requires absorption with subsequent pulmonary excretion for removal from the body. Therefore, significant subcutaneous emphysema associated with CO_2 insufflation could result in prolonged CO_2 absorption. The significance of the subcutaneous emphysema probably depends on its extent, so that the more extensive subcutaneous emphysema results in a higher $PaCO_2$ peak and lower nadir pH than less severe subcutaneous emphysema. However, the time required for CO_2 and pH to return to baseline values does not depend on the extent of emphysema [24]. If minute ventilation is fixed — as could be the case for patients with severe chronic obstructive pulmonary disease or in patients with ventilatory dysfunction due to depressant drugs — prolonged hypercapnia and respiratory acidosis would result from the subcutaneous emphysema.

Even if postoperative ventilation is required in only very few cases, patients with subcutaneous emphysema after laparoscopic surgery should be monitored in the recovery room until $PaCO_2$ and pH values approach baseline. Generally, subcutaneous emphysema is not associated with significant changes in arterial pressure, but an increase in cardiac output may be observed, probably as a result of vasodilatation due to elevated $PaCO_2$.

The incidence of pneumomediastinum and pneumothorax in patients undergoing extraperitoneal insufflation is not surprising, since the potential routes of gas into the thoracic spaces are more easily exposed to extraperitoneal gas. Direct passage of gas into the pleural cavity, as reported by some investigators, is less likely than passage from the mediastinum through the pulmonary hilus.

As might be expected with pneumothorax due to CO_2, thoracostomy is not required in the absence of direct surgical injury. Therefore, chest X-rays after extraperitoneal laparoscopy are necessary only in cases of suspected high trocar insertion or pulmonary symptoms, since all other thoracic gas collections appear to be clinically insignificant.

Other severe complications include visceral or vascular injuries, more commonly the result of laceration by the Veress needle or trocar insertion than due to the actual surgical procedures [25].

A more serious, but less frequent, complication is CO_2-related pulmonary embolism, which may be differentiated from pneumothorax and subcutaneous emphysema not only by clinical examination, but also by means of the rapid decrease in $ETCO_2$ [26].

Anaesthetic Management

Preoperative Considerations

Contraindications to laparoscopic surgery include severe coagulopathy, intracardiac shunt defect, and inability to tolerate general anaesthesia and hypercarbia (poor cardiopulmonary function, impaired intracranial compliance).

Obesity cannot be considered a real contraindication to anaesthesia, even if anaesthetic management may be challenging in patients with morbid obesity.

Data collected from a retrospective audit in members of the French Association of Anaesthetists in Paediatrics (ADARPEF) show that contraindications to laparoscopic surgery include respiratory disability, cardiopathy and age under 5 years when surgical instruments of the correct size are not available [26].

Although it has been reported that patients with preoperative cardiopulmonary disease show significant increases in $PaCO_2$ and decreases in pH during CO_2 insufflation [27], the theory that patients with severe cardiovascular or pulmonary diseases should not be submitted to transperitoneal laparoscopic surgery [28] does not apply to extraperitoneal laparoscopy, since the negative pathophysiological effects of transperitoneal gas insufflation on the haemodynamic and respiratory systems are more marked than those observed during extraperitoneal laparoscopy.

Newborns and infants under 6 months of age should be considered patients at high risk as much as their foramen ovale or their ductus arteriosus is patent, pulmonary arterial resistance is increased and bronchodysplasia is present [26].

In this age group, contraindications for laparoscopic surgery also include hypovolaemia, heart diseases, increased intracranial pressure and alveolar distension.

Monitoring

Monitoring should be tailored according to the clinical conditions of the individual patient and the extraperitoneal procedure used.

Invasive monitoring is not clinically indicated in ASA I or II patients, but intraoperative monitoring should include an electrocardioscope, non-invasive arterial pressure, pulse oximetry, capnography, neuromuscular function, inspired O_2 fraction, peak airway pressure, oesophageal temperature and urinary output.

$PETCO_2$ is useful for evaluating the effectiveness of ventilation in eliminating the extra "load" of CO_2. However, this parameter may not be reliable in some instances, such as in ventilation—perfusion mismatching, since it does not reflect the true arterial level of CO_2. Thus, arterial blood gas analysis should be performed in patients presenting with cardiopulmonary diseases in order to modify adequately the ventilatory pattern [29].

Likewise, $ETCO_2$ may not be valid in infants, since the decrease in Functional Residual Capacity (FRC) leads to an increase in ventilation—perfusion mismatching and alveolar deadspace; it may also not be valid in children with rapid respiratory and low tidal volume. P(a–ET) CO_2 values are often negative in healthy ventilated children during general anaesthesia, especially during laparoscopic procedures. Several factors, such as the gas sampling site, rebreathing, the increasing level of CO_2, may contribute to these negative values. Overestimation of $PaCO_2$ by $PETCO_2$ (reaching high levels) may lead to hyperventilation which can be deleterious. To prevent this situation, arterial blood gas analysis should be repeatedly performed during long laparoscopic procedures [30].

Anaesthetic Technique

General endotracheal anaesthesia is the anaesthetic technique of choice in extraperitoneal laparoscopy, because it allows one to obtain a secured airway as well as to modulate ventilation according to the hypercarbic level. In contrast, regional anaesthesia is very rarely used for laparoscopic urological surgery, mainly because it does not assure patient comfort, especially in the case of kidney position.

Although it has been suggested that ventilation should be increased by 15%–30% to compensate for the extra "load" of CO_2, intraoperative adjustments of minute ventilation by the anaesthesiologist are necessary to keep blood CO_2 levels in a steady state, despite occasional increases in $ETCO_2$ [31]. When an increase in $ETCO_2$ levels is observed during an extraperitoneal procedure, tidal volume and respiratory rate should be increased immediately.

Furthermore, since significantly greater peak airway pressures are required with intraperitoneal than with retroperitoneal insufflation to obtain the same tidal volume, the neuromuscular blockade is not strictly necessary during extraperitoneal laparoscopy.

The choice of the anaesthetic agent has no significant bearing on the overall CO_2 absorption during laparoscopic surgery, but it is important to provide an adequate level of anaesthesia throughout the procedure.

Some anaesthesiologists prefer to use total intravenous anaesthesia during laparoscopic surgery because it offers better control of cardiovascular function than the volatile anaesthetic agents, which may cause myocardial depressant effects [14, 31]. Moreover, in some institutions, halothane has been abandoned because of cardiovascular concern, while in others, N2O is no longer used so as to limit the risk of potential gas embolism [7].

Anaesthesiological management should also include warming measures to prevent hypothermia, bearing in mind that during laparoscopy, the gas cycled in and out of the patient induces relevant evaporative heat losses [26].

During anaesthesia, problems may arise, which the anaesthesiologist must be trained to recognize and treat. Thus, if an increase in end-tidal CO_2 is associated with an increase in airway pressure, dislocation of the endotracheal tube or pneumothorax should be suspected.

Subcutaneous emphysema should be considered, however, when hypercarbia occurs in the absence of an increase in airway pressure [7].

Hypoxaemia may also be encountered and several different causes have been held responsible. Excluding a pre-existing cardiopulmonary disease, the most frequent events causing hypoxaemia during laparoscopic procedures are: (a) pneumothorax [7] or (b) venous CO_2 embolism [26]. Pulmonary oedema should be suspected when large quantities of fluids are used to irrigate.

Postoperative Management

After long laparoscopic procedures, the extra "load" of CO_2 will gradually be excreted during the postoperative period, leading to increases in ventilatory requirements even after laparoscopy is completed. Therefore, bearing in mind that the patient's postoperative ability to increase minute ventilation may be compromised by residual inhalation, after laparoscopy, patients (particularly those with pre-existing cardiopulmonary diseases) should be observed in the recovery room until $PaCO_2$ and pH values approach baseline, even if postoperative ventilation is required in only very few cases.

To obtain adequate postoperative analgesia, it is important that surgeons deflate CO2 as much as possible at the end of the surgical procedure, since it has been demonstrated that residual CO_2 represents a relevant causative factor of postoperative pain [26].

Moreover, infiltration of the incision sites with local anaesthetics associated with opioids by parenteral or patient-controlled analgesia allows for the adequate control of postoperative pain. The intramuscular administration of Ketorolac before the end of surgery also appears to be adequate for postoperative analgesia; however, its use is limited due to surgeons' fear concerning increased risk of bleeding.

References

1. Tobias JD (1993) Anesthetic considerations for endoscopic procedures in children. Semin Pediatr Surg 2:190-194
2. Tobias JD (1998) Anesthetic considerations for laparoscopy in children. Semin Pediatr Surg 5:60-66
3. Baird JE, Granger R, Klein R, Warriner CB, Phang PT (1999) The effects of retroperitoneal carbon dioxide insufflation on hemodynamics and arterial carbon dioxide. Am J Surg 177:164-166
4. Bannenberg JJ, Rademaker BM, Froeling FM, Meijer DW (1997) Hemodynamics during laparoscopic extra- and intraperitoneal insufflation. An experimental study. Surg Endosc 11:911-914
5. Wolf JS Jr, Carrier S, Stoller ML (1995) Intraperitoneal versus extraperitoneal insufflation of carbon dioxide as for laparoscopy. J Endourol 9:63-66
6. Mullet CE, Viale JP, Sagnard PE, Miellet CC, Ruynat LG, Counioux HC, Motin JP, Boulez JP, Dargent DM, Annat GJ (1993) Pulmonary CO2 elimination during surgical procedures using intra- or extraperitoneal CO2 insufflation. Anesth Analg 76:622-626
7. Wolf JS Jr, Monk TG, McDougall EM, McClennan BL, Clayman RV (1995) The extraperitoneal approach and subcutaneous emphysema are associated with greater absorption of carbon dioxide during laparoscopic renal surgery. J Urol 154:959-963
8. Hall D, Goldstein A, Tynan E, Braunstein L (1993) Profound hypercarbia late in the

course of laparoscopic cholecystectomy: detection by continuous capnometry. Anesthesiology 79:173-174

9. Wolf JS Jr, Clayman RV, Monk TG, McClennan BL, McDougall EM (1995) Carbon dioxide absorption during laparoscopic pelvic operation. J Amer Coll Surg 180:555-560
10. Gueugniaud PY, Abisseror M, Moussa M, Godard J, Foussat C, Petit P, Dodat H (1998) The hemodynamic effects of pneumoperitoneum during laparoscopic surgery in healthy infants: assessment by continuous esophageal aortic blood flow echo-Doppler. Anesth Analg 86:290-293
11. Hsing Ch, Hseu SS, Tsai SK, Chu CC, Chen TW, Wei CF, Lee TY (1995) The physiological effect of pneumoperitoneum in pediatric laparoscopy. Acta Anaesthesiol Sin 33:1-6
12. Diemunsch P, Becmeur F, Meyer P (1999) Retroperitoneoscopy versus laparoscopy in piglets: ventilatory and thermic repercussions. J Pediatr Surg 34:1514-1517
13. Chiu AW, Chang LS, Birkett DH, Babayan RK (1995) The impact of pneumoperitoneum, pneumoretreoperitoneum, and gasless laparoscopy on the systemic and renal hemodynamics. J Am Coll Surg 181:397-406
14. Giebler RM, Behrends M, Steffens T, Walz MK, Peitgen K, Peters J (2000) Intraperitoneal and retroperitoneal carbon dioxide insufflation evoke different effects on caval vein pressure gradients in humans. Evidence for the Starling resistor concept of abdominal venous return. Anesthesiology 92:1568-1580
15. Giebler RM, Kabatnik M, Stegen BH, Scherer RU, Thomas M, Peters J (1997) Retroperitoneal and intraperitoneal CO2 insufflation have markedly different cardiovascular effects. J Surg Res 68:153-160
16. Dexter SP, Vucevic M, Gibson J, McMahon MJ (1999) Hemodynamic consequences of high- and low-pressure capnoperitoneum during laparoscopic cholecystectomy. Surg Endosc 13:376-381
17. Guyton AC, Adkins LH (1954) Quantitative aspects of the collapse factor in relation to venous return. Am J Physiol 77:523-527
18. Marathe US, Lilly RE, Silvestry SC, Schauer PR, Davis JW, Pappas TN, Glower DD (1996) Alterations in hemodynamics and left ventricular contractility during carbon dioxide pneumoperitoneum. Surg Endosc 10:974-978
19. Tobias JD, Holcomb GW III, Brock JW III, Deshpande JK, Lowe S, Morgan WM III (1995) Cardiorespiratory changes in children during laparoscopy. J Ped Surg 30:33-36
20. Mann C, Boccara G, Pouzzeratte Y, Eliet J, Serradel-Le Gal C, Vergnes C, Bichet DG, Guillon G, Fabre JM, Colson P (1999) The relationship among carbon dioxide pneumoperitoneum, vasopressin release, and hemodynamic changes. Anesth Analg 89:278-283
21. Mikami O, Kawakita S, Fujise K, Shingu K, Takahashi H, Matsuda T (1996) Catecholamine release caused by carbon dioxide insufflation during laparoscopic surgery. J Urol 155:1368-1371
22. Bozkurt P, Kaya G, Yeker Y, Tunali Y, Altinaz F (1999) The cardiorespiratory effects of laparoscopic procedures in infants. Anaesthesia 54:831-834
23. Ng CS, Gill IS, Sung GT, Walley DG, Graham R, Schweizer D (1999) Retroperitoneoscopic surgery is not associated with increased carbon dioxide absorption. J Urol 162:1268-1272
24. Rudson-Brown BCD, MacLennan D, Warriner CB, Phang PT (1996) Effect of subcutaneous carbon dioxide insufflation on arterial pCO2. Am J Surg 171:460-463
25. Ono Y, Katoh N, Kinukawa T, Matsuura O, Oshima S (1996) Laparoscopic nephrectomy via the retroperitoneal approach. J Urol 156:1101-1104
26. Sfez M (1993) Cœliochirurgie en pédiatrie: le point de vue de l'anesthésiste. Cah d'Anesth 41:237-244
27. Matsuda T, Fujise K, Matsumoto S, Mikami O, Uchida J, Shingu K (1996) Respiratory effects of CO2 pneumoperitoneum during transperitoneal laparoscopic urological surgery. Eur Urol 30:484-489

28. Junghans T, Böhm B, Gründel K, Schwenk W, Müller JM (1997) Does pneumoperitoneum with different gases, body positions, and intraperitoneal pressures influence renal and hepatic blood flow? Surgery 121:206-211
29. Iwasaka H, Mijakawa H, Yamamoto H, Kitano T, Taniguchi K, Honda N (1996) Respiratory mechanics and arterial blood gases during and after laparoscopic cholecystectomy. Can J Anaesth 43:129-133
30. Laffon M, Gouchet A, Sitbon P, Guicheteau V, Bijick E, Duchalais A, Mercier C (1998) Difference between arterial and end-tidal carbon dioxide pressures during laparoscopy in paediatric patients. Can J Anaesth 45:561-563
31. Manner T, Aantaa R, Alanen M (1998) Lung compliance during laparoscopic surgery in paediatric patients. Paed Anaesth 8:25-29

Chapter 9

Indications for Retroperitoneal Laparoscopic Surgery in Pediatric Patients

Paolo Caione, Nicola Capozza

Retroperitoneal laparoscopic surgery has recently become available to urologists and pediatric urologists as a new surgical technique and a different approach for an increasing variety of clinical conditions that can develop in the retroperitoneal organs. After the first urological application presented by Wickham [1] on retroperitoneal endoscopic ureterolithotomy in 1979, surgical technique and the dissection of the retroperitoneal space were standardized by Gaur [2] and Gill [3] in the first half of the 1990s. Since then, retroperitoneal laparoscopy has attracted interest and progressively become known among urologists and laparoscopic surgeons.

The application of retroperitoneal laparoscopic approaches in pediatric patients with urological problems has only followed with some hesitation [4,5]. Even now, children represent a critical group of patients in employing laparoscopic urological procedures, except for cases of nonpalpable testes, ovarian pathology in girls, and, lastly, the internal genitalia examination in intersexual patients. Finding the proper indications for retroperitoneal laparoscopic procedures in children is an even more uncertain endeavor.

The question of the advantages and limitations of retroperitoneoscopy in pediatric urology is still under debate, if compared with the results of well-standardized open surgery. In fact, the advantages of any laparoscopic technique seem to be less evident in children than in adult patients. In the pediatric age group, wound healing is more rapid than in adults or in the elderly, and it is associated with less severe scarring. Further criticism to the use of laparoscopic procedures in pediatrics has also been raised considering the better and quicker ability of young children to recovery after open surgery. Infants and young children return to their normal activities more promptly than adult patients [6]. If we consider that a large number of pediatric urological operations are mostly carried out in early childhood or in infancy, the clinical use and the need for laparoscopic approaches may seem smaller in pediatric than in adult patients.

A questionable point to be discussed is the possible higher risk of complications from minimally invasive surgery, and particularly from laparoscopic procedures, in pediatrics compared with the adulthood experience. A review of the results of an American study of pediatric urological laparoscopy was presented by Peters [7] in 1996. Actually, there is a lack of large series in the published literature that analyze the results in adults versus those in children. Nevertheless, it is common knowledge that endoscopic surgical maneuvers must be carried out with

Table 1. Limitations of retroperitoneal laparoscopic procedures in pediatrics, compared with adult patients

More rapid wound healing
Less severe tissue scarring
Quicker recovery after open surgery
Prompt return to normal activities
Higher rate of reconstructive rather than ablative procedures
Surgery in early pediatric age or in infancy
Lack of working space in retroperitoneoscopy
No adequate laparoscopic instrumentation for the young child
Need for laparoscopic experience and skill
Higher risk of complications? (not confirmed)

much more accuracy and delicacy in young patients. Furthermore, the laparoscopic instrumentation is often not adequate for use in very young children.

A last point to be considered in pediatric transperitoneal or retroperitoneal laparoscopy is the fact that children need a higher number of reconstructive procedures: pyeloplasty, ureteral tapering, vesicoureteral reimplantation, and bladder augmentation are almost always required in infancy and childhood. Conversely, reconstructive urological procedures are quite uncommon in adulthood and surgery is mostly ablative: simple or radical nephrectomy and nephroureterectomy, renal cyst marsupialization, radical prostatectomy or cystectomy, and stone removal are just examples. Undoubtedly, ablative surgery is simpler and easier to perform with minimally invasive techniques, if compared with reconstructive procedures (Table 1).

Nevertheless, the increased capability of laparoscopic techniques to delicately handle tissues and the properties of video-assisted surgery in providing significant amplification of the operative field may play a positive role in enhancing its application in pediatric patients.

As a further consideration, retroperitoneal laparoscopic procedures may offer the benefit of less postoperative pain and a reduced physical and psychological impact in pediatric patients, too, allowing a quicker return to working activities for their parents [6].

We believe that the near future will demonstrate further progress and technical advances, such as the miniaturization of laparoscopic instrumentation, that can be applied to pediatric patients. It will be possible to widen the field of application of retroperitoneal or extraperitoneal laparoscopic surgery in pediatric patients, even to reconstructive surgery. Here, the progressive gain in clinical experience on the part of urologists is a critical point (Table 2).

It must be stressed that the results of minimally invasive procedures, such as retroperitoneoscopic surgery, have to compare with the well-established open operations that presently represent the gold standard. The Anderson-Hynes dismembered pyeloplasty is the first choice procedure to correct Ureteropielic Junction (UPJ) obstruction in the pediatric age group because of the high safety and efficacy rate. Any other technique, including retroperitoneal laparoscopic procedures, must compare with the standardized results of the Anderson-Hynes "open" pyeloplasty. Only when the new technology and the surgeon's skill can replicate the results of

Table 2. Possible advantages of retroperitoneal laparoscopic procedures in the pediatric age group

Delicate tissue handling
Significant amplification of the operative field
No violation of the peritoneal cavity in retroperitoneoscopy
Decreased postoperative pain
Reduced physical and psychological impact
Quicker return of parents to working activities

the gold standard open operations in terms of efficacy and security can we definitively modify our current surgical options in favor of the new minimally invasive procedures, among which retroperitoneal laparoscopy must be considered

Indications for Retroperitoneal Laparoscopic Procedures in the Pediatric Age Group

Definite indications for retroperitoneoscopic laparoscopy in children are still being debated and differ partially from those in adult patients. It is interesting to recall that laparoscopy in urologic procedures was first initiated by pediatric urologists in patients with nonpalpable, undescended testes for diagnostic purposes almost two decades ago, and for single-stage or staged orchiopexy at the beginning of the 1990s [8]. Since then, many other transperitoneal laparoscopic procedures have been proposed and performed for urological indications in the pediatric age group. Nephrectomy and nephroureterectomy for benign diseases, heminephrectomy for dysplastic hydronephotic upper or lower renal moiety, orchiectomy, and one- or two-stage orchidopexy for intraabdominal testicles, ovarian cysts, and pubertal varicocele have become the most commom transperitoneal laparoscopic indications in childhood.

The retroperitoneal access to laparoscopy was proposed only recently in pediatric patients [4, 9, 10] and the extension of indications has been episodical up to now, often with simple reports from different authors.

Confirmed Indications

A few indications are now well established and probably will represent the new gold standard for the pediatric urology centers where retroperitoneal laparoscopic procedures are currently available (Table 3). Concerning renal surgery, nephrectomy and nephroureterectomy for benign disease, upper pole or lower pole heminephrectomy in double systems, renal biopsy, and cyst marsupialization can be performed through a retroperitoneal laparoscopic access as a valid alternative to the standardized open procedures. In 1996, Valla et al. [4] presented their initial six cases of retroperitoneal laparoscopic nephrectomy. El-Ghoneimi [9] reported on nephrectomy in high-risk childen with pretransplant end-stage renal disease. The technique for retroperitoneoscopic nephrectomy is described elsewere in this book by M. Franks et al. (Chap. 11. "Retroperitoneoscopy in Children," this volume) . Borer et al. [11] described a posterior access with the patient in prone position, using 2-mm instrumentation. The real advantage of using the miniscope, however, must be proven with respect to the commonly used 5- to 10-mm ports.

Polar heminephroureterectomy is a reliable indication in double systems with a nonfunctioning hydronephrotic or dysplastic atrophic pole, as may be found in ureteroceles or in refluxing ureters associated with complete ureteral duplication. Janetschek et al. [12] pointed out the indications and the technique with tranperitoneal laparoscopic access. Other authors [9, 11] stressed the retroperitoneal laparoscopic access. Partial duplex heminephrectomy involves careful identification of polar or accessory vessels to the pathological moiety. Borzi [13] presented his experience with posterior retroperitoneoscopic access, recently comparing it with the lateral approach: he did not find statistically significant differences in the operative time, bleeding, and complications. He concluded that the posterior approach gives easier vascular control for nephrectomy or heminephrectomy, but the lateral approach is preferred if extended ureterectomy is needed, as in the case of a refluxing ureter, or in the presence of renal ectopia or fusion.

Renal cyst marsupialization [5] and renal biopsy [14] represent other minor procedures in the kidneys, not seen very frequently in children, that benefit from the minimal invasiveness of retroperitoneoscopic access. We believe that if surgery is indicated, it should be performed via a retroperitoneal laparoscopic approach.

Controversial Indications

Several different indications for retroperitoneoscopy have been proposed in the last few years. Although the number of possible utilizations is increasing quickly in the pediatric age group, too, there is not yet a general consensus for all of them, as there is still too little experience in children (Table 3). We could attempt to separate the confirmed indications mentioned above from numerous others that are not fully accepted or only episodically proposed in the pediatric age group. Retroperitoneal laparoscopic procedures must prove to be as efficient as the open techniques. We believe that some of them may become standardized and accepted in the near future, after their advantages have been proven by controlled studies.

Dismembered pyeloplasty for UPJ obstruction has been mostly performed via the transperitoneal approach [15] or in adult patients [16]. One of the critical points is the lack of working space in the retroperitoneal approach in pediatric patients, as discussed above. Only recently have reports of extraperitoneal laparoscopic repair of UPJ obstruction in adults been published [17]: the authors conclude that retroperitoneoscopy, by providing easy and rapid access to the retroperitoneal space, seems to be a valuable alternative treatment for UPJ obstruction. In pediatrics experience through the retroperitoneal approach is still limited.

There are episodical indications for ureterolithotomy and pyelolithotomy ([5], J.S. Valla, personal communication) in pediatrics, but laparoscopic technique can be used with positive results in preschool-aged patients, too. Spermatic vessel obliteration for varicocele [18, 19] represents a simple but controversial indication in pediatric urology, because the cost-benefit ratio compared with other percutaneous or open techniques is still to be defined.

Table 3. Retroperitoneal laparoscopy in the pediatric age group

Procedure	Indications
Confirmed	
Nephrectomy	Poorly functioning kidney with : - Reflux - UPJ obstruction - Renal calculus disease - Renal hypertension - Chronic pyelonephritis
Kidney	Symptomatic dysplastic, multicystic - - pre-transplant end-stage nephropathy with: - Refractary hypertension - Severe nephrotic syndrome - Hemolytic-uremic syndrome
Nephroureterectomy	- Severe reflux nephropathy - Atrophic kidney with megaureter
Upper or lower heminephrectomy	Double system with dysplastic renal moiety - Ureterocele - Megaureter - Ectopic ureter
Cyst marsupialization	Giant renal cyst
Renal cortical biopsy	- Nephrological indications if percutaneous needle biopsy not safe or effective
Controversial	
Adrenalectomy	Adrenal benign pathology
Dismembered pyeloplasty	UPJ obstruction, Fenger or Y-V pyeloplasty
Pyelolithotomy	Large pyelic stone (cystine)
Nephrolithotomy	
Calycostomy	Calyceal diverticula
Ureterolithotomy	Ureteric stone (cystine)
Spermatic vessel obliteration	Varicocele

Other retroperitoneal laparoscopic procedures have been reported occasionally that may be performed by utilizing the extraperitoneal mini-invasive access. Retroperitoneoscopic access in lymphadenectomy, cutaneous ureterostomy, and bladder diverticula has been proposed episodically, but, due to the lack of experience, these indications are still experimental.

Contraindications

A relative contraindication for retroperitoneal laparoscopic procedures is any previous retroperitoneoscopic laparoscopy, as well as the presence of dense retroperitoneal fibrosis, as a result of local inflammatory processes [20]. As in adult patients, moderate obesity could increase the difficulty in identifying anatomical structures

Table 4. Absolute or relative contraindications to retroperitoneal laparoscopic surgery

Urological malignancy (Wilms tumor)
Renal or ureteral trauma
Sepsis
Severe cardiopulmonary disease
Significant coagulopathy
Previous retroperitoneal inflammations or infections
Previous retroperitoneoscopic procedures
Age less than 2 years, body weight below 15 kg
(Obesity)

in the retroperitoneal space, but this is not an absolute contraindication [21]. Retroperitoneal laparoscopy procedures have been demonstrated to be safe in both adult patients [21] and children [9, 14] with chronic renal failure.

Young age and body weight of young patients may represent a limiting factor to applying retroperitoneal laparoscopic procedures in the pediatric population, but retroperitoneoscopic surgery has been effectively carried out in infants aged less than 2 years [5, 13, 14]. The short distance between the ports and the conflict of movements of the laparoscopic instrumentation is a practical problem during operative retroperitoneoscopy in small babies. The miniaturization of the laparoscopic instrumentation and the overall increasing experience will help pediatric urologists who would like to consider these procedures in the youngest patients (Table 4).

Conclusions

Retroperitoneal laparoscopy surgery has developed relatively quickly in the past few years, gaining more acceptance in urology. The direct access to retroperitoneal structures and the limited invasiveness represent the rationale for adopting retroperitoneoscopic procedures in urological clinical practice [22]. It has been recently calculated that retroperitoneoscopy accounts at this time for half of all laparoscopic procedures in adult urology [23]. Retroperitoneoscopic procedures for benign renal diseases seem to represent an effective, safe. and viable alternative to conventional open surgery with reasonable complication and conversion rates [24].

In pediatrics, the implementation of retroperitoneoscopic surgery has been more limited so far, because of the difficulties in reconstructive procedures due to the smaller space in the retroperitoneum, and the less evident advantages versus open surgery compared with adult patients. Moreover, when considering the application of any laparoscopic technique in pediatric urology, we must be concerned about the safety and the economics of the new procedure, if compared with standardized open surgery. Several reports [7, 23] have been presented concerning the low rate of complications when transperitoneal or retroperitoneal laparoscopic procedures are carried out by trained, experienced surgeons.

We are basically optimistic that the demand for less invasive procedures together with increased experience and the documented improvement in results and safety will help to establish retroperitoneoscopy and laparoscopy in pediatrics.

References

1. Wickham JEA (1979) The surgical treatment of renal lithiasis. In: Wickham JEA (ed) Urinary calcolus disease. Churchill Livingstone, New York, pp 145-198
2. Gaur DD, Agerwal DK, Purhoit KC (1993) Retroperitoneal laparoscopic nephrectomy: initial case report. J Urol 149:103-105
3. Gill IS, Clayman RV, Albala DM et al. (1998) Retroperitoneal and pelvic extraperitoneal laparoscopy: an international perspective. Urology 52:566-571
4. Valla JS, Guilloneau B, Montupet P et al (1996) Retroperitoneal laparoscopic nephrectomy in children :preliminary report of 6 cases. J Laparoendosc Surg 6:S55-S59
5. El-Gonheimi A, Valla JS, Steyaert H, Aigrain Y (1998) Laparoscopic renal surgery via a retroperitoneal approach in children. J Urol 160:1138-1141
6. Ross JH, Gill IS, Kay R (2001) Optimizing minimally invasive surgery for the pediatric patient. Dialogues Pediatr Urol;24(7):4-6
7. Peters CA (1996) Complications in pediatric urological laparoscopy: results of a survey. J Urol 155:1070-1073
8. Bloom DA (1991) Two-step orchiopexy with pelviscopic clip ligation of spermatic vessels. J Urol 145:1030-1033
9. El-Ghoneimi A, Sauty L, Maintenant J, Macher M, Lottmann H, Aigrain Y (2000) Laparoscopic retroperitoneal nephrectomy in high risk children. J Urol 164:1076-1079
10. Kobashi K., Chamberlain D, Rajpoot D, Shanberg A (1998) Retroperitoneal laparoscopic nephrectomy in children. J Urol 160:1142-1144
11. Borer J, Cisek L, Atala A, Diamond D, Retik A, Peters C (1999) Pediatric retroperironeoscopic nephrectomy using 2 mm instrumentation. J Urol 162:1725-1730
12. Janetschek G, Seibold J, Radmayr C, Bartsch G (1997) Laparoscopic heminephroureterectomy in pediatric patients. J Urol 158:1928-1930
13. Borzi P (1998) Retroperitoneoscopic partial nephrectomy in infants and children. J Pediatr 3(2):646-649
14. Caione P, Micali S, Rinaldi S, Capozza N, Lais A, Matarazzo E, Maturo G, Micali F (2000) Retroperitoneal laparoscopy for renal biopsy in children. J Urol 164:1080-1083
15. Moore RG, Kavoussi LR, Adams JB (1995) Laparoscopic pyeloplasty. J Urol 153:515 A
16. Janetschek G, Peschel R, Altarac S, Bartsch G (1966) Laparoscopic and retroperitoneoscopic repair of ureteropelvic junction obstruction. Urology 47(3):311-316
17. Ben Slama MR, Salomon L, Hoznek A, Cicco A, Saint Free Net, Alame Web, Antiphon P, Chopin DK, Abbou CC (2000) Extraperitoneal laparoscopic repair of ureteropelvic junction obstruction: initial experience in 15 cases. Urology 56(1):45-48
18. Gaur DD, Agarwal DK, Purohit KC (1994) Retroperitoneal laparoscopic varicocelectomy. J Urol 151:895-897
19. Valla JS (1999) Videosurgery of the retroperitoneal space in children. In: Bax NMA, Georgeson KE, Najmaldin A, Valla JS (eds) Endoscopic surgery in children. Springer, Berlin Heidelberg New York, pp 379-392
20. Rassweiler JS, Seemann D, Frede Target, Henkel TO, Atken P(1998) Retroperitoneoscopy: Experience with 200 cases. J Urol 160:1265-1268
21. Gaur DD, Rathi SS, Ravandale AV, Gopichand M (2001) A single-centre experience of retroperitoneoscopy using the balloon technique. BJU Int 87:602-606
22. Capelouto CC, Moore RG, Silverman S G, Kavoussi LR (1994) Retroperitoneoscopy: anatomical rationale for direct retroperitoneal access. J Urol 152:2008-2010
23. Kumar M, Kumar R, Hemal AK, Gupta NP (2001) Complications of retroperitoneoscopic surgery at one centre. BJU Int 87:607-612
24. Hemal AK (2001) Retroperitoneoscopic nepthrectomy for benign diseases of kidney. Urol Int 67:121-129

Chapter 10

Retroperitoneal Laparoscopic Adrenalectomy

Vincenzo Disanto, Gino Scalese

A number of surgical approaches may be used when operating on the adrenal gland and often the surgeon's choice is determined by factors such as the type of disease present, tumor bulk and side, the constitutional features of the patient, and the surgeon's own experience and preference.

Given the anatomical position of the gland, there is no doubt that open surgery is particularly invasive, irrespective of the type of incision made (Figs. 1, 2). The advent of laparoscopy has brought into being the most advantageous solution for adrenal gland excisions, and laparoscopic adrenalectomy is nowadays commonly considered the gold standard in this field.

Retroperitoneoscopy was first performed in 1992 [1] and then retroperitoneal laparoscopic adrenalectomy in 1994 [2, 16, 17]. There is still controversy over which of the two techniques is to be preferred; the transperitoneal approach is unquestionably simpler to perform because of the larger space available but it also requires greater mobilization of the viscera, with a greater risk of iatrogenic injury.

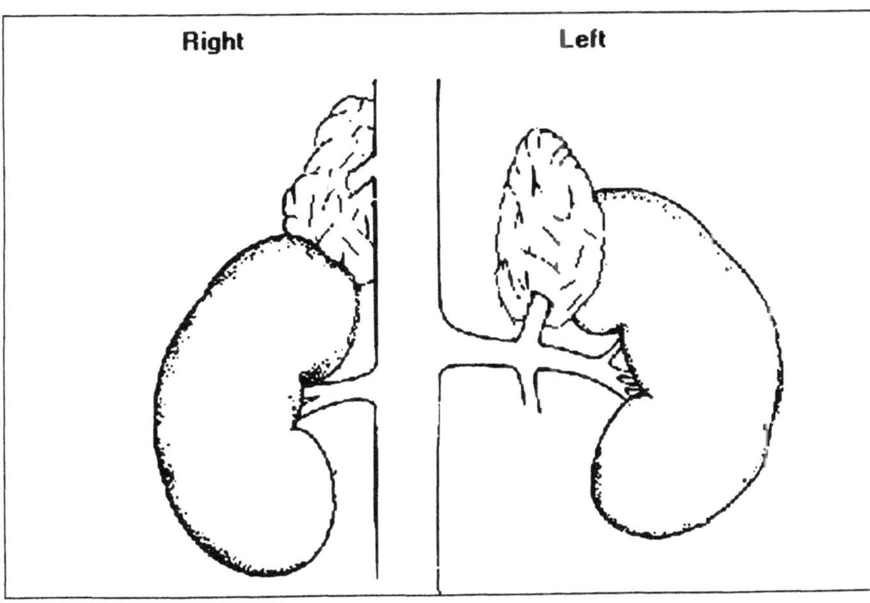

Fig. 1. Venous vascularization of the adrenal glands

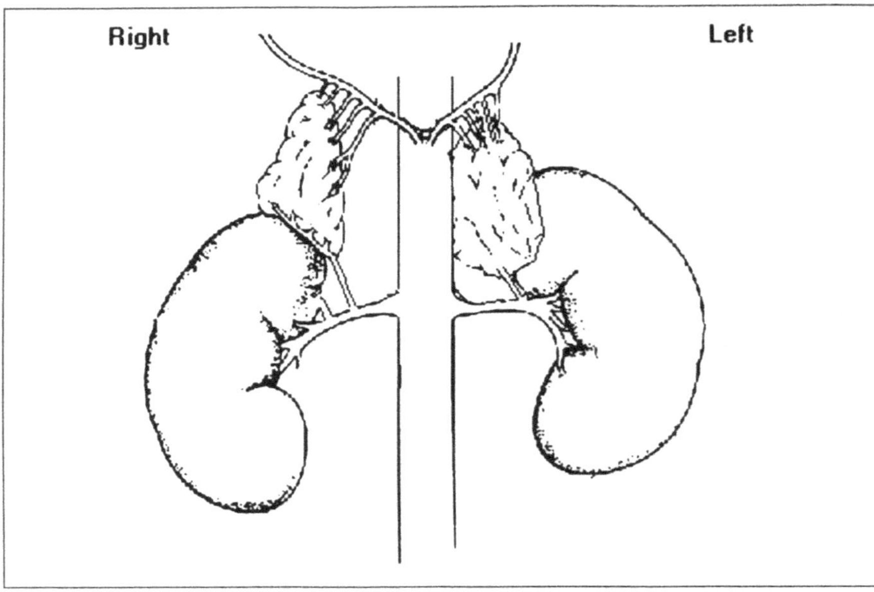

Fig. 2. Arterious vascularization of the adrenal glands

The retroperitoneal approach offers a smaller space and is technically more difficult, but direct access to the gland — without passing through the peritoneal cavity — makes it less invasive and traumatic, thus promoting a quicker recovery postoperatively [13].

Benign tumors smaller than 5 cm in diameter represent a clear indication for laparoscopic adrenalectomy although numerous cases of laparoscopic procedures on larger tumors [4] or even malignancies [5] have been reported in the literature. Indeed, there is no contraindication to laparoscopy in these conditions and the indication is directly related to the operator's skill. Age is not a discriminating factor. Kuriansky et al. [6] examined the outcome of a group of patients over 65 and concluded that age does not constitute a contraindication to laparoscopy. A relative contraindication most likely exists for children because of the smaller working space available [7, 8].

Patient Preparation

Preparation, in terms of hormone therapy, depends on the adrenal disease and is performed practically in the same way as it is for open surgery or transperitoneal laparoscopy, especially in patients with a hyperfunctioning neoplasm.

Unlike transperitoneal procedures, for which bowel preparation is recommended over several days, there is no need for special preparation in retroperitoneal procedures; the patient is only given an enema the night before surgery with no prophylactic antibiotic therapy. Blood loss is 50 ml on average so no blood transfusion is required. The retroperitoneal approach we use is performed with the patient in a lateral recumbent position and does not create any particular problems in patients with respiratory failure or who are obese as may occur when the patient is kept prone.

The procedure is well tolerated by the patients since the substantial technical difficulties the surgeon meets with are well compensated by the minor surgical stress to the patient and the quick postoperative recovery, requiring on average 2-3 days of hospitalization. Patients can eat and leave their beds on day 1 after surgery and complications occur only very rarely. Retroperitoneal laparoscopic adrenalectomy may be performed with a lateral or posterior approach.

Positioning the Patient

For the lateral retroperitoneal approach the patient is kept in a lateral recumbent position with the operating table tilted to broaden the lumbar space (Fig. 3). The position is practically the same as for a subcostal lumbotomy. The head surgeon stands dorsal to the patient; his assistant is positioned ventrally while the camera operator stands behind the head surgeon. The scrub nurse stands alongside the assistant (Fig. 4). The head surgeon and the assistant both face the patient, which makes vision on a single screen awkward; therefore, two monitors have to be used, one on each side of the patient's head, to allow the whole team a direct and unhampered view. During the surgical procedures it sometimes becomes necessary

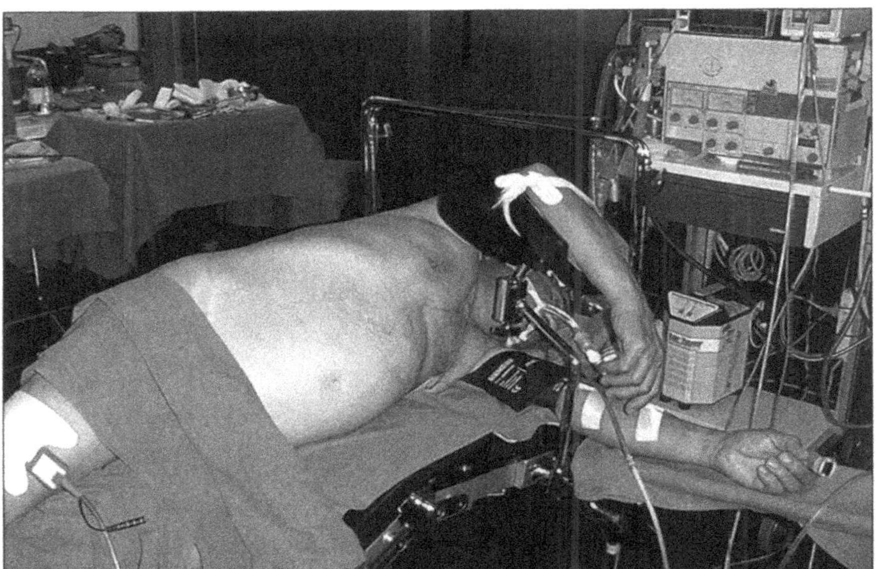

Fig. 3. The patient is kept in a lateral recumbent position with the operating table tilted to broaden the lumbar space

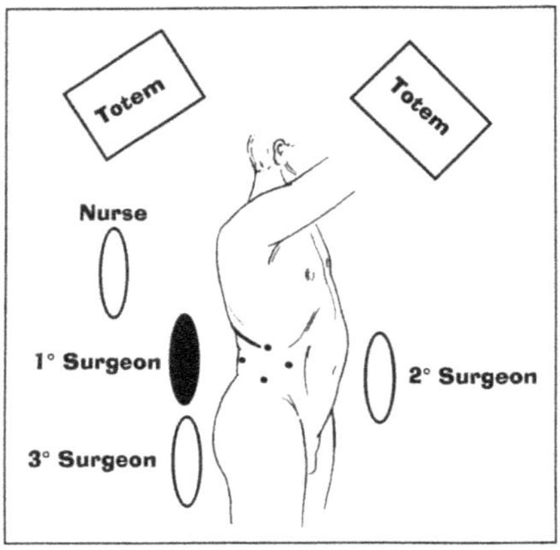

Fig. 4. Position of the surgeons

to broaden the retroperitoneal space. In such cases it is useful to turn the operating table anteriorly, along the longitudinal axis of the patient's body, to displace the intestinal viscera and peritoneum anteriorly.

Instrumentation

No particular instrumentation is required except for a camera with a 0° optical lens (some authors prefer a 30° lens), a CO_2 pump , forceps, clamp, shears, a suction device, a clip applier, and a dissector. A unipolar electrosurgical cutting device should be available with a bipolar or hemostatic device such as Ultracision. Four 10-mm trocars comprising an Asson are used. The retroperitoneal space is created by means of a trocar fitted with a balloon (Fig. 5), or by means of a surgical glove connected to a catheter as a more economical solution.

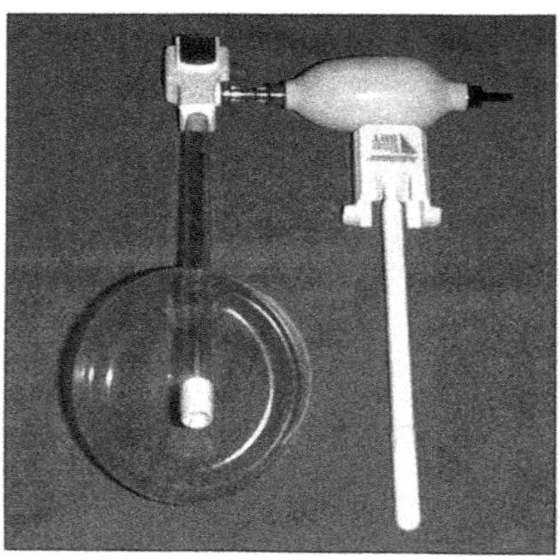

Fig. 5. Inflatable balloon for the dissection of the retroperitoneum

Creating the Surgical Space and Dissection of the Retroperitoneum

The first phase of the procedure consists in creating the retroperitoneal space. The space posterior to Gerota's capsule is accessed by displacing the capsule anteriorly to the peritoneum. With the patient in a lateral recumbent position, a 2-cm incision is made along the lower border of the tip of the 11th rib and the end of the 12th; the shears are placed perpendicular to the patient and are gently pushed inside to dissect the muscle planes without tearing them (Fig. 6). The scissors are open when passing through the various planes and then closed when they are pushed deeper. The muscle planes are thus progressively dissected. This is a safe and smooth maneuver when it is performed gently. The surgeon can clearly feel that the retroperitoneal space has been accessed. No complication has ever been registered in this phase in over 500 retroperitoneoscopic procedures. Digital and then balloon dissections of the retroperitoneum are performed [3]. Some trocars fitted with a balloon are currently available on the market. A more economical solution consists in using a surgical glove connected to a catheter. The retroperitoneum is distended with 500–800 ml of air.

Such a step is useful to medially displace the retroperitoneal fat and create a sufficiently large cavity with no tongues of fat hanging into the space to reduce the operator's view into the field (Figs. 7, 8). In this phase special care must be taken to avoid opening the peritoneum. Such an incident would allow gas to pass into the peritoneal cavity and thus reduce the retroperitoneal space. Should this occur, the opening needs to be closed with a stitch or fat once the trocars are positioned.

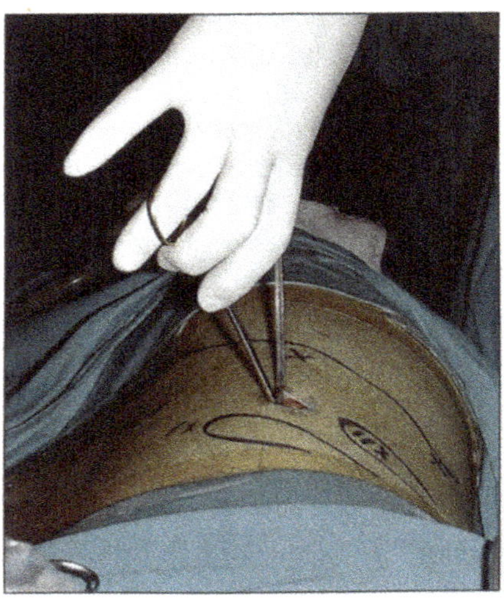

Fig. 6. Incision dissection to the apex of the 12th rib

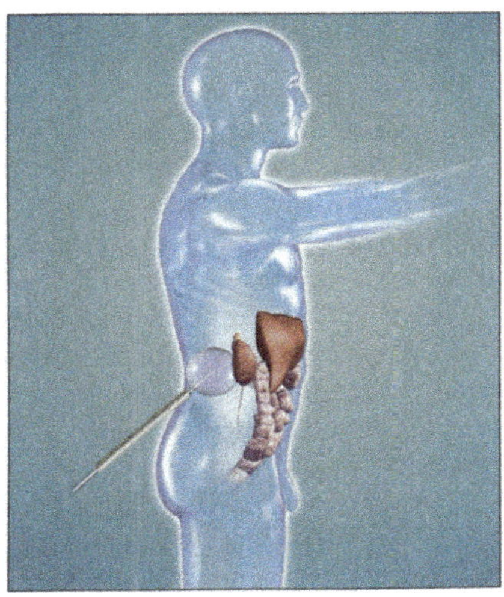

Fig. 7. Schematic balloon dissection of the retroperitoneum (sagittal)

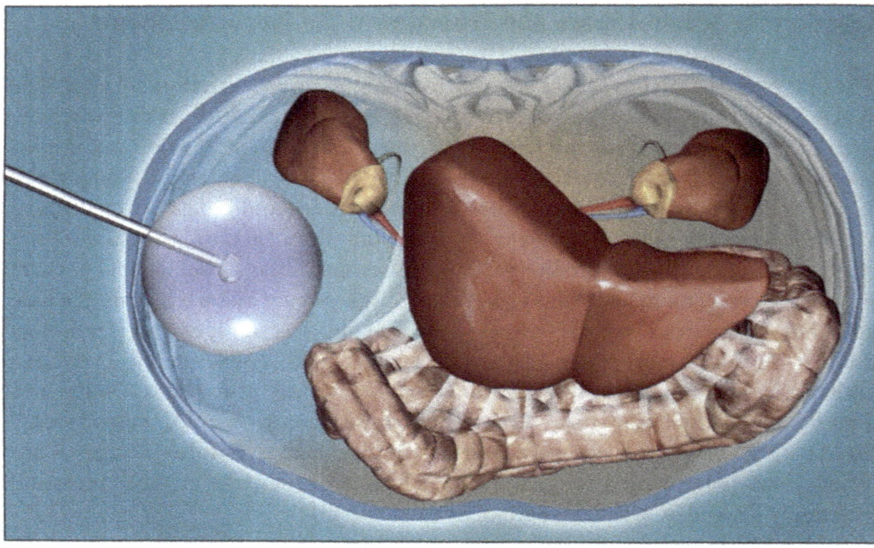

Fig. 8. Schematic balloon dissection of the retroperitoneum (transverse)

Three ports are created on the anterior, middle and posterior axillary lines at the transverse umbilical line (Fig. 9). After putting his index finger through the incision to check whether the peritoneal sac has been adequately displaced with the dissection, the surgeon can correctly insert the three trocars, carefully avoiding injury to the viscera (special care must be taken not to hurt one's finger).

An Asson trocar is used to close the incision. Accurate and correct positioning of the ports is of utmost importance to make the surgeon's task less taxing since the available space to operate in is small and deep and the instruments often reach their stop limit. The anterior trocar is inserted at an angle of about 45° to the longitudinal axis of the kidney and is used to stretch the structures to be dissected while the posterior trocar is positioned at an angle of about 20° to the longitudinal axis of the kidney.

The next phase consists in pumping about 3 l of CO_2 at a rate of 1.5 l/min to distend the retroperitoneum, which thus becomes a proper cavity. The maximum pressure should not exceed 12 mmHg so as to minimize problems of CO_2 being reabsorbed into the circulation. The camera with the 0° lens is inserted through the port on the mid-axillary line.

In our opinion placing the camera through the lower sleeve gives more leeway in the operating space by limiting soiling of the camera through contact with the fat investing the kidney.

After appropriately heating the camera to avoid fogging of the lens and having attained an optimal distention of the retroperitoneum, the camera is inserted into the sleeve. The first technical step is orientation. Recognizing the various structures not only means safeguarding the patient but also not having to swim through the fat surrounding the kidney. The main landmark is the psoas muscle,

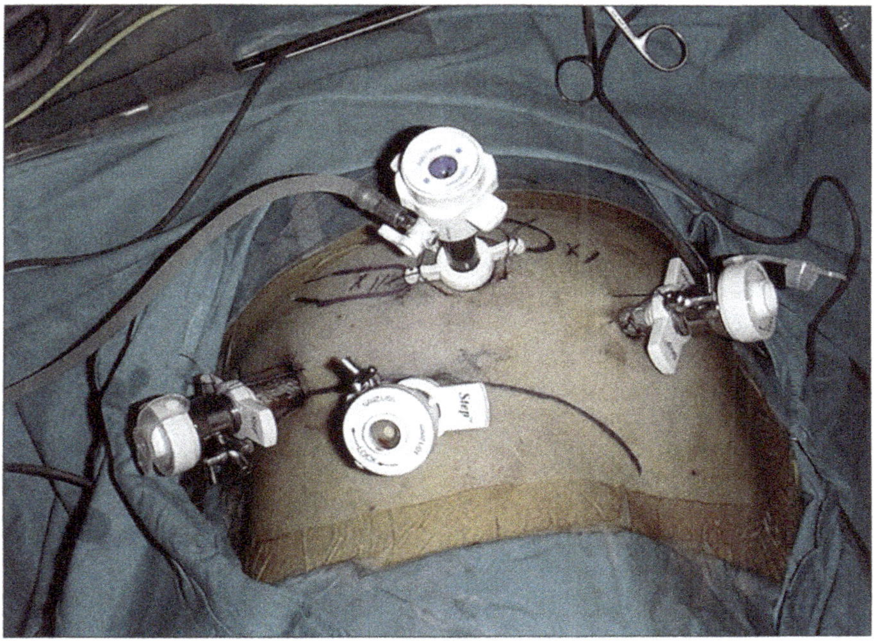

Fig. 9. Position of the trocars

which can be visualized posteriorly by elevating Gerota's capsule. Anteriorly the other landmark is the reflection of the peritoneum.

Gerota's capsule is dissected from the psoas muscle along an avascular plane leading to the dome of the diaphragm. In this phase only the two trocars on the anterior and posterior axillary lines are used. The dissection is extremely easy to perform with two forceps. Some tiny vessels may be encountered and easily cauterized with the bipolar device. The dissection is continued upward to the dome of the diaphragm. At this point Gerota's capsule is opened at the upper pole of the kidney. Up to this phase the procedure is identical for both the right and left side. The main difference between right and left adrenalectomies emerges in the subsequent steps of the operation and is linked to the different anatomy and vasculature of the two glands.

Right Retroperitoneal Adrenalectomy

The right adrenal gland covers the anterior surface of the upper pole of the kidney and receives arterial blood from the renal artery (inferior suprarenal artery) and the phrenic artery (superior suprarenal artery). There is generally only one vein of an appreciable caliber which opens directly into the vena cava and is almost always short. Anomalies in the vasculature are the norm so one should never count on finding a classical vascular anatomy and always proceed with greater caution, unveiling the patient's anatomy step by step. In my experience two or even three adrenal veins are often found when entering the vena cava. Identifying arteries and veins, even atypical vessels, is not a difficult task but one should always act as if one were walking through a minefield.

In retroperitoneoscopic surgery, a clean operating field is always necessary to ensure optimal vision. This means that even the smallest vessels will have to be cauterized before being cut in order to avoid minor, unimportant and yet troublesome bleeding. This rule should be borne in mind especially when performing a retroperitoneal laparoscopic adrenalectomy because the operating field is small and very deep and the structures are highly vascularized.

After opening Gerota's capsule the dissection is continued upward until the adrenal gland is disconnected from the dome of the diaphragm. At this point, the operator moves downward to disconnect the anterior surface of the upper pole of the kidney. Up to this point the ports on the anterior and posterior axillary lines have been used while the camera is still in the trocar on the mid-axillary line. Once the upper pole of the kidney is disconnected, it is pulled downwards with a forceps inserted through the trocar on the anterior axillary line and is then taken care of by the assistant surgeon. The unipolar scalpel and the bipolar device are now used in the Asson trocar and in the trocar on the posterior axillary line to continue the operation. This is the standard procedure, but even if four 10-mm trocars are available, one may sometimes need to change the position of either the lens or the instruments, or both.

When the upper pole of the kidney is pulled downwards, the vena cava becomes clearly visible. The adrenal gland is pushed very gently, especially in patients with a hyperfunctioning tumor. The inferior suprarenal artery – a branch of the renal artery – can easily be found between the vena cava and the upper pole of the kidney. A clip is applied and the artery cut. At this point the vena cava can easily be dissected. The adrenal gland is lifted, thereby stretching the lymphatics vessels, which are cauterized and cut.

The suprarenal vein is higher up. Great care must be taken while looking for it since it is a very short vein (1 cm) with a wide caliber (Fig. 10): if torn or badly clipped, a massive hemorrhage would occur. The vein is thus isolated with the dissector and two clips conveniently applied distally and two proximally. Before cutting the vein, the surgeon must ensure that the entire vein has been caught in the clips.

It is mandatory that clips are applied on the adrenal side of the vein to avoid any reflux hemorrhage from the superior suprarenal artery, which is the last to be cut because of its position. In some cases I was able to clamp the superior suprarenal artery in the first phase while dissecting the gland immediately after disconnecting the suprarenal body from the diaphragm. This is a very favorable circumstance, which may occur only in patients with a small tumor (2-3 cm). For larger tumors the superior suprarenal artery is isolated after dissecting the suprarenal body and should always be accurately isolated and clipped. Often there is not only one artery but several small arteries. The adrenal gland is placed into an endobag and pulled out through the small lumbar incision.

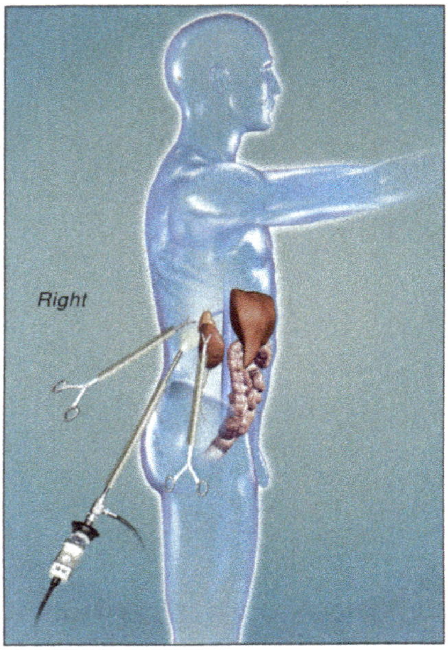

Fig. 10. Approach to the right suprarenal gland

Left Retroperitoneal Adenalectomy

Similarly to the right adrenal gland, the left gland is situated on the upper pole of the kidney where it partially covers the anterior surface of the pole. The anterior surface of the of the gland is in contact with the left colonic flexure, the tail of the pancreas, and the spleen. These relations are of utmost importance in transperitoneal laparoscopic procedures because an incision has to be made on the peritoneum and these structures will be dissected and displaced to access the retroperitoneum and the adrenal gland. The neighboring organs (pancreas, colon, and spleen) do not interfere with the retroperitoneal approach and the adrenal gland only needs to be gently dissected.

The medial surface of the left adrenal gland is in relation with the aorta: three arterial peduncles originate from the renal artery, the aorta, and the inferior diaphragmatic artery.

Analogously to the right, the vasculature on the left is extremely variable so great care must be taken when dissecting the small arteries. Venous flow almost constantly occurs through a 1- to 1.5-cm vein which opens at a right angle into the renal vein.

The procedure in the left adrenal gland is performed following the same steps as in the right, up to the incision of Gerota's capsule and disconnection of the upper pole of the kidney. The upper pole of the kidney is pulled downwards and laterally using a flat-tipped forceps inserted through the trocar on the anterior axillary line. The surgeon works through the ports on the posterior axillary line and the Asson trocar using the unipolar device with the right hand and the bipolar device with the left. The downward displacement of the upper pole of the kidney creates a larger

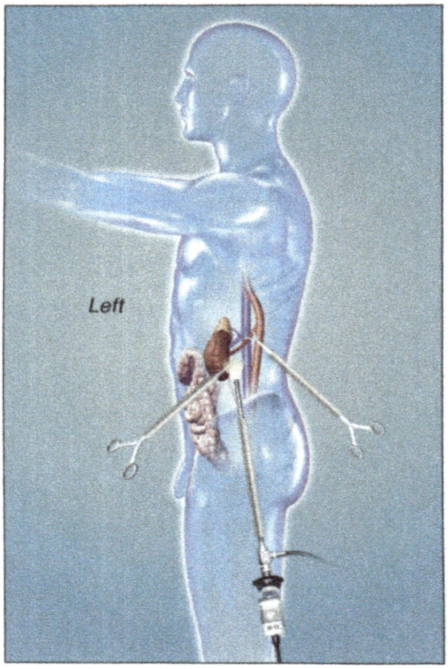

Fig. 11. Approach to the left suprarenal gland

space to work in around the adrenal gland. By gently lifting the suprarenal body, the renal artery and vein become visible, together with the inferior suprarenal artery, which arises from the renal artery, and the suprarenal vein, which opens into the renal vein (Fig. 11). Clips are applied both upstream and downstream to the vessels, which are then cut. The adrenal gland is gently pulled downward following the dome of the diaphragm. The small arteries originating from the inferior diaphragmatic artery or directly from the aorta are either clamped with clips or cauterized with the bipolar forceps. The adrenal gland with its surrounding fat is put into an endobag and removed through the incision made at the Asson trocar.

Retroperitoneal Laparoscopic Adrenalectomy Through the Posterior Approach

With the posterior approach, the patient is in a prone position, with his arms stretched upwards and two beanbags under his chest and hips. The legs of the operating table are tipped to extend the patient's abdomen and easily create the retroperitoneal space to work in [10]. Access to the retroperitoneum is attained as in the lateral approach. A 2-cm incision is made lateral to the sacrospinal muscles; the planes are dissected using the shears, and digital dissection of the retroperitoneum is then perform while the operating space is created using a balloon. The 10-mm trocars are placed on the subcostal area under the surgeon's direct control and, if necessary, a fourth trocar inserted at the angle between the iliac crest and the posterior axillary line. The surgical technique is the same as in the lateral approach. The advantages of using the posterior approach consist in attaining direct access to the posterior surface of the adrenal gland and its vessels and the possibility of performing a bilateral procedure. The main drawbacks of this approach are the very small operating space and the difficulties of working with ports that are situated close together. Adequate training, however, enables surgeons to perform correct procedures even with this approach and with excellent results [11, 12]. There are no differences between the two approaches in terms of blood loss, use of analgesics, or length of hospital stay for the patient following the operation [9]

Similarly, there seems to be no difference between trans- and retroperitoneal laparoscopic adrenalectomies in terms of the time required for surgery, blood loss, use of analgesics, and length of postoperative hospital stay for the patient [14]. The retroperitoneal procedure certainly presents the advantage of not accessing the peritoneum or manipulating the intestine and can thus be used in patients who have undergone abdominal surgery.

Postoperative Treatment

Postoperative recovery is rapid with a good prognosis. On day 1 after surgery the patient can walk and start eating. Analgesics are necessary only for a short time after surgery and no antibiotics are required. Replacement therapy is necessary only in cases of bilateral adrenalectomy. The drainage system is removed on day 2 and the patient can be discharged from the hospital on day 3.

Concluding Considerations

Retroperitoneoscopic adrenalectomy is an elegant procedure with exceptionally favorable results for the patient.

It is certainly not an easy procedure and it requires extensive training in laparoscopy because of the depth of the area to work in and the dense vasculature supplying the adrenal gland. It is not sensible to start retroperitoneoscopic surgery with this procedure unless one is ready to accept the inevitable complications and the strong likelihood of having to convert to open surgery. Once a surgeon has mastered the technique, however, procedures can be easily performed in a short time and with minimal complications.

Laparoscopy unquestionably offers several advantages, namely, a magnified view of all the anatomical structures and their details, thanks to the close-up potentials of the camera, the possibility of performing accurate dissections of the cleavage planes, and a very careful hemostasis.

Hemostasis is of great importance in laparoscopy because the operating field must be clean at all times to precisely identify the correct cleavage plane. Even minimal bleeding, which creates no problem in open surgery, has to be avoided as it restricts visibility in laparoscopy.

There seems to be no difference between trans- and retroperitoneal laparoscopic adrenalectomies in terms of the time required for surgery, blood loss, use of analgesics, and length of postoperative hospital stay for the patient [14]. The retroperitoneal procedure certainly presents the advantage of not having to access the peritoneum or manipulate the intestine and can thus be used in patients who have undergone abdominal surgery [15]. The different anatomical situation between right and left should perhaps be borne in mind. The transperitoneal approach is easier on the right because the suprarenal vein is immediately found on the anterior surface of the vena cava. On the left, in contrast, the retroperitoneal approach appears to be more accessible since the transperitoneal approach requires mobilization of the colon, spleen and tail of the pancreas. Obesity is a factor which favors recourse to the retroperitoneal procedure.

Only few series of patients who have undergone retroperitoneoscopic adrenalectomies have been reported in the literature and fewer yet have been compared with series of patients submitted to open surgery while a greater number have been compared with cases of transperitoneal adrenalectomies.

At present there is no indication for open surgery of the adrenal gland, except in tumors larger than 10 cm and especially if malignancies are suspected.

References

1. Gaur DD (1992) Laparoscopic operative retroperitoneoscopy. Use of a new device. J Urol 148:1137-1142
2. Mandressi a. Buizza C, Antonelli D, Chisena S, Servadio G (1995) Retroperitoneoscopy. Ann Urol 29: 91-96
3. Gill IS, Munch LC, Grune MT (1996) Access for retroperitoneal laparoscopy. J Urol:156:1120-1124
4. Henry JF, Defechereux T, Gramatica.L, Raffaelli M (1999) Should laparoscopic approach be proposed for large and or potentially malignantadrenal tumors Langenbecks Arch Surg 384:366-369
5. Heniford BT, Arca MJ, Walsh RM, Gill IS (1999) Laparoscopic adrenalectomy for cancer. Semin Surg Oncol 6:293-306
6. Kuriansky J, Saenz A, Astudillo E, Ardid J, Cardona V, Fernandez-Cruz L (1999) Laparoscopic adrenalectomy in the elderly. J Laparoendosc Adv Surg Tech (A) 9:317 - 320
7. Clerments RH, Golostein RE,Holcomb GW 3rd (1999) Laparoscopic left adrenalectomy for pheochromoytoma in a child. J Pediatr Surg 34: 1408-1409
8. Azal W, Mitre AL, Castilho LN, Denes FT, Arap S (1999) Laparoscopic adrenalectomy in children and adolescents. J Urol 161 [Suppl]: 20 (abstract V13)
9. Baba S, Miyajima A, Uchida A, Asanuma H, Miyakawa A, Murai M (1997) A posterior lumbar approach for retroperitoneosopic adrenalectomy: assessment of surgical efficacy. Urology 50: 19-23
10. Duh QJ, Siperstein AE, Clarck OH, Shecter WP, Horn JK, Harrison MR, Hunt TK, Way LW (1996) Laparoscopic adrenalectomy, comparison of the lateral and the posterior approaches. Arch Surg 131: 870-875
11. Walz MK, Peitgen K, Hermann R, et al (1996) Posterior retroperitoneoscopy as a new minimally invasive approach for adrenalectomy: results of 30 adrenalectomies in 27 patients .World J Surg 20: 769-774
12. Siperstein AE, Berber E, Engle KL, et al (2000) Laparoscopic posterior adrenalectomy: technical considerations. Arch Surg 135:967-971

13. Takeda M (2000) Laparoscopic adrenalectomy: transperitoneal vs retroperitoneal approaches. Biomed Pharmacother 54: 207s-210s
14. Sung GT, Gill IS, Hobart M, Soble J, Schweizer D, Bravo EL (1999) Laparoscopic adrenalectomy: prospective,randomized comparision of transperitoneal approaches. J Urol 161 [Suppl]: 21 (abstract 69)
15. Guazzoni G,Cestari A, Montorsi F, Lanzi R, Nava L, Centemero A, Rigatti P (2001) Eight-year experience with transperitoneal laparoscopc adrenal surgery. J Urol 166:820-824
16. Whittle DE, Schroeder D, Purchas SH, Sivakumaran P, Conaglen JV (1994) Laparoscopic retroperitoneal left adrenalectomy in a patient with Cushing's syndrome. Aust NZJ Surgery 64(5): 375-376
17. Uccida M, Imaide Y, Yoneda K, Uehara H, Ukimura O, Itoh Y, Nakamura M, Watanabe H, Fujito A (1994) Endoscopic adrenalectomy by retroperitoneal approach for primary aldosteronism. Hinyoka Kiyo 40(1):43-46. Japanese

Chapter 11

Retroperitoneoscopy in Children

MICHAEL FRANKS, FRANCIS X. SCHNECK, STEVEN G. DOCIMO

Introduction

In this era of minimally invasive surgery, pediatric urologists are becoming more adept with laparoscopic techniques, due mainly to having gained familiarity with transperitoneal laparoscopy in the management of cryptorchidism. More recently, retroperitoneoscopic techniques have gained popularity in the treatment of benign renal disease in adults [1]. With further refinement in instrumentation and techniques, retroperitoneoscopy has naturally found a place in the armamentarium of many pediatric urologists at academic centers.

Compared to transperitoneal laparoscopy, the retroperitoneoscopic approach to the kidney offers several potential advantages. Most urologists are familiar with the retroperitoneal flank approach to the kidney in children, and with initial retroperitoneal dissection, the renal hilum is typically encountered first. Less retroperitoneal fat present in children also improves exposure to the kidney [2]. Previous abdominal surgery is not a contraindication to retroperitoneal laparoscopy. In contrast to the transperitoneal route, retroperitoneoscopy does not require colon mobilization, and without entering the peritoneal cavity, risk of visceral injury or intraperitoneal contamination from urinoma, hematoma, or infection is theoretically reduced [3]. Drawbacks to retroperitoneal laparoscopy include the steep learning curve, the limited working space, more difficult access and port placement (compared to transabdominal approaches), and subcutaneous emphysema [3, 4].

Although still in its infancy without controlled studies, retroperitoneoscopy in children appears to be an alternative to open renal surgery. Retroperitoneoscopic techniques commonly utilized in the pediatric population at this time include: nephrectomy for benign disease, nephroureterectomy, heminephroureterectomy or partial nephrectomy, and renal biopsy. The indications, technical aspects, results, and complications of these procedures will be discussed in detail. At this time, too little experience exists with laparoscopic retroperitoneal pyeloplasty, partial nephrectomy, adrenalectomy, cyst marsupialization, nephropexy, cutaneous ureterostomy, lymphadenectomy, and pyelolithotomy in the pediatric population to warrant inclusion in this chapter. To date, many of the aforementioned procedures have been performed via the transperitoneal laparoscopic approach in children or by retroperitoneal means in the adult population. However, we will focus on the retroperitoneal laparoscopic technique as it applies to children exclusively.

Patient Preparation

Bowel preparation, placement of a ureteral stent, or preoperative renal embolization are not routinely performed prior to retroperitoneoscopic renal surgery. Routine blood work is typically unnecessary in low-risk patients. Blood should be typed and crossed at the time of the procedure. Ureteral catheter placement prior to heminephroureterectomy has been advocated by some to improve identification of the lower pole moiety of a duplicated system. Informed consent is absolutely essential in the pediatric population, as the reported benefits of the laparoscopic approach have not been firmly established. The surgeon's experience as well as the risk of conversion to open procedures should be disclosed to patients and their families, who should be counseled accordingly.

Anesthetic Considerations

General endotracheal anesthesia is recommended with monitoring of end-tidal CO^2 in children undergoing retroperitoneoscopy. Nitrous oxide (N2O) is generally withheld to reduce bowel distension. Hypercapnia associated with subcutaneous emphysema and minor hemodynamic changes have been documented in humans and in animal models of retroperitoneoscopy [4–6]. However, no significant adverse sequelae of CO_2 insufflation have occurred to date in the pediatric population [5–8]. We recommend paying special attention to ventilatory parameters and reduced insufflation pressures in children (<12 mmHg) to minimize potential pulmonary risks.

Retroperitoneoscopic Nephrectomy

Indications and Contraindications

Generally, indications for retroperitoneoscopic simple nephrectomy or nephroureterectomy in children are analogous to those of open surgery. Table 1 demonstrates indications for nephrectomy or nephroureterectomy, which include poorly functioning kidneys with reflux, Ureteropelvic Junction (UPJ) obstruction or hydronephrosis, renal calculous disease, hypertension, and chronic pyelonephritis. Many believe that nephrectomy with multicystic-dysplastic kidneys should be limited to symptomatic patients, given that these kidneys may involute with time and are not associated with significant development of hypertension or tumors [9]. Additionally, El-Ghoenimi and Sauty [6] advocate nephrectomy in pretransplant patients with renal disease associated with refractory hypertension, severe nephrotic syndrome, or hemolytic-uremic syndrome. Surgery was safely performed in this "high-risk" group, most of whom had qualitative platelet dysfunction. Contraindications to the retroperitoneoscopic approach at this time include renal tumors, trauma, coagulopathy, sepsis, and limiting cardiopulmonary disease. Caution has also been recommended in children with

Table 1. Indications and contraindications for retroperitoneoscopic nephrectomy/nephroureterectomy in children

Indications
- Reflux nephropathy
- Hydronephrosis with nonfunctioning kidney
- Calculous renal atrophy
- Symptomatic multicystic dysplastic kidney
- Renovascular atrophy
- Chronic pyelonephritis
- Pretransplant end-stage renal disease
  - Refractory hypertension
  - Severe nephrotic syndrome
  - Hemolytic—uremic syndrome
- Nonfunction, infection, or dysplasia in duplicated moiety secondary to ureterocele, ectopic ureter, reflux, megaureter

Contraindications
Absolute
- Tumors
- Trauma
- Coagulopathy
- Sepsis
- Acute retroperitoneal inflammation or infection
- Significant cardio-pulmonary risk

Relative
- Prior renal surgery
- Renal tuberculosis
- Xanthogranulomatous pyelonephritis
- Obesity

acute or subacute retroperitoneal inflammation or infections (pyelonephritis, calculous disease, renal TB or XGP), where difficulty with retroperitoneal balloon dissection has been found [10, 11]. Obesity is considered by most to be a relative contraindication, as experience is limited. However, Gill reports that the retroperitoneal approach is preferred in this subset of adult patients [3, 11].

Surgical Technique of Retroperitoneoscopic Nephrectomy in Children

Positioning

Standard positioning for retroperitoneoscopic nephrectomy is full flank with the kidney rest up to maximize working space between the iliac crest and lower ribs. Special padding is necessary on all pressure points to avoid skin breakdown. The location of the lateral peritoneal reflection in this position is the most anterior, allowing a larger window to the retroperitoneum with the first port placement [12]. Borer et al. [13] have also described retroperitoneoscopy in the prone position, which may provide specific advantages over the flank position. In the prone position, the abdominal contents and peritoneum fall away from the operative field, improving access, retroperitoneal dissection, and eventual hilar exposure as reported by the authors.

Retroperitoneal Access

After sterile preparation and draping, anatomical landmarks are palpated (11-12th ribs, iliac crest, sacrospinalis muscle) and port placement is planned. As do others, we favor an open technique for primary retroperitoneal access. A 1.0- to 1.5-cm incision is made below the 12th rib at the posterior axillary line. A muscle splitting dissection is used to gain access deep to the thoracodorsal fascia into the retroperitoneal space. In larger children, S-retractors facilitate observation of these layers. A 3-= polygalactin suture is placed in this fascia in a U-configuration to allow closure and sealing of the primary cannula. Using the finger or a cotton-tipped instrument, the peritoneal reflection is gently swept medially, and the retroperitoneal space is developed as shown by Gill [14]. Often, the psoas muscle and the lower pole of the kidney can be palpated at this time, as the retroperitoneal fat is sparse in children.

Retroperitoneal Dissection and First Port Placement

Two techniques have previously been described to dissect the retroperitoneum - the Gaur ballon technique [15] and the videoendoscopic balloon dilator (Origin Medsystems, Menlo Park, CA) method as described by Gill [14]. We find that in children, reliable dissection can be accomplished the Gaur technique, which uses one or two fingers of a surgeon's glove tied to a rubber catheter for balloon dissection [15]. Saline volumes of 250-800 cc are generally necessary for adequate dissection with this method, depending on the size of the child. At these volumes, rupturing of the finger balloon using the Gaur technique has not been a problem. No specific weight/volume guidelines have been proposed. Advantages of the videoendoscopic balloon dilator include direct visual inspection of the pneumoretroperitoneal dissection, which may allow earlier hilar landmark identification. Not uncommonly, a second dissection is necessary to ensure adequate mobilization. In children, who have a paucity of retroperitoneal fat, it is not necessary to initially develop the space within Gerota's fat with initial retroperitoneal dissection.

After balloon deflation and removal, the primary port (blunt, 10-mm disposable) is placed and secured with the suture through the lumbodorsal fascia to create a seal for the pneumoretroperitoneum. A 0° or 30° lens is inserted after CO_2 insufflation to observe signs of bleeding or injury before proceeding. At this time, landmarks should be visualized, and the surgeon should be oriented to the retroperitoneal anatomy, including the psoas muscle, ureter, renal hilum, and great vessels. Generally, the pneumoretroperitoneal pressure is safe at 12-14 mmHg in children, but can be reduced to <10 mmHg in younger children with maintenance of adequate vision of vital structures.

Placement of Accessory Ports

Two additional 5-mm ports can be placed under direct vision. In older children we recommend the port placement described in detail by Gill [3, 11, 16], which maximizes distance between instruments. This port configuration is generally in line with an open flank incision (Fig. 1a). Caveats in accessory port placement include maximizing distance between instruments, avoidance of a working port too

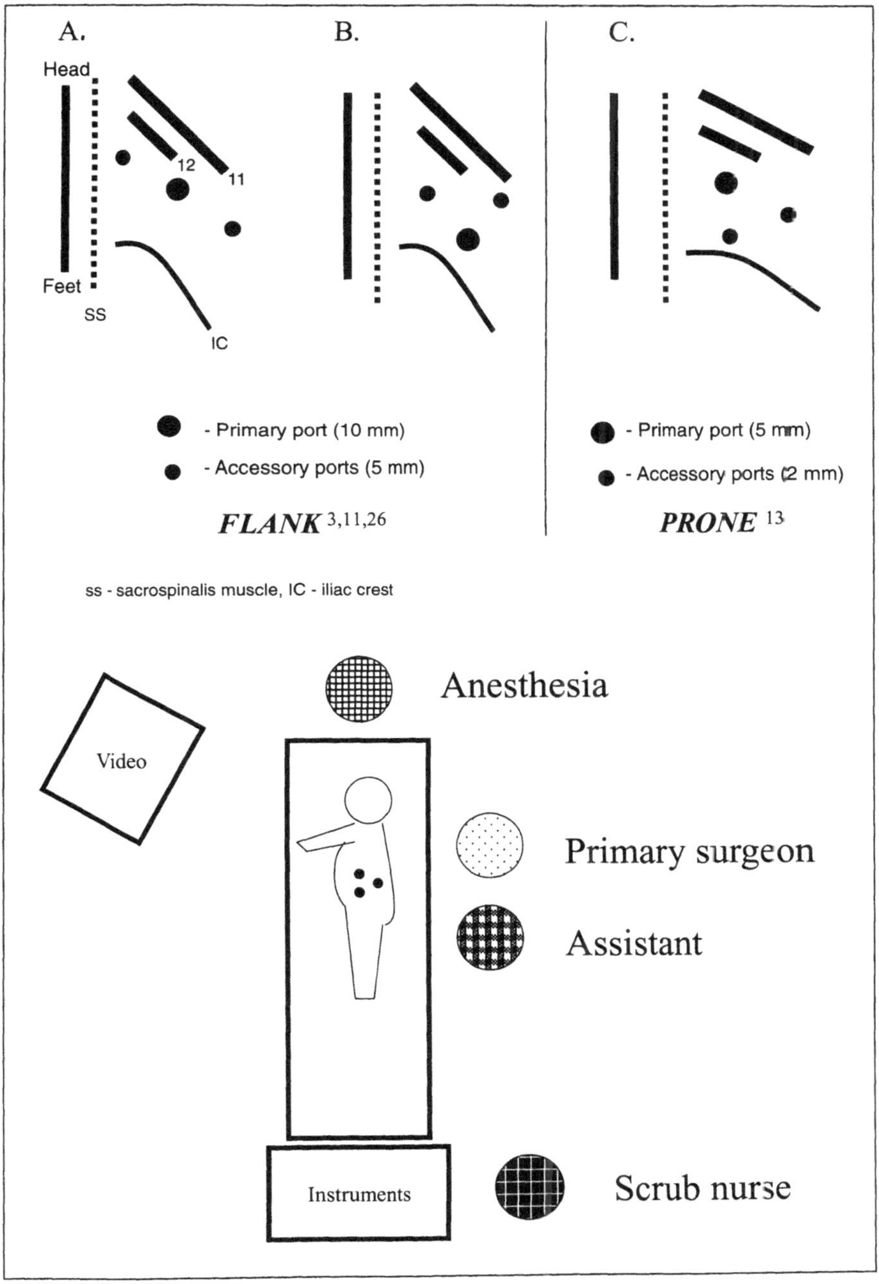

Fig. 1. Port placements for pediatric retroperitoneoscopic nephrectomy

A B

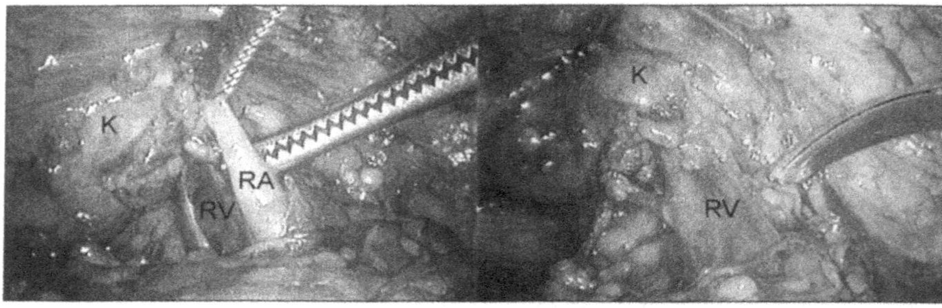

Fig. 2A, B. Intraoperative picture of right retroperitoneoscopic nephrectomy. A Exposure of the solitary renal artery (*RA*) with apical kidney (*K*) and underlying renal vein (*RV*). B A large renal vein (*RV*) after the renal artery has been clipped and divided

close to the iliac crest, and occasional use of the bimanual port placement technique [14] if retroperitoneal space is limited. In neonates or toddlers, triangulation of port placement also maximizes exposure and minimizes instrument conflict in a tighter working space [13]. Alternative port placements are also shown for the flank and prone positions (Fig. 1b, c) [13]. If the peritoneum is entered during accessory port placement, pressure equilibration between spaces occurs almost instantly. Needle decompression of the peritoneal space with simple suture closure of the peritonotomy allows further dissection to continue by retroperitoneoscopy [17]. Alternatively, a combined transperitoneal approach can be used by introducing a peritoneal trocar [18]. Inspection for visceral injury after peritoneal transgression is a must.

Initial Dissection and Control of the Renal Hilum

A unique advantage to retroperitoneal laparoscopic nephrectomy is the early presentation of the renal hilum after retroperitoneal balloon dissection as described above. If the hilum is not visible, posterior dissection should proceed to identify the lower pole of the kidney, using the psoas muscle as a landmark. Anterior traction with a fan retractor or blunt instrument facilitates this maneuver, and initial dissection, once oriented properly, will often reveal the renal hilum. Dissection with a blunt right angle or electrocautery scissors cleans the artery and vein (Fig. 2a, b). Taking time to perform more proximal dissection is often worthwhile to avoid the segmental artery branches. Countertraction using the nondominant hand is essential to provide safe windows for vascular control. Once the renal artery is isolated, two or three proximal and one distal vascular clip is applied to secure the renal artery. The vessel is cut under direct vision. The more anterior and caudad vein can often be managed with 10-mm vascular clips in small children. In older children, an Endo GIA stapler (12-mm) is often necessary to secure the larger renal vein.

Specimen Dissection

Dissection using electrocautery continues from caudal to cephalad in the posterior plane. Lymphatics at the hilum are cauterized or clipped. Upper pole dissection in proximity to the adrenal bed requires cautery to avoid significant venous bleeding. Anterior dissection should be limited at this time to prevent the kidney from flopping ventrally. Polar vessels, if encountered, should be clipped and cut. Significant bleeding from a polar artery is the usual cause for conversion to open nephrectomy in the pediatric series to date. The ureter is then taken between clips, and the rest of the kidney is completely freed from surrounding fat. Reduction of the pneumoretroperitoneum at this time will reveal any significant bleeding.

Specimen Removal

Atrophic kidneys can often be removed through the 1.5-cm incision in a child. Occasionally, increasing the incision size in an older child is necessary to facilitate removal. Many endoscopic retrieval bags are now available for kidney removal. Blunt fragmentation within the bag or formal morcellation will allow removal of these larger kidneys. The benign nature of pediatric renal disease enables more rigorous removal without concern for spillage as with tumor specimens in adults.

Exit

After confirmation of hemostasis at low pressure, ports are removed under direct vision, and the pneumoretroperitoneum is evacuated. The fascia is closed in ports 5 mm or greater with 3-0 polygalactin suture. Injection of incisions with an equal mixture of 0.5% bupivicaine and 1% lidocaine provides some postoperative incisional pain relief. Lastly, the skin is closed with subcuticular stitches or adhesive strips. Table 2 lists the general steps in surgical technique.

Special Circumstances

Giant Hydronephrosis

Care must be taken to avoid entering the renal pelvis during the initial or accessory trocar placement, as the distended pelvis aids in dissection, especially of the often adherent parietal peritoneum. Hemal and Gupta [19] have described needle decompression of the enlarged renal pelvis under laparoscopic vision using a

Table 2. Retroperitoneoscopic nephrectomy operative steps

1. Patient positioning (Flank or Prone)
2. 1st trocar placement (Open, Hasson technique)
3. Retroperitoneal balloon dissection (Gaur balloon or videoendoscopic balloon)
4. Accessory trocar placement (2nd, 3rd, 4th)
5. Kidney mobilization
6. Hilar dissection (clip artery, staple vein)
7. Superior dissection (cauterize @ adrenal)
8. Ureter
9. Specimen removal (in situ or bag retrieval)
10. Exit

Veress needle. As much as 750 cc of urine has been removed, which greatly improves exposure and dissection of the ureter and blood vessels. The decompressed renal pelvis also serves as a handle for countertraction in this case.

Horseshoe/Ectopic Kidneys

A modified 45° flank position with more anterior placement of trocars was used by Hemal and Aron [20] to approach the horseshoe or ectopic kidney. Additional ports along the margin of the iliac crest enabled dissection of the ectopic kidney by the retroperitoneal approach. Hemal also performed retroperitoneoscopic nephrectomy and isthmusectomy in a horseshoe kidney. Intracorporeal methods utilized a GIA stapler or loop suture ligature to control the isthmus. In a particularly thin patient, the kidney and isthmus were mobilized and brought extracorporeally to where the isthmusectomy was performed. Aberrant vascular anatomy is commonplace in these cases, but did not pose any considerable problem as reported by the authors [20].

Other

Nephrostomy tubes do not limit retroperitoneal laparoscopy, but care should be taken in dissection of the often dense associated adhesions. Adjunctive open procedures after Retroperitoneal nephrectomy (RPN), retroperitoneal nephroureterectomy (RPNU), namely, ureteral reimplantation via standard Pfannenstiel incision or excision of an ectopic ureter or ureterocele, are also commonly done. Bilateral retroperitoneal nephrectomies have been performed by El-Ghoneimi et al. [6].

Nephroureterectomy

The main indication for retroperitoneoscopic nephroureterectomy in the pediatric age group is reflux nephropathy or an atrophic kidney associated with an ectopic ureter or megaureter. Advantages and disadvantages of this approach mirror that of simple nephrectomy. The more retroperitoneal location of the distal ureter and bladder in young children may enable more complete ureterectomy in this group of patients by retroperitoneal laparoscopic approach. The surgical technique is similar to that described for retroperitoneal laparoscopic simple nephrectomy with the exception of management of the ureter. Most surgeons dissect the ureter distally to the level of the bladder before transection. At the ureterovesical junction, care should be taken to avoid injuring the ovaries or fallopian tubes in females, or the vas deferens in boys. If concern exists regarding reflux into the ureteral stump, alternative methods have been described, including cystoscopic bugbee fulguration of the intravesical ureter, the double balloon technique described by Gill, Grune, and Munch [18], or open removal via a small incision. The gonadal vessels can generally be spared with careful technique.

Heminephrectomy

Heminephrectomy is a much more demanding procedure in the pediatric population, given that the blood supply to the functional kidney and ureter must be preserved. A nonfunctioning or dysplastic renal moiety of a duplex system, often associated with recurrent urinary infections, is the typical indication for this procedure. These renal units often have ectopic ureters, megaureters, or ureteroceles, which may require adjunctive open management at the level of the bladder. Janetscheck [21] and Jordan [22] initially described this technique transperitoneally in children, and since then, groups have reported series in which retroperitoneoscopic techniques have been used [6, 13]. Ureteral stent placement in the lower pole ureter, with removal at the end of the case, has been described but is not mandatory. An additional fourth port has been used to improve exposure to the middle and distal ureter.

In contrast to retroperitoneal nephrectomy, dissection begins with the middle portion of the upper pole ureter, which is freed close to its wall to avoid injury to the adjacent lower pole ureter. Distal dissection is carried down to the level of the bladder, where the ureter is transected. If no reflux is present, a more proximal ureteral division can be done. Proximal ureteral dissection is facilitated by upper pole ureter traction, and the ureter is pulled beneath the renal vessels. Care is taken not to injure the renal vessels to the functional segment. The upper pole vessels are often small and either singly clipped or coagulated. Monopolar or bipolar diathermy is used to coagulate the upper pole from the lower pole. Adjunctive hemostatic techniques, such as argon beam coagulation, oxidized cellulose, or fibrin glue, have also been described [21]. Changes in color after vessel ligature or cystic dysplasia often aid in distinguishing between upper and lower pole segments. After ablation of the upper pole, specimen removal via a 10-mm port is performed, with exit as previously described.

Renal Biopsy

The percutaneous needle approach is used in most children today for diagnostic renal biopsy. Indications include renal failure associated with proteinuria, hematuria, or idiopathic nephrotic syndrome resistant to steroids. Biopsy under direct vision by a retroperitoneal laparoscopic technique has been popularized in children by Caione et al. [23]. This technique is indicated when percutaneous renal biopsy is high risk — that is, in children less than 7 years old, children with uncontrolled hypertension or a solitary kidney, and children on anticoagulants or with a bleeding disorder. Potential advantages to the retroperitoneoscopic approach compared to the percutaneous method include improved hemostasis and a greater degree of certainty in kidney biopsy specimen identification.

A two-port technique is used in the full flank position with a Foley catheter in place. A 12-mm port is placed at the posterior axillary line, midway between the 12th rib and iliac crest. Caione [23[, like Giminez et al. [24] used the Visiport (US Surgical, Norwalk, Conn.) device to advance into the retroperitoneal space under direct vision, where retroperitoneal insufflation with CO_2 is performed. Alternatively, standard incisional exposure with retroperitoneal dissection using the Gaur balloon technique can be done as well. In general, less retroperitoneal insufflation or dissection is needed to ex-

Table 3. Summary of pediatric retroperitoneoscopic renal surgery series

Author	N	Diagnosis	Procedures	Port Size
Kobashi 1992	20	Reflux - 5, MCDK - 8, Hydro/pyelo 5, Chronic pyelo - 10, HTN - 2	Nephrectomy - 15, Nephroureterectomy - 5	1 - 10 mm, 2,3,4 5 mm
Valla 1996	18	Reflux - 6, MCDK - 6, UPJO w/ atrophy - 2, HTN - 2, Ureterocele - 2	Nephrectomy - 16 Partial - 2	1 - 10 or 5 mm, 2,3-5 or 3 mm
El Ghoneimi 1998	42	Reflux - 8, MCDK - 8, Obstructive nephropathy - 8, HTN - 2, Pre-transplant - 4, XGP - 1, Obstructed upper pole - 1	Nephrectomy - 31 Partial - 8	1 - 10 or 5 mm, 2,3 - 5 or 3 mm 153 minutes
Hemal 1999	11	Reflux - 2, UPJO - 2, others not mentioned	Nephrectomy 8 Nephroureterectomy - 2 Nephrectomy w/ isthmusectomy - 1	1 - 10 mm, 2,3,4 - 5 mm
Borer 1999	14	Reflux - 5, MCDK - 4, Chronic pyelo - 3, HTN - 2, Ureterocele - 1, Ectopic ureter - 1	Nephrectomy - 14	1 - 5 or 10 mm, 2,3 - 2 or 5 mm
El Ghoneimi 2000	12	All pre-transplant ESRD	Nephrectomy - 12 (2 bilateral)	1 - 10 or 5 mm, 2,3 - 5 or 3 mm

pose the lower pole of the kidney to allow renal biopsy. Working insufflation pressure of 8-10 mmHg is recommended. Laparoscopic cup biopsy forceps with teeth (5-mm) are used to grasp two cortical areas under direct vision. The biopsy sites are coagulated with monopolar or bipolar electrocautery. Oxidized cellulose or argon beam coagulation have also been described as adjuncts to effective hemostasis [24]. Inadequate hemostasis is the most serious complication in these high-risk patients. Insufflation pressure is slowly evacuated under direct vision to inspect for venous bleeding, and ports are removed.

Mean or time	EBL	Mean LOS (days)	Return to activity	Complications	Remarks
102 min	5-10 cc	17/20 as outpatient	5-7 days	Vena caval laceration - 1, peritoneal tearing - 3, 1conversion to open (bleeding)	1st series - now 45 patients
106 min	N/A	2.3 days	6 days	Peritoneal tear - 8, 1converion to open (unidentified polar vessels in partial Nx)	
Nephrectomy - 104 minutes, partial -	N/A	2 days	N/A	Peritoneal tear - 8, duodenal perf. - 1, 2 conversions to open (both partial Nx)	3 other procedures included: 2 cyst ablation, 1 pyelolithotomy
149 min	82 cc	2.25 days	12 days	Peritoneal tear - 2	1st to describe extracorporeal isthmusectomy and management of giant hydronephrosis
142 min	< 15 cc	2 days	N/A	None	Use 2mm instrumentation, prone position, additional open surgery (ureter reimplant)
N/A	120 min		5.2 days	N/A	Peritoneal tear - 3, hematoma - 1 All "high-risk" patients with ESRD

Results and Complications

Nephrectomy, Nephroureterectomy, and Heminephrectomy

Table 3 shows the results of the six pediatric retroperitoneoscopy series to date [6, 13, 17, 19, 25, 26]. These data include nephrectomy, nephroureterectomy, and partial nephrectomy procedures. Operative times in general were less than 2 h, blood loss was minimal, and length of stays were short (1–5 days). Kobashi [25] noted that these surgeries could be performed as outpatient procedures in most children (17 of 20). El-Ghoneimi [17] also showed that there is a distinct learning curve to retroperitoneoscopic nephrectomy — the second group of 21 patients had significantly improved operative times versus the first 21. They were also able to safely perform retroperitoneal laparoscopic nephrectomy (sometimes bilateral) in high-risk patients with end-stage renal disease [6]. Additionally, Borer et al. [13] describe the use of smaller instrumentation and the prone position to perform nephrectomy, with no acute complications. The distinct advantage of reduced trocar size has yet to be determined, but the prone position appears to have some utility with regard to facilitating exposure and dissection of the hilum. Lastly, Hemal [19] expands the use of retroperitoneal nephrectomy in children to include ectopic or pelvic kidneys or horseshoe kidneys, although experience is limited.

In summary, the most common complication reported was a peritoneal tear, which was found in up to 20% of patients. This did not impact conversion rates or result in visceral injury. The most common indication for conversion to open procedure was uncontrolled bleeding, which occurred in only one of 101 nephrectomies or nephroureterectomies, but two of ten heminephrectomies. The culprit in most cases was a polar vessel or accessory renal vessel when performing heminephrectomy. Duodenal perforation was also the consequence of partial nephrectomy, although this was the first performed by the surgical group. This underscores the fact that heminephrectomy is a more technically demanding procedure. In high-risk children with end-stage renal disease, no bleeding complications occurred either. Overall, major complications occurred in four of 117 patients (3.4%), and minor complications, excluding peritoneal tears, in 8%.

Renal Biopsy

Caione et al. [23] are the only authors who have described a formal retroperitoneoscopic series of renal biopsies in children. Their indications were somewhat liberal, as most biopsies were done because of patient age and uncontrolled hypertension rather than anticoagulation or bleeding diathesis.

Retroperitoneoscopic renal biopsy was successful in 19 of 20 cases. One obese patient required conversion to open biopsy because of poor visualization and bleeding. Biopsy specimens were adequate for interpretation in all cases, compared to insufficient specimens in 11% of percutaneous specimens obtained during the same period. No bleeding complications occurred, although serial hematocrit or hemoglobin levels were not measured. Mean length of stay was 1.2 days. This approach is reliable and apparently safe with little morbidity. It appears to be an acceptable alternative to open renal biopsy.

Discussion

Pediatric retroperitoneoscopic renal surgery is evolving rapidly, mainly through the advances that have been made in adult laparoscopy. Retroperitoneoscopic renal surgery must be considered an alternative to the transperitoneal approach, with no proven superiority at this time. In fact, many pediatric urological laparoscopists are more comfortable with a transperitoneal approach, and this should not be discouraged. Although no prospective studies have been conducted in the pediatric age group, data from the aforementioned series on retroperitoneal laparoscopic nephrectomy, nephroureterectomy, and renal biopsy demonstrate an acceptable margin of safety and efficacy. It is important to note that these data are generated by endoscopic centers of excellence.

There are considerably more data available about adult retroperitoneoscopy than about pediatric procedures. Retrospective studies comparing retroperitoneal laparoscopic nephrectomy to open nephrectomy for benign disease reveal that the retroperitoneal approach compares well to open surgery in a number of areas [14, 27, 28]. A recent prospective study by Hemal et al. [29] evaluated 43 open and 43 retroperitoneal laparoscopic nephrectomies and found minimal postoperative analgesic requirement, reduced length of stay, with a nearly 2-week improved convalescence time in the retroperitoneal laparoscopic group. Complication rates were similar and an increased operative time in the laparoscopic group compared to the open group did not translate into increased morbidity. Subset analysis also demonstrated significant improvement in operative time in the second group of 21 laparoscopic patients with refinement in operative technique (from 137 to 90 min), emphasizing the learning curve of retroperitoneal laparoscopic nephrectomy.

Comparisons in the adult literature of the transperitoneal laparoscopic versus retroperitoneoscopic simple nephrectomy showed little difference in operative times, complications, length of hospitalization, and recovery [10, 30, 31]. Only McDougall's retrospective review [10] demonstrated a trend favoring the retroperitoneal approach, with fewer complications, shorter operating time, and less postoperative pain. Guilloneau's limited study [31], which included some children, showed a modest reduction only in operative time in the retroperitoneal group (173 versus 210 min) with similar morbidity. Overall, based on the limited conclusions that can be drawn from retrospective studies, it appears that in adults the retroperitoneoscopic nephrectomy is at least comparable to the transperitoneal approach.

The pediatric retroperitoneum is significantly different than the adult retroperitoneum. The smaller space may turn out to be a limiting factor, especially if reconstructive procedures are to be considered. One cannot assume that efficacy similar to that in adults will be demonstrated for retroperitoneoscopy, especially in young children. More experience will need to be documented before retroperitoneoscopy can be considered the approach of choice for anything beyond renal biopsy. Because children recover more quickly than adults and are not lost to the work force during their convalescence, issues of operative morbidity carry less weight in this population. In the long run, it may be cosmetic considerations and their impact on children's self image that drive the demand for endoscopic flank procedures [32]. It will be the responsibility of endoscopic surgeons to document improvement in technique and operative time and to carefully document outcomes. Only in this way will the value of retroperitoneoscopy and laparoscopy be verified.

References

1. Gill I, Clayman R, Albala D, Aso Y, Chiu A, Das S, Donovan J, Fuchs G, Gaur D, Go H, Gomella L, Grune M, Harewood L, Janetschek G, Knapp P, McDougall E, Nakada S, Preminger G, Puppo P, Rassweiler J, Royce P, Thomas R, Urban D, Winfield, H (1998) Retroperitoneal and pelvic extraperitoneal laparoscopy: an international perspective. Urology 52: 566
2. Gill I, Das S (1998) Retroperitoneoscopic nephrectomy and nephroureterectomy. In: Graham SD Jr (ed) Glenn's urologic surgery, 5th edn. Lippincott-Raven, Philadelphia
3. Kaouk J, Gill I (2000) Laparoscopic retroperitoneal nephrectomy (simple). Atlas Urol Clin North Am 8(2): 103-114
4. Wolf J, Monk T, McDougall E, McClennan B, Clayman R (1995) The extraperitoneal approach and subcutaneous emphysema are associated with greater absorption of carbon dioxide during laparoscopic renal surgery. J Urol 154: 959-963
5. Geibler R, Walz M, Peitgen K, Scherer R (1996) Hemodynamic changes after retroperitoneal CO^2 insufflation for posterior Retroperitoneoscopic adrenalectomy. Anesth Analg 82: 827-831
6. El Ghoneimi A, Sauty L, Maintenant J, Macher M, Lottmann H, Aigrain Y (2000) Laparoscopic retroperitoneal nephrectomy in high risk childen. J Urol 164: 1076-1079
7. Diemunsch P, Becmeur F, Meyer P)1999) Retroperitoneoscopy versus laparoscopy in piglets: ventilatory and thermic repercussions. J Pediatr Surg 34(10): 1514-1517
8. Ng C, Gill I, Sung G, Whalley D, Graham R, Schweizer D (1999) Retroperitoneoscopic surgery is not associated with increased carbon dioxide absorption. J Urol 162: 1268-1272
9. Wacksman J, Phipps L (1993) Report of the multicystic kidney registry: preliminary findings. J Urol 150: 1870-1872
10. McDougall E, Clayman R (1996) Laparoscopic nephrectomy for benign disease: comparison of transperitoneal and retroperitoneal approaches. J Endourol 10: 45-49
11. Hsu T, Sung G, Gill I (1999) Retroperitoneoscopic approach to nephrectomy. J Endourol 13(10): 713-720
12. Capelouto C, Moore R, Silverman S, Kavoussi L (1994) Retroperitoneoscopy: anatomical rationale for direct retroperitoneal access. J Urol 152: 2008-2010
13. Borer J, Cisek L, Atala A, Diamond D, Retik A, Peters C (1999) Pediatric Retroperitoneoscopic nephrectomy using 2 mm instrumentation. J Urol 162: 1725-1730
14. Gill I (1998) Retroperitoneal laparoscopic nephrectomy. Urol Clin North Am 25: 343-359
15. Gaur D (1992) Laparoscopic operative retroperitoneoscopy: use of a new device. J Urol 148: 1137-1139
16. Gill I, Rassweiler J (1999) Retroperitoneoscopic renal surgery: our approach. Urology 54: 734-738
17. El Ghoneimi A, Valla J, Stayaert H, Aigrain Y (1998) Laparoscopic renal surgery via a retroperitoneal approach in children. J Urol 160: 1138-1141
18. Gill I, Grune M, Munch L (1996) Access technique for retroperitoneoscopy. J Urol 156: 1120-1124
19. Hemal A, Gupta N, Wadhwa S (1999) Modified minimal cost Retroperitoneoscopic nephrectomy with isthmusectomy and nephroureterectomy in children: a pilot study. BJU Int 83(7): 823-827
20. Hemal A, Aron M, Gupta N, Seth A, Wadhwa S (1999) The role of retroperitoneoscopy in the managementof renal and adrenal pathology. BJU Int 83: 929-936
21. Janetschek G, Seibold J, Radmayr C, Bartsch G (1997) Laparoscopic heminephroureterectomy in pediatric patients. J Urol 158, 1928-1930
22. Jordan G, Winslow B (1993) Laparoendoscopic upper pole partial nephrectomy with ureterectomy. J Urol 150: 940-943
23. Caione P, Micali S, Rinaldi S, Capozza N, Lais A, Matarazzo E, Maturo G, Micali F (2000) Retroperitoneal laparoscopy for renal biopsy in children. J Urol 164: 1080-1083
24. Giminez L, Micali S, Chen R, Moore R, Kavoussi L, Scheel P (1998) Laparoscopic renal biopsy. Kidney Int 54: 525-529

25. Valla J, Guilloneau B, Montupet P, Geiss S, Steyaert H, El Ghoneimi A, Jordana F, Volpe P (1996) Retroperitoneal laparoscopic nephrectomy in children. Eur Urol 30: 490–493
26. Kobashi K, Chamberlain D, Rajpoot D, Shanberg A (1998) Retroperitoneal laparoscopic nephrectomy in children. J Urol 160: 1142-1144
27. Ono Y, Katoh N, Kinukawa T, Matsuura O, Ohshima S (1996) Laparoscopic nephrectomy via the retroperitoneal approach. J Urol 156: 1101-1104
28. Doublet J, Barreto H, Degremont A, Gattegno B, Thibault P (1996) Retroperitoneal nephrectomy: comparison of laparoscopy with open surgery. World J Surg 20: 713-716
29. Hemal A, Talwar M, Wadhwa A, Gupta N (1999) Retroperitoneoscopic nephrectomy for benign diseases of the kidney: prospective nonrandomized comparison with open surgical nephrectomy. J Endourol 13(6): 425-431
30. Rassweiler J, Fomara P, Weber M, Janetschek G, Fahlenkamp D, Henkel T, Beer M, Stackl W, Boeckmann W, Recker F, Lampel A, Fischer C, Humke U, Miller K (1998) Laparoscopic nephrectomy: the experience of the laparoscopy working group of the German Urologic Association. J Urol 160: 18-21
31. Guillonneau B, Ballanger P, Lugagne P, Valla AJ, Vallencien G (1996) Laparoscopic versus lumboscopic nephrectomy. Eur Urol 29: 288-291
32. Docimo S (1999) Editorial: pediatric endourology — coming into focus. J Urol 162: 1732-1732

Chapter 12

Laparoscopic Renal, Pelvic and Ureteral Surgery

John G. Pattaras, Robert G. Moore

Introduction

Over the last decade, genitourinary surgery has experienced a revolution in minimally invasive procedures. Urology as a surgical subspecialty has experienced unparalleled changes in applying laparoscopy to some of the most common urologic procedures. Urologic laparoscopic techniques, originally developed and perfected for diagnostic and extractive genitourinary procedures, now have been expanded to the field of reconstructive urologic surgery. The addition of improved laparoscopic suture instruments has made a variety of laparoscopic ureteral surgeries feasible. At several centers, including our own, laparoscopic genitourinary reconstructive surgery is a first-line therapy offered as treatment for ureteropelvic obstruction, impacted ureteral and renal calculi, retrocaval ureter, and retroperitoneal fibrosis with excellent success rates.

Renal and Ureteral Anatomy

A detailed and comprehensive knowledge of ureteral anatomy is imperative when contemplating a laparoscopic procedure. The ureter is described radiologically in terms of three segments: upper (renal pelvis to upper border of sacrum), middle (down to lower border of sacrum), and lower or pelvic (extends to the bladder). Surgically, the ureter can be described in terms of abdominal and pelvic segments. The abdominal ureter extends from the renal pelvis to the iliac vessels and the pelvic ureter extends then down to the bladder. The ureter receives its blood supply in a segmental distribution, depending on its level. The ureter receives vascular branches from the renal artery, gonadal artery, abdominal aorta, and common iliac artery and finally branches of the internal iliac artery. The feeding arterial branches approach the ureter medially in the upper ureter and laterally in the pelvis. This anatomic relationship is important to establish laparoscopic and endoscopic approaches to the ureter.

The ureter is a tubular extension of the renal pelvis that courses along the anterior surface of the psoas muscle before encountering the genitofemoral nerve around the fourth lumbar vertebral body. The gonadal vessels traverse over the ureter medially to laterally as the ureter enters the pelvis. The ureter continues towards the pelvic brim to cross over the external iliac vessels on the right and the common iliac vessel on the left. In the pelvis it courses medially and posteriorly to the medial umbilical ligament and enters the detrusor muscle just behind the superior vesicle artery. Midline retroperitoneal masses, such as massive lymphadenopathy or aortic aneurysms, may push and laterally deviate the ureters. The disease process of retroperitoneal fibrosis may contract and pull the ureters medially.

Patient Selection and Preparation for Laparoscopy

Preoperative evaluation includes identification of patients who are unsuitable candidates for a laparoscopic approach (i.e., coagulopathies, intrauterine pregnancy, and severe cardiopulmonary disease). Relative contraindications include large abdominal aortic aneurysms, multiple prior transperitoneal surgeries or renal trauma. However, experienced laparoscopists have successfully completed complex laparoscopic procedures in these patients [1]. Laparoscopic expertise of the surgeon is also the major determinant when considering such technically challenging cases. Informed consent should always be obtained and understood that there is the possibility of converting to an open approach because of difficult dissection or for safety issues.

Laboratory testing should include: a complete blood count, standard electrolyte panel, prothrombin time and partial thromboplastin time, urine analysis, culture/sensitivity, and a blood type and screen. Patients should be advised to discontinue any use of aspirin or aspirin-like compounds (such as nonsteroidal anti-inflammatory drugs, NSAIDs) at least 7 days before surgery. Patients should take nothing orally after midnight prior to the procedure. A mechanical bowel preparation (such as clear liquid diet and magnesium citrate) should be performed in any patients with a prior history of intra-abdominal operations. A single intravenous dose of a first-generation cephalosporin or a combination of ampicillin and gentamicin should be administered 1 h prior to arriving to the operating room.

Laparoscopic Pyeloplasty

Indications

Open pyeloplasty has been considered the "gold standard" for the treatment of ureteropelvic junction obstruction (UPJ). Success rates as high as 99% have been reported in large series [2]. The incisional morbidity associated with the open procedure has led urologists to explore less invasive alternatives to UPJ repairs [3]. Retrograde repairs, such as the Acucise (Applied Medical Resources, Laguna Hills, California, USA) ureteral cutting balloon, have made UPJ surgery an outpatient procedure but only has reported success rates of 70%-80% and an increased risk of hemorrhage compared to an open or laparoscopic approach]3,4]. Several unusual complications with the Acucise device have recently been reported in a recent series of 52 patients over 5 years, which included: device malfunction and breakage, ovarian vein laceration, and lower pole accessory renal artery lacerations [5]. The laparoscopic pyeloplasty, initially introduced in 1993, was conceived to combine the decreased morbidity of laparoscopy with a direct visual repair of obstructed UPJ [6]. The goal was to maintain the success level of the open procedure with the minimal morbidity of the endopyelotomy. Laparoscopic pyeloplasties have been performed in all age groups, pediatric through adult population. Patients as young as 2 1/2 years have been reported to have successful laparoscopic dismembered laparoscopic pyeloplasties [7].

Laparoscopic pyeloplasty should be considered in patients with UPJ obstruction secondary to a crossing vessel, a high ureteral insertion, failed prior procedures [8,9], high-grade hydronephrosis or marginal differential (less than 35%) renal function. Hynes-Anderson dismembered [7-10] and Foley Y-V [8] and Fenger nondismembered [10] pyeloplasties have all been described laparoscopically.

Evaluation of patients should include a diuretic renal scan (MAG-3) with furosemide washout as well as an intravenous urogram (IVU). A diuretic renal scan will quantify the degree of obstruction and split renal function by documenting the clearance half-time and relative percent function of the two kidneys. An IVU outlines the upper collecting system anatomy, rules out renal calculus disease, and provides information about the contralateral side. A retrograde ureteropyelogram also provides essential information. The level and length of obstruction as well as distal pathology are evaluated by retrograde ureteropyelography and should ideally be performed at the time of laparoscopic intervention. If the patient has had a stent placed for symptomatic obstruction, it should be removed at least 1 week prior to surgery to reduce ureteral edema and friability which facilitates laparoscopic suturing.

Surgical Technique

The patient is admitted the same day of surgery. After administration of antibiotics and induction of general anesthesia, an orogastric tube and sequential compression devices are placed on the lower extremities. All pertinent radiological studies confirming operative side and location of the obstruction should be available and visible in the operating room.

Step 1: Cystoscopy

Flexible (or rigid) cystoscopy is first performed and, if necessary, retrograde ureteropyelography. Any previously placed stents should have been removed at least 1 week before surgery. Initially, a 7-Fr internal double pigtail ureteral stent is placed. The stent should be one size (2 cm) longer than the measured appropriate length and placed in an upper pole calyx to facilitate closure of the renal pelvis. This also prevents direct contact of the coiled proximal stent with the newly reconstructed anastomosis.

Step 2: Repositioning and Room Setup

A Foley catheter is then inserted and the patient is placed in a 45° lateral decubitus position. The patient's umbilicus should be centered at the table break level in the event that an open repair would be performed. The break (flexion) in the table

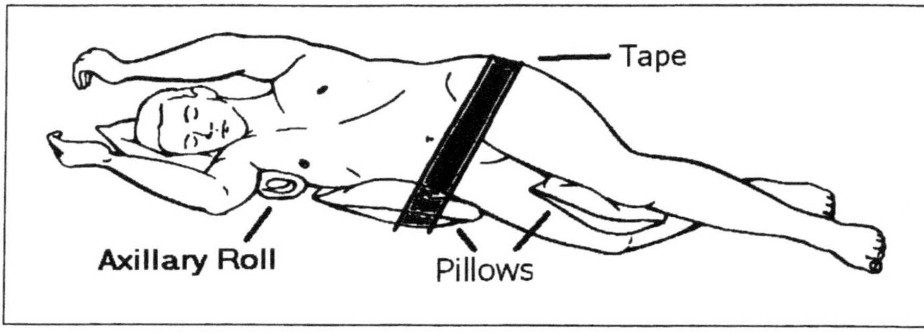

Fig. 1. The patient is positioned in a flank (60°) position with the arms in a "praying" position

should be kept to a minimum to reduce torque on the laparoscopic equipment. An axillary role (1,000 cc intravenous fluid bag wrapped in a towel) is placed under the lower arm, which is brought out perpendicular to the patient. The arms are then positioned parallel in a "praying position" near the patient's head and separated by padding. The lower knee is bent at 90° and the upper leg is kept straight with pillows or foam placed in between them (Fig. 1). Wide cloth tape is placed across the upper shoulder/arm and hip and secured to the operative table. The entire abdomen and flank from the xiphoid to the genitalia are shaved, then scrubbed. The surgeon is positioned on the contralateral side of the table (opposite side of affected renal unit). The assistant stands on the same side of the table as the surgeon as well as the scrub nurse (Fig. 2). An additional assistant may be positioned on the contralateral side to help with exposure, if necessary.

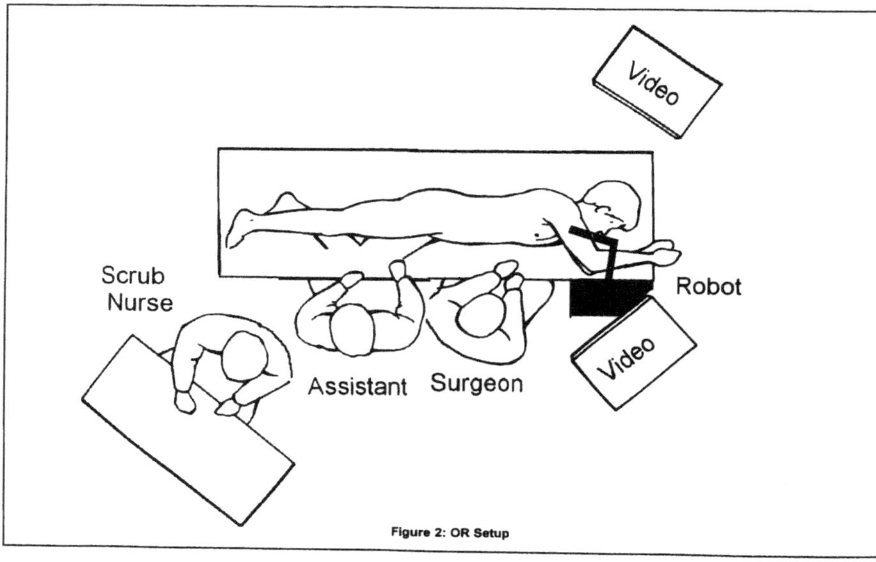

Fig. 2. Room setup for laparoscopic pyeloplasty or upper ureteral surgery

Step 3: Pneumoperitoneum

Laparoscopic pyeloplasty is performed via the transperitoneal approach. Pneumoperitoneum is established by inserting a Veress needle into the lower abdomen just lateral to the rectus muscle at the level of the anterior superior iliac crest.

Step 4: Initial Trocar Placement

After an insufflation pressure of 20 mmHg is obtained, the first trocar is placed using a 12-mm Visiport (U.S. Surgical, Norwalk, CT, USA) or Optiview (Ethicon Endo-Surgery, Inc. Cincinnati, Ohio, USA) under direct vision at the level of the anterior superior spine in the midclavicular line (MCL). The pneumoperitoneum can now be lowered to a working pressure of 12-15 mmHg.

Step 5: Remaining Trocars

The remaining trocars include 12-mm ports at the umbilicus and in the upper midline halfway between the xyphoid and umbilicus (Fig. 3). The sheaths are positioned 2 cm within the peritoneal cavity and secured to the skin with a heavy suture. The surgeon operates through the MCL and epigastric ports. The assistant manipulates the camera via the umbilical port.

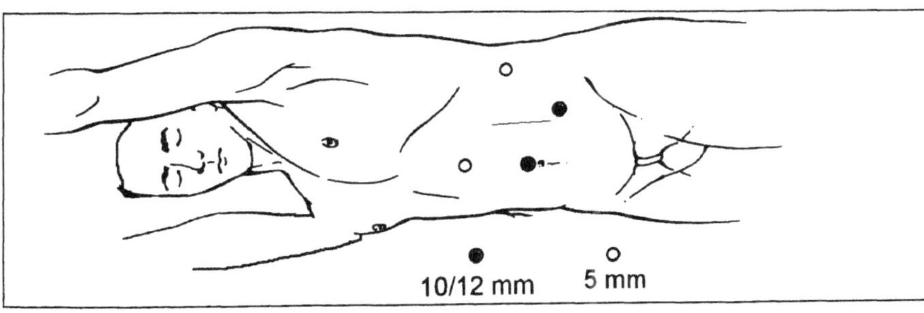

Fig. 3. Port placement for laparoscopic pyeloplasty

Step 6: Entering the Retroperitoneum

The lateral peritoneum reflection overlying the kidney is incised with laparoscopic harmonic scalpel (Ultracision Inc., Smithfield, RI, USA or Ultrasonix - U.S. Surgical, Norwalk, CT, USA) or bipolar forceps (Everest Medical Corporation, Minneapolis, MN, USA) from the upper pole to approximately 3 cm below the lower pole using the 0° laparoscopic lens. The harmonic scalpel and bipolar forceps reduces the risk of a transmitted electrocautery injury to the bowel. The colon is then retracted medially with a medial sweeping motion, further exposing the retroperitoneum.

Step 7: Lateral Trocar Placement

An additional 5-mm trocar may now be inserted in the anterior axillary line (AAL) at the level of the umbilicus. The assistant uses this trocar to retract during the UPJ repair but this is not always necessary. This will be the eventual site for external drain placement.

Step 8: UPJ Exposure

The laparoscopic lens is now switched from a 0° to a 30° lens. The psoas muscle is identified and followed cranially until the medial aspect of Gerota's fascia at the lower pole of the kidney is encountered. The ureter is identified by retracting the lower pole upward and sweeping the soft tissue medial and below Gerota's fascia from a caudal to cranial motion. The gonadal vessels lie in close proximity and can be confused with the ureter. Using a gentle sweeping motion parallel to the ureter with the graspers allows the surgeon to bluntly dissect and define the UPJ obstruction. Any crossing vessels will be identified at this point. Gentle palpation of the indwelling stent confirms the structure to be the ureter. The UPJ and renal pelvis are gently separated from the crossing vessels and surrounding tissue with atraumatic grasper or a right angle laparoscopic forceps. Careful attention should be made not to disrupt or injure the upper ureteral blood supply. This is achieved by keeping the mobilization of the proximal ureter to a minimum.

Step 9: Hynes-Anderson Dismembered Pyeloplasty

Laparoscopic scissors (Endoshears – Ethicon Endo-Surgery, Inc. Cincinnati, Ohio, USA) are utilized to transect the UPJ, taking care not to spiral this incision or damage the ureteral stent (Fig. 4 A-D). The renal pelvis is first circumferentially incised above the stenotic area and the stent is identified and delivered through this incision. Again, care must be taken to avoid transecting the internal stent. The posterior wall is transected and this frees the ureter from the renal pelvis. The ureter distal to the area of obstruction is then cut circumferentially and the ring of residual ureteral tissue is manipulated off the stent. The proximal ureter is spatulated on the lateral aspect for 1 cm using laparoscopic scissors. An anterior (or less commonly a posterior) crossing segmental renal vessel can be encountered in close proximity to the UPJ. This vessel may be identified as the cause of the obstruction and is reported to occur 25%-67% of the time [8,11,12]. In this case of anterior crossing vessels, the ureter must be transposed anteriorly to these vascular structures for the reanastomosis to the renal pelvis. A stitch of 4-0 polyglactin (SH needle) is placed at the apex of the spatulated ureter and then through the most dependent portion of the reduced renal pelvis. After tying this knot, the long stay suture (from the apically placed stitch) is passed under the new UPJ with a right angle laparoscopic forceps to expose the posterior pyelotomy. The cephalad portion of the pyelotomy is closed with several interrupted 4-0 polyglactin sutures utilizing the Endostitch (U.S. Surgical, Inc., Norwalk, CT, USA). The posterior row is finished using two or three additional interrupted sutures; the stent is then replaced back into the renal pelvis and then the anterior interrupted sutures are placed. Interrupted 4-0 sutures are used to tailor the anterior segment of the anastomosis to the spatulated ureter. The sutures are placed and tied intracorporeally where all knots are to be located outside the urinary tract in a square knot fashion. The Endostitch has been advantageous in improving accuracy of stitch placement and achieving faster knot tying when compared to conventional laparoscopic suturing [13,14]. After reconstruction of renal pelvic ureteral anastomosis is completed, the excess renal pelvis may be excised (reduction pyeloplasty), if necessary, and the remaining pyelotomy is closed, utilizing the Endostitch with a running 4-0 polyglactin suture. This suture is secured with a Lapratye (Ethicon Endo-Surgery, Inc., Cincinnati, Ohio, USA) or fishing knot. Most recently, we have been using fibrin glue in addition to the sutures, which has decreased urinary leakage.

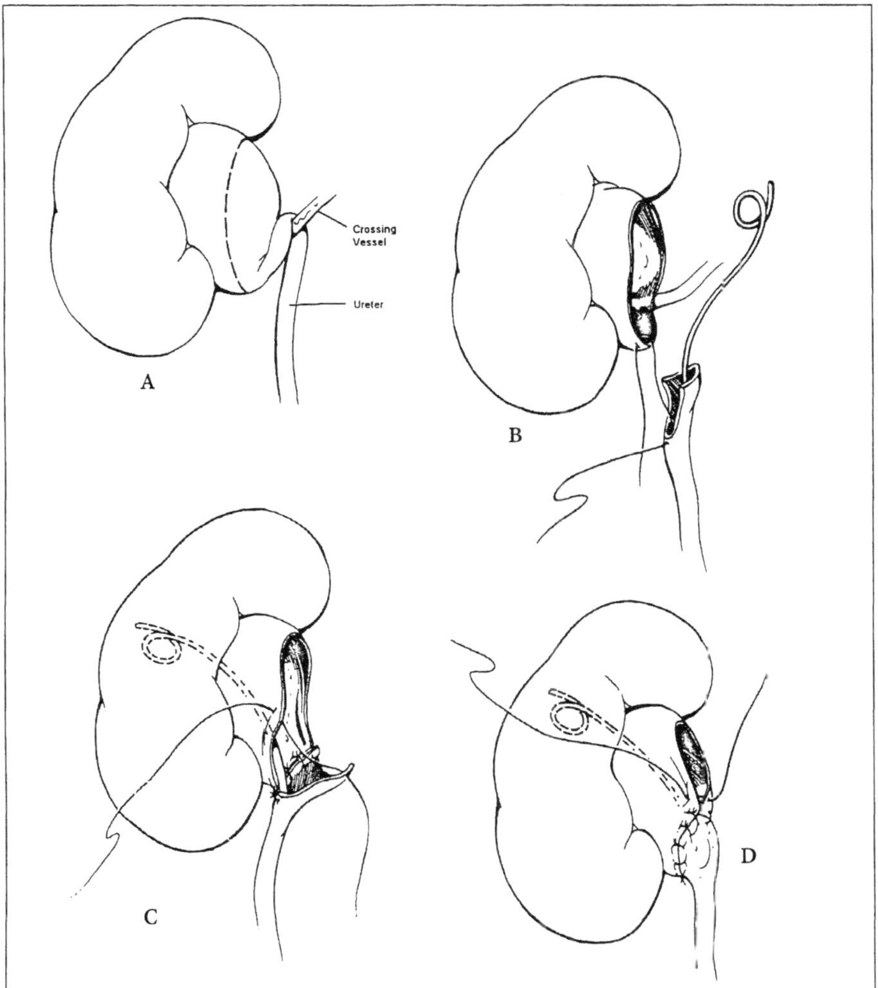

Fig. 4A-D. Steps of a Hynes-Anderson dismembered pyeloplasty

Step 10: Encountered Renal Calculi

If renal stones are encountered when performing the pyeloplasty, they are removed by placing a flexible cystoscope through a 10- to 12-mm port and extracting the stones with a stone basket via the pyelotomy incision. This is done prior to any suture placement.

Step 11: Drains and Closure

A small closed bulb suction drain is introduced and back-loaded through a 12-mm cannula and extracted with straight graspers with the 5-mm port and carefully placed in the retroperitoneum to lie adjacent (but not in direct contact) to the newly completed anastomosis (Fig. 5). The pneumoperitoneal pressure is lowered to 5 mmHg and the operative sites are re-examined to look for hemorrhage. All the trocars are removed under direct vision. Interrupted 2-0 polyglactin or PDS suture is used to close the abdominal fascia of the 10/12-mm port sites. The drain is secured to the skin with a nonabsorbable stitch. The CO_2 pneumoperitoneum is fully expunged to decrease postoperative diaphragmatic irritation. The skin incisions are closed with subcuticular 4-0 polyglactin suture and adhesive skin tape.

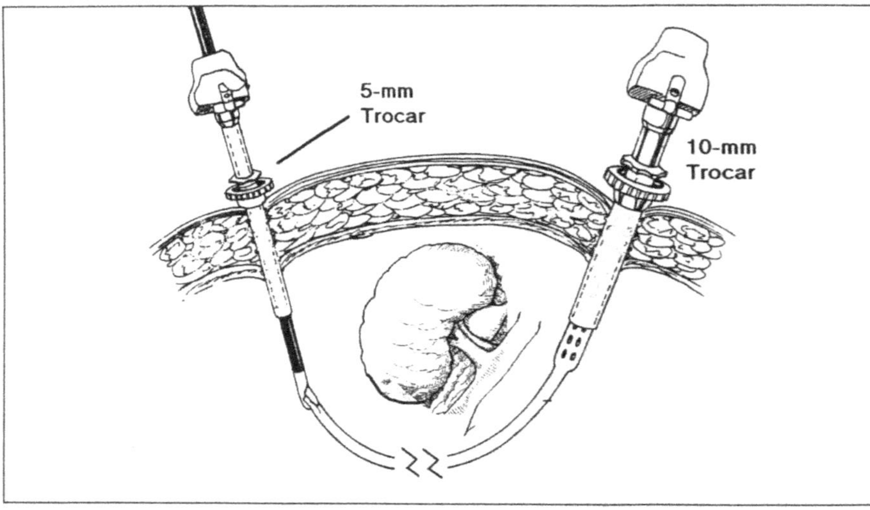

Fig. 5. Drain placement in through 10-mm port and out lateral 5-mm port

Step 12: Postoperative Care

The orogastric tube is removed immediately before extubation. The Foley catheter is removed the first or second day. A drain fluid creatinine is obtained on postoperative day 1. The drain may be removed only after the Foley catheter is removed and the drainage is negligible and/or the drain fluid creatinine is equal to the serum creatinine (i.e., drain fluid=peritoneal fluid), which is usually postoperative day 2. A clear liquid diet is started the night of surgery and advanced as tolerated. The intravenous antibiotics are continued for 24 h, then switched to an oral agent. The oral antibiotic is continued until the stent is removed at the surgeon's preference, usually 4 weeks postoperatively. The stent is removed 3-6 weeks postoperatively. At that time, a guide wire is passed through the stent prior to removal and a retrograde ureteropyelogram is performed to confirm ureteral patency and exclude extravasation. The anastomosis is radiologically then re-evaluated with an IVU 6 weeks after stent removal. A follow-up diuretic renal scan is obtained at 6 months postoperatively and compared to the previous study. Thereafter, an IVU or renal scan is obtained at yearly intervals.

Alternatives to Dismembered Pyeloplasty

Two alternative methods of performing pyeloplasties, the Foley Y-V [8] and Fenger non-dismembered [9], have both been described laparoscopically. Similar trocar placement and dissection to the renal pelvis are utilized.

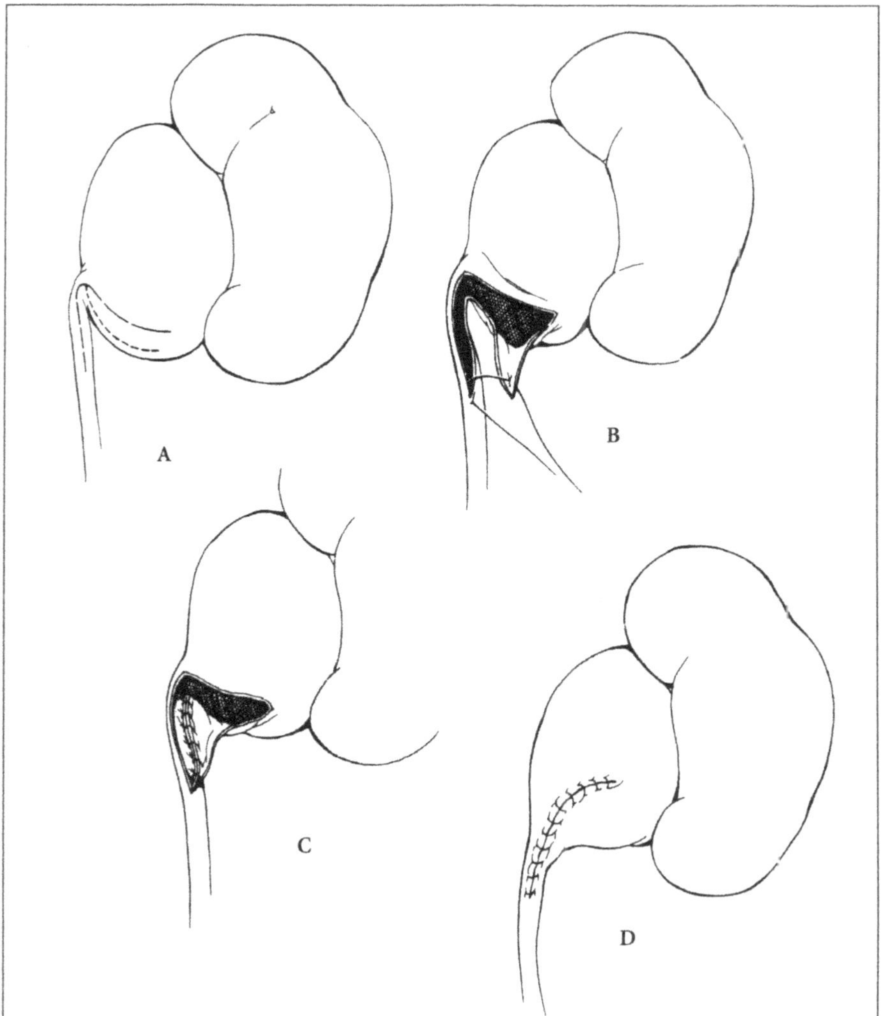

Fig. 6A-D. Steps of a Foley Y-V pyeloplasty

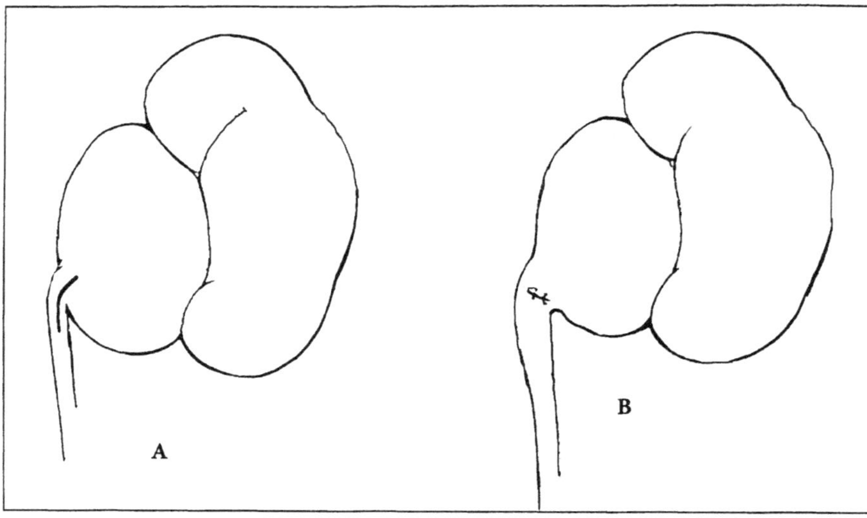

Fig. 7A, B. Steps of a Fenger pyeloplasty

The Foley Y-V pyeloplasty (Fig. 6 A-D) may be an alternative approach when no crossing vessel, a small renal pelvis, and/or a high ureteral insertion into the renal pelvis are encountered. Using laparoscopic scissors, a wide-based V-shaped flap is constructed from the anterior pelvis. The proximal ureter is spatulated anteriorly for 1 cm. Using 4-0 polyglactin suture, the apex of the V flap is sutured to the apex of the spatulated ureteral incision and tied intracorporeally with the Endostitch. The lower wall is completed first utilizing the Endostitch or conventional suturing to place two to four interrupted sutures. Several more interrupted sutures are placed from the apex out towards the upper pelvis to complete the anastomosis.

A Fenger pyeloplasty (Fig. 7 A,B) can be performed for the same indications as Foley Y-V pyeloplasty. The principle behind this procedure is a longitudinal incision and transverse closure (Heineke-Mikulicz). This technique has the advantage of a shorter operative time because less intracorporeal sutures are needed [10]. The longitudinal incision is made with laparoscopic scissors from the renal pelvis distally 1 cm below the UPJ segment. The initial pyelotomy incision (just above the UPJ) can be made with a laparoscopic knife (#15 or #11 blade on a needle holder). This maneuver will facilitate scissors incisions through the UPJ. The longitudinal incision is then closed transversely in a Heineke-Mikulicz fashion over the stent using one to three interrupted 4-0 polyglactin sutures.

Results

Overall, laparoscopic pyeloplasty outcomes have been excellent. Different age groups, techniques, and even histories of previous interventions have still resulted in symptomatic and radiologic relief of obstruction. Seven complications are reported in the literature from over 60 cases. Five of the seven were minor complications. One major complication was readmission for an adynamic ileus which responded to conservative therapy [8]. Another was a pulmonary embolism which required anticoagulation and prolonged hospitalization [10]. A reported intraoperative complication involved the clipping of a colonic diverticulum which was immediately recognized and subsequently resected with a GIA stapler with no adverse sequelae [8]. Postoperative distal ureteral narrowing treated with successful balloon dilation [6], severe flank pain after balloon calibration of the UPJ at time of stent removal of two patients (no longer performed), and thrombophlebitis at the antecubital intravenous site are also reported as minor complications [7].

Laparoscopic Pyelolithotomy

Indication

Extracorporeal shock wave lithotripsy for renal calculi larger than 2 cm has had disappointing outcomes. These larger calculi may be managed by retrograde ureteroscopy, percutaneous nephrolithotomy, or laparoscopic pyelolithotomy in the presence of an extrarenal pelvis. Large renal pelvic stones may be quickly and efficiently managed by laparoscopic techniques similar to those utilized for the pyeloplasty. Preoperative evaluation should include IVU or computed tomography (CT) to diagnose an extra-renal pelvis. A MAG-3 renal scan may also be considered to rule out a co-existing UPJ obstruction but results may be altered because of an obstructing calculus or secondary edema.

Surgical Technique

The technique is verbatim to the dismembered pyeloplasty previously described (Steps 1-8). After cystoscopy, stent placement, repositioning, and laparoscopy to the retroperitoneum is performed, the affected renal pelvis is exposed.

Step 9: Pyelotomy

A longitudinal incision is made into the renal pelvis. This can performed by placing a #11 or #15 knife blade in a laparoscopic needle driver. The incision may then be extended using the laparoscopic scissors.

Step 10: Calculus Removal

If the calculus is visualized, it may be removed using laparoscopic spoon graspers. If there is any difficulty in visualization, or multiple calculi are present, a flexible cystoscope and tipless stone basket may be utilized.

Step 11: Pyelotomy Closure

The incision is closed using interrupted 4-0 vicryl sutures in a watertight fashion. A small bulb suction drain is placed through the lateral 5-mm port and positioned in the retroperitoneum.

Laparoscopic Repair of the Retrocaval Ureter

Indications and Preoperative Evaluation

A circumcaval or retrocaval ureter is an anomalous development of the inferior vena cava (IVC). The fetal posterior cardinal vein does not regress and leads to the IVC becoming anterior to the ureter and displacing it medially. If this obstruction is below the third lumbar vertebrae, the result is an obstructed ureter from kinking. A similar procedure to a dismembered pyeloplasty is utilized to correct this congenital anomaly [15]. Indications for reconstruction of the retrocaval ureter include recurrent infection, obstruction, and flank pain. Preoperative evaluation and preparation for laparoscopic reconstruction of the retrocaval ureter are identical to the laparoscopic dismembered pyeloplasty.

Surgical Technique

A similar procedure to a dismembered pyeloplasty is utilized to correct this congenital anomaly.

Step 1: Cystoscopy

A 7-Fr internal double pigtail ureteral stent is placed after general anesthesia is induced. A lubriguide (hydrophilic) guide wire is often needed to negotiate the reverse "s" shaped deformity of the retrocaval ureter.

Steps 2–7: Trocar Placement and Retroperitoneal Exposure

Laparoscopic technique includes the same steps (2-7) and trocar configuration as the previously described laparoscopic dismembered pyeloplasty. The respective peritoneal reflection is incised from the lower pole of the kidney to the iliac vessels. The colon is reflected toward the midline via a medial sweeping motion.

Step 8: IVC Exposure

The upper portion of the retrocaval ureter has an atypical course (Fig. 8). It is located much more medially and closer to the IVC. At the level of lumbar vertebrae number three (L3), the retrocaval ureter generally goes under the IVC. Lifting the lower pole of the kidney upward and laterally can facilitate founding the retrocaval ureter. The ureter is freed from its surrounding tissue for 3 cm above and below the IVC crossing.

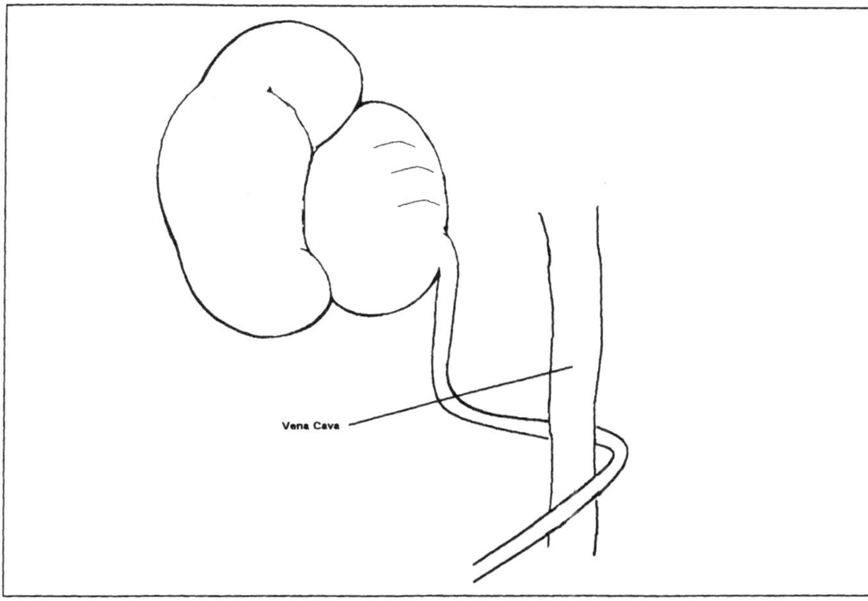

Fig. 8. Course of retrocaval/circumcaval ureter

Step 9: Ureteral Transection and Reanastomosis

The ureter is transected 2 cm above the IVC ureteral crossing. The distal ureteral portion is then brought under the IVC. The lower ureteral segment is then spatulated laterally for 1 cm. The sutured anastomosis is performed identically to the earlier description of laparoscopic dismembered pyeloplasty. This maneuver is often easier than the laparoscopic reconstruction of the UPJ because of the excess length of the retrocaval ureter. The anastomosis is drained with a closed suction drain, as previously described. Postoperative care and complications are also the same as described in the previous pyeloplasty section.

Laparoscopic Ureterolithotomy

Indications

With the advancing technology of ureteroscopy, extracorporeal shock wave lithotripsy (ESWL), and medical therapy, open calculus surgery has become a rare occurrence. Indications for ureterolithotomy are failure of ureteroscopy or ESWL (i.e., inability to localize or access the stone, inability to focus the shock waves, or inability to fragment a hard stone or an impacted stone). Since the advent of the holmium laser, almost all ureteral stones (including an impacted stone) can be fragmented. This almost negates the need to perform ureterolithotomy in these patients. The presence of ureteral strictures or congenital anomalies or urinary diversions may also require an open ureterolithotomy but may be considered relative contraindications for laparoscopy, depending on experience. Raboy et al., using a similar technique to laparoscopic pelvic lymph node dissection, described the first laparoscopic ureterolithotomy on a cystinuric patient [16]. Since then several others have advocated the laparoscopic approach [17, 18].

Preoperative Evaluation

An IVU must be obtained prior to the procedure to clearly delineate the ureteral anatomy. If there is insufficient visualization of the distal ureter, a retrograde ureterogram should be obtained in the operating room to rule out a concomitant stricture. Laparoscopic ureterolithotomy with ureteral reconstruction has been successfully completed in the presences of an ureteral stricture [16].

Surgical Technique

Step 1: Cystoscopy and Stent Placement

The patient is placed in a supine position and general anesthesia is induced. A nasogastric or orogastric tube should be placed after intubation and continued on continuous low wall suction to decompress the stomach. Flexible cystoscopy is performed and a 0.035-in. floppy-tip or hydrophilic guide wire is manipulated past the calculus under fluoroscopic guidance. A 7-Fr double pigtail stent of the appropriate length is passed over the wire and positioned in the renal pelvis; then a Foley catheter is placed. If necessary, an open-ended catheter may be inserted at the level of the stone to help direct the tip of the wire past the stone. If a retrograde wire or stent cannot be passed, an external ureteral catheter is passed up to the large ureteral stone and brought out through a Council catheter, which is then secured to a Tuohy-Bokz side arm adapter.

Step 2: Repositioning

Patient positioning on the operating room table is customized according to stone location. A fluoroscopic operative table must be used. A stone in the upper half of the ureter is approached from a lateral decubitus position.

Step 3: Laparoscopic Entrance

Pneumoperitoneum is established by a Veress needle either placed lateral to the rectus muscle in patients positioned in the flank or in the umbilicus for the supine position to treat lower ureteral stones. Carbon dioxide insufflation is performed to an abdominal pressure of 18-20 mmHg to facilitate trocar placements and then can be lowered to a working pressure of 15 mmHg.

Step 4: Trocar Placement

Laparoscopic technique and trocar sites include the same steps (2-7) and trocar configuration as the previously described laparoscopic dismembered pyeloplasty. The re-

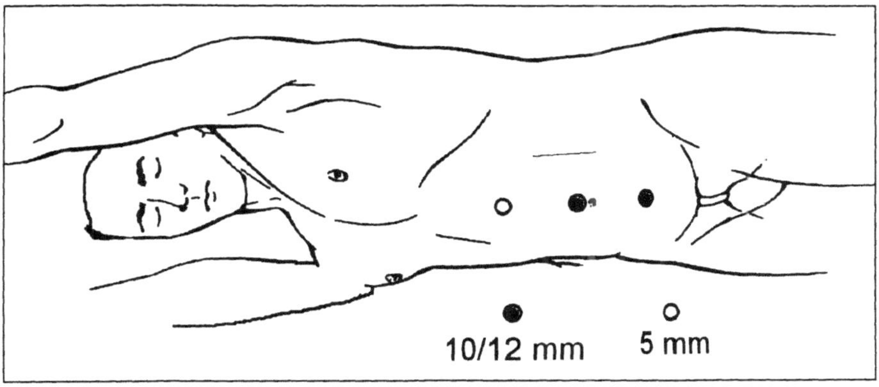

Fig. 9. Port placement for ureterolithotomy

spective peritoneal reflection is incised from the lower pole of the kidney to the iliac vessels. The colon is reflected toward the midline via a medial sweeping motion.

For lower ureteral stones, the patient is in the flank position. The 12-mm ports are placed at the umbilicus and subumbilical midline. A 5-mm port is then placed in the midline between the umbilicus and xyphoid (Fig. 9).

Step 5: Entering the Retroperitoneum

Incising the line of Toldt is performed, as previously described, starting near the estimated stone position. The colon is then reflected medially, exposing the retroperitoneum.

Step 6: Ureter

Identification of the ureter and stone positioning is then performed by gentle transverse sweeping motion made parallel to the ureter with atraumatic graspers. Proximal ureteral dilation from the calculus obstruction is not usually seen and therefore fluoroscopy or X-rays may be needed to pinpoint the actual location. Often, the ureteral stone is visually seen by a bulge in the ureter and by palpation with large laparoscopic Cril forceps.

Step 7: Incision

Once the stone is located, a longitudinal incision is made with scissors or laparoscopic knife. The stone is milked out through the ureterotomy and extracted from the peritoneal cavity, either grasped by forceps or delivered into an entrapment sack.

Step 8: Closure

The ureterotomy is then loosely reapproximated over the ureteral stent by using 4-0 polyglactin sutures. Several interrupted sutures are spaced out 3-4 mm (Fig. 10). If the incision is less than 1 cm, the ureterotomy can be left open to heal around the stent but the authors prefer closure of the ureterotomy in the above-stated fashion.

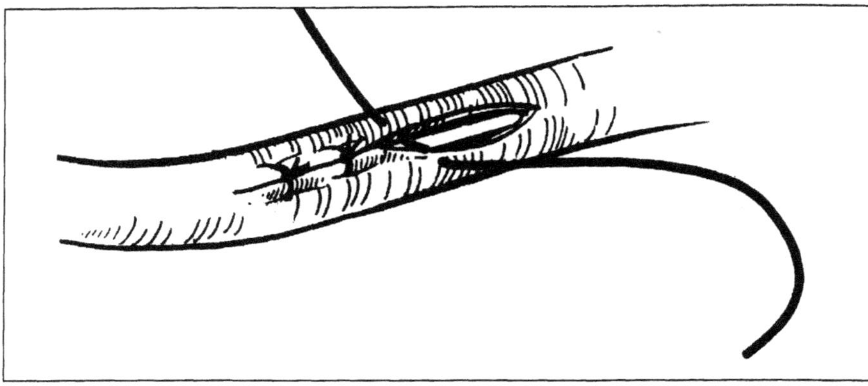

Fig. 10. Suture closure of ureteral incision

Retroperitoneal Approach

An alternate method of performing a laparoscopic ureterolithotomy is via the retroperitoneal route. Techniques of creating the extraperitoneal space differs by location (flank and pelvis) and by closed and open methods of creation of the retroperitoneal/extraperitoneal space.

The following depiction is one description of obtaining extraperitoneal/retroperitoneal access. For extraperitoneal access of the lower ureter, a 2-cm vertical midline skin incision is made 3 cm below the umbilicus. The subcutaneous fat is spread until the underlying fascia is exposed. The rectus fascia is incised vertically and deepened until the properitoneal space is exposed. Utilizing blunt finger dissection, the extraperitoneal space is created. Stay sutures (2-0 polyglactin) are placed on each side of the fascia. A 10- to 12-mm cannula is back loaded onto a 0° lens and is placed through the incision directly into the properitoneal space under direct vision. Once in the extraperitoneal space, the laparoscopic cannula is advanced over the lens into the dissected cavity. The extraperitoneal space can be expanded by visually directed blunt lens dissection. A homemade balloon is created from the cut middle finger of a size 8 glove and affixed to the end of a 16-Fr red rubber Robinson catheter with 2-0 silk free ties. A catheter guide is placed within the red rubber Robinson catheter and the whole apparatus is passed through the 10- to 12-mm cannula into the extraperitoneal space. The balloon is then filled with saline solution up to 800 cc via a 60 cc catheter-tip syringe. The expansion of the balloon can be seen and palpated in the lower abdomen. A laparoscopic irrigator/aspirator is utilized to decompress the balloon. The balloon is then extracted and a pneumoretroperitoneum is initiated. Alternatively, commercially available balloons (Origin Medsystems, Inc., Menlo Park, CA, USA) allow rapid expansion of the preperitoneal space under direct laparoscopic visualization.

The same aformentioned technique is utilized to create a retroperitoneal space. The initial skin incision is placed 2 cm below the tip of the 12th rib. The ureterolithotomy is then carried out as previously described. While the concept of extraperitoneal/retroperitoneal ureterolithotomy is attractive, the shortcoming of this approach is that ureteral suturing is difficult, if not impossible, because of small retroperitoneal/extraperitoneal space. For this reason the authors prefer the much more direct transperitoneal approach.

Postoperative Care

The postoperative care is similar to the previously described pyeloplasty. An IVU should be obtained at 3 months to assess ureteral patency and rule out obstruction.

Laparoscopic Ureterolysis

Introduction and Indications

Idiopathic retroperitoneal fibrosis or Ormond's disease is a benign fibrous process that aggressively envelops the ureters and great vessels. This fibrous encasement leads to a mechanical obstruction, resulting in hydronephrosis, pain, and renal deterioration. The radiographic hallmark of this process is hydronephrosis and severe medial deviation of the mid-ureters. Several conditions, such as inflammatory bowel disease, endometriosis radiation therapy, drug therapy (i.e., methysergide), and malignancy may all result in secondary retroperitoneal fibrosis. The two goals of ureterolysis surgery are to release the ureteral entrapment, thus relieving the obstruction, to preserve renal function, and also to prevent any recurrent obstruction by placing the ureters intraperitoneally and away from the disease process.

Preoperative Evaluation

The proper evaluation of retroperitoneal fibrosis involves determining the extent of the disease and excluding the possibility of malignancy. An abdominopelvic CT scan with oral and intravenous contrast is the most appropriate study and must be obtained prior to surgery. Retroperitoneal malignancies should be evaluated with a digital rectal exam, prostate-specific antigen level, stool examination and chest X-ray. Women should also have pelvic and breast examinations with a mammogram. A diuretic renal scan (MAG-3) should also be obtained to assess residual renal function and quantitate the degree of obstruction. Even with a CT scan, an IVU or coronal 3D reconstruction of the CT scan can be obtained to determine the degree of ureteral displacement. A retrograde ureteropyelogram just prior to the procedure can replace the IVU and also be helpful in mapping the ureteral courses and ruling out distal obstruction.

Preparation

A mechanical bowel preparation may be useful to facilitate exposure transperitoneally by decompressing the bowel. A first-generation cephalosporin should be given prior to surgery.

Surgical Technique

Step 1: Cystoscopy and Stent Placement

Indwelling ureteral stents are first placed with a flexible cystoscope and the patient is positioned similarly to the laparoscopic pyeloplasty. An assistant can manipulate the stent while the surgeon observes for motion. Lighted and infrared stents are now available and may help facilitate identification and outline the course of the ureter. If a bilateral approach is anticipated, the patient can be placed in a supine fashion,with the table being rotated to allow the bowel to fall away from the operative field.

Step 2: Pneumoperitoneum

Pneumoperitoneum is then established via a Veress needle, either through the umbilicus in the supine position or lateral to the ipsilateral rectus muscle, as previously described.

Step 3: Trocar Placement

Using a Visport, the initial trocar is placed in the umbilicus. Under direct vision, the remaining ports are placed. Another two 10- to 12-mm ports are placed above and below the umbilicus in the midline with an optional 5-mm port placed in the AAL at the umbilical level which can help in retraction of the ureter during the dissection (Fig. 11). The peritoneal cavity, including all visible organs, should then be inspected for any signs of gross malignancy and biopsied appropiately.

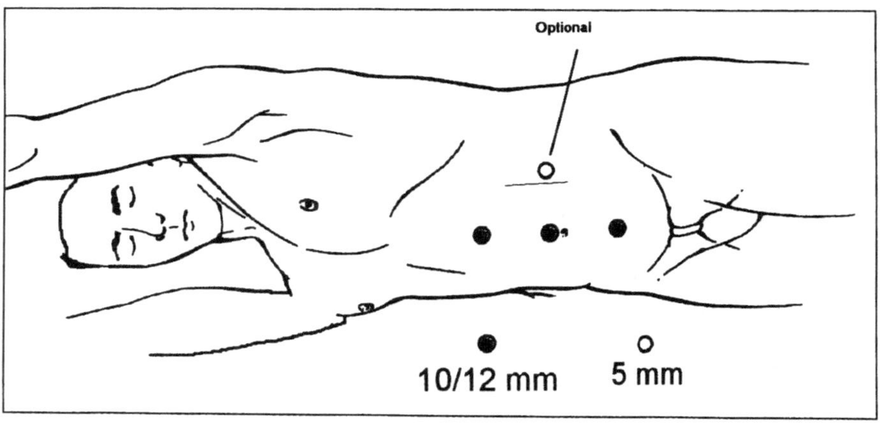

Fig. 11. Port placement for ureterolysis

Step 4: Entering the Retroperitoneum

The surgeon uses a grasping forceps or Babcock clamp to retract the colon medially and the peritoneal reflection (white line of Toldt) is incised at the level of the iliac vessels. The incision is then extended cephalad to the hepatic flexure on the right or splenic flexure on the left. A gentle sweeping motion with graspers or scissors frees up the colon and mobilizes it medially, exposing the psoas muscle.

Step 5: Ureteral Identification

The ureter should be identified in a proximal portion that is uninvolved by the fibrotic process, which may be as high as the UPJ. Distally, the ureter may be found in proximity to the bladder just medial to the medial umbilical ligament. These authors prefer to begin their ureteral dissection proximally up at the UPJ. It is always important to remember the abnormal anatomical relationship the retracted ureter may have with either the vena cava or aorta.

Step 6: Biopsy

Once these relationships are established, multiple biopsies for frozen and permanent pathology should be taken of the surrounding tissue to rule out a neoplastic process.

Step 7: Exposing the Ureter

Once the ureter is clearly identified, the assistant retracts the periureteral tissues laterally while the surgeon develops a window around and behind the ureter. Using a right angle forceps, a single 4-in. piece of umbilical tape is passed around the freed area and the ends are fastened together using a 9-mm clip. The umbilical tape aids in retracting the ureter for further dissection and is stronger than a vessel loop.

Step 8: Dissecting the Ureter

With minimal cauterization, a combination of sharp and blunt dissection is employed to detach and shell out the ureter from its hard fibrotic encasement. All attempts to maximize the ureteral blood supply should be made. The gonadal vessels should be noted to be in close approximation and even cross the ureter on the right side. These vessels should be dissected free of the ureter and, if necessary, may be clipped and transected. This careful dissection is continued until the ureter is freed and mobilized from the renal pelvis to below the fibrotic process (usually just below the iliac vessels).

Step 9: Peritonealizing the Ureter

Once the ureter is freed, it is mobilized and transposed into the peritoneal cavity by reapproximating the medial and lateral cut edges of the posterior peritoneum behind the ureter. This maneuver is performed to isolate the ureter from the fibrotic process and prevent any further obstruction. The reapproximation of the peritoneal edges may be done with either a hernia stapler passed through the umbilical port or by running absorbable sutures (Fig. 12). If an omental wrap is desired, an endo-GIA stapler can be inserted to split the omentum into a length sufficient to be positioned loosely around the ureter and clipped to itself using 9-mm clips or interrupted 3-0 polyglactin sutures. The CO_2 is evacuated; the ports are

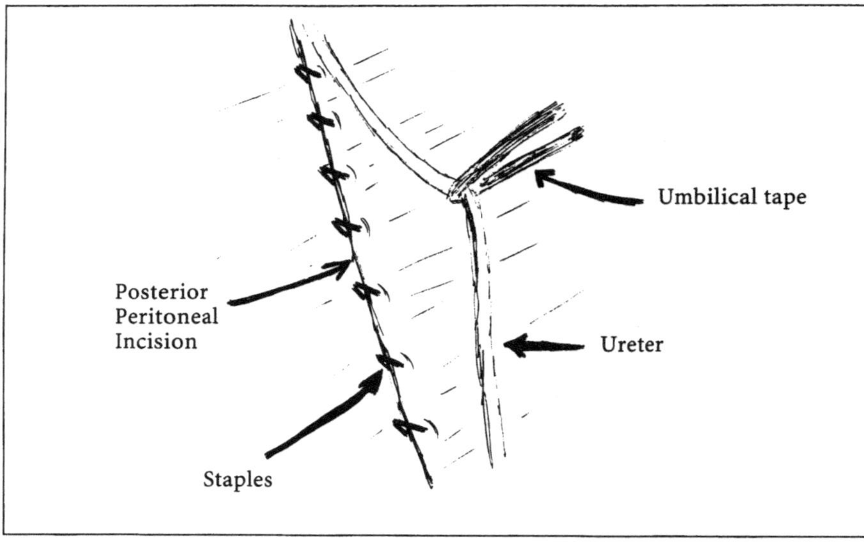

Fig. 12. Closure of posterior peritoneum with staples

removed under direct vision, then closed. A drain is not necessary unless the ureter is inadvertently entered.

Postoperative Care

The orogastric tube is immediately removed postoperatively. The Foley catheter and pneumatic compression boots are continued until the patient is fully ambulatory. Parenteral antibiotics are usually continued for 24 h; then the patient is switched to an oral agent of choice as a prophylactic measure until the stents are removed. A clear liquid diet, which is advanced as tolerated, is either started on the day of surgery or postoperative day 1, depending on the length of the surgery. An IVU is performed to assess the course of the ureter(s) 2-3 weeks postoperatively. If the ureter(s) remains laterally displaced, the stent(s) is removed. Follow-up IVUs are performed at 3, 6, and 12 months. Full activity may be resumed after the stent is removed.

Postoperative Complications

Though there are few case reports, ureteral injury, stricture, re-obstruction, infection, and severe bleeding are all possible complications of laparoscopic ureterolysis.

Conclusion

Long-term outcomes for laparoscopic ureteral surgery are being shown to be comparable to its open surgical counterpart. The laparoscopic pyeloplasty has the greatest degree of follow-up at this time. In a comparison study of laparoscopic open and endourologic procedures, laparoscopic and open patients experienced a 100% success rate in relief of obstruction versus 78% for the Acucise retrograde approach and 77% for the antegrade percutaneous approach [3]. The laparoscopic patients were also found to have better tolerance of the procedure, less hospital stay, and a quicker recovery time than the open pyeloplasty group. Laparoscopic ureterolithotomy has a limited but favorable follow-up according to the data from three different centers [16-18]. Though not compared to open counterparts, the laparoscopic technique seems to have reliable results.

However, laparoscopic pyeloureteral surgery requires advance laparoscopic skills currently only obtained during an endourology fellowship. Thus, for now, reconstructive laparoscopic procedures are performed primarily at select university urologic centers. The ongoing advances in surgical instruments and refinements of technique have decreased operative times over the last few years, making laparoscopy a more attractive option for renal surgery.

References

1. Chen RN, Moore RG, Kavoussi LR (1998) Laparoscopic renal surgery in patients at high risk for intra-abdominal or retroperitoneal scarring. J Endourol 12(2):143
2. Rushton HG, Salem Y, Belman AB et al (1994) Pediatric pyeloplasty: is routine retrograde pyelography necessary? J Urol 152: 604
3. Brooks JD, Kavoussi LR, Preminger GM, Schuessler WW (1995) Comparison of open and endourological approaches to the obstructed ureteropelvic junction. Urology 46:791
4. Chandhoke PS, Clayman RV, Stone AM et al (1993) Endopyelotomy and endoureterotomy with the Acucise ureteral cutting balloon device: preliminary experience: J Endourol 7:45
5. Schwartz BF, Stoller ML (1999) Complications of retrograde balloon cautery endopyelotomy. J Urol 162: 1594
6. Schuessler WW, Grune MT, Tecuanhuey LV, Preminger GM (1993) Laparoscopic dismembered pyeloplasty. J Urol 150: 1795
7. Tan HL, Roberts JP (1996) Laparoscopic dismembered pyeloplasty in children: preliminary results. Br J Urol 77:909
8. Moore RG, Averch TD, Schulam PG, Adams II JB, Chen RN, Kavoussi LR (1997) Laparoscopic pyeloplasty: experience with the initial 30 cases. J Urol 157:459
9. Nakada SY, Mc Dougall EM, Clayman RV (1995) Laparoscopic pyeloplasty for secondary ureteropelvic junction obstruction: preliminary experience. Urology 46: 257
10. Janetschek G, Peschel R, Altarac S, Bartsch G (1996) Laparoscopic and retroperitoneoscopic repair of ureteropelvic junction obstruction. Urology 47: 311
11. Sampaio FJB, Favorito LA (1993) Ureteropelvic junction stenosis: vascular anatomical background for endopyelotomy. J Urol 150:1787
12. Gupta M, Smith AD (1996) Crossing vessels at the ureteropelvic junction: do they influence endopyelotomy outcomes? J Endourol 10:183
13. Adams JB, Schulam PG, Moore RG, Partin AW, Kavoussi LR (1995) New laparoscopic suturing device: initial clinical experience. Urology 46:242
14. Pattaras JG, Smith GS, Landman J, Moore RG (2000) A comparison and analysis of laparoscopic intracorporeal suturing devices: preliminary results. J Endourol 14 [Suppl 1]: A69
15. Baba S, Oya M, Miyahara M et al (1994) Laparoscopic surgical correction of circumcaval ureter. Urology 44:122
16. Raboy A, Ferzli GS, Ioffreda R et al (1992) Laparoscopic ureterolithotomy. Urology 39: 223

17. Bellman GC, Smith AD (1994) Special considerations in the technique of laparoscopic ureterolithotomy. J Urol 51:146
18. Harewood LM, Webb DR, Pope AJ (1994) Laparoscopic ureterolithotomy: the results of an initial series and an evaluation of its role in the management of ureteric calculi. Br J Urol 74: 170

Chapter 13

Renal Surgery in Adults

Peter A. Pinto, Thomas W. Jarrett

Introduction

The field of minimally invasive surgery has developed from endoscopic and percutaneous techniques to now encompass laparoscopic surgery. Adult renal surgery that traditionally required large flank or abdominal incisions can today be routinely performed laparoscopically. In 1990, Clayman, Kavoussi, and colleagues pioneered this field by performing the first laparoscopic nephrectomy [1]. Further advances have led to laparoscopic nephroureterectomy and partial nephrectomy.

Mimicking open techniques, the approach to laparoscopic renal surgery has been both transperitoneal and retroperitoneal. The latter has become more popular since 1992, when Gaur described balloon dissection of the retroperitoneal space [2]. Both techniques have advantages and disadvantages, with the decision of which to perform often being dependent on patient factors, such as body habitus and prior surgery and surgeon preference. In this chapter, techniques for laparoscopic retroperitoneal nephrectomy, nephroureterectomy, partial nephrectomy, and renal cyst decortication will be discussed in detail.

Nephrectomy

Indications

Simple or radical nephrectomy can be performed via a retroperitoneal laparoscopic approach. Indications for simple nephrectomy are benign renal diseases. This includes poorly or nonfunctioning kidneys secondary to long-standing obstruction or infection, dysplastic or cystic kidneys, and renovascular hypertension not amenable to reconstructive surgery. Relative contraindications include prior inflammatory processes such as xanthogranulomatous pyelonephritis or tuberculous kidneys.

Indications for radical nephrectomy include organ-confined tumors (clinical stage T1 or T2) not amenable to nephron-sparing surgery. Some investigators have demonstrated that even large masses (12 cm) can be removed in this fashion [3]. Tumors spreading beyond Gerota's fascia or involving the renal vein or inferior vena cava are contraindicated. Metastatic disease is not contraindicated provided the tumor is not locally invasive.

Technique

Setup and Patient Position

The patient is placed on the operating table in the standard flank position with the side of pathology facing up. The top arm is draped over a padded Mayo stand or multiple pillows. An axillary roll is placed. The bottom leg is flexed and bent while the top leg is straight. The kidney rest is elevated and the table is flexed in order to maximize the working space between the ribs and iliac crest (Fig. 1). The skin between the iliac crest and the ribs should be taut on palpation. The patient is then secured to the table with tape at the shoulders, hips, and legs. The table is rotated left and right to make sure the patient does not shift during the procedure.

The surgeon and camera assistant are positioned facing the patient's back. The scrub nurse stands on the opposite side at the end of the table (Fig. 2). Two monitors are used to provide all personnel with an unobstructed view. Alternatively, the camera assistant can be replaced by a robotic arm. The AESOP® robot (Computer Motion, Santa Barbara, Calif., USA) can be fixed to the operating table to hold the camera. The robot is controlled by the surgeon through voice commands or a foot pedal.

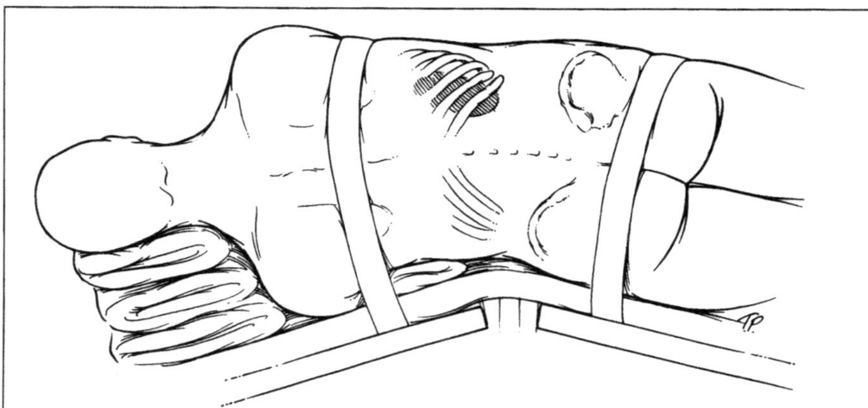

Fig. 1. The patient is placed in a full flank position with the kidney rest elevated and the table flexed. This increases the distance between the costal margin and iliac crest, thus maximizing the working space

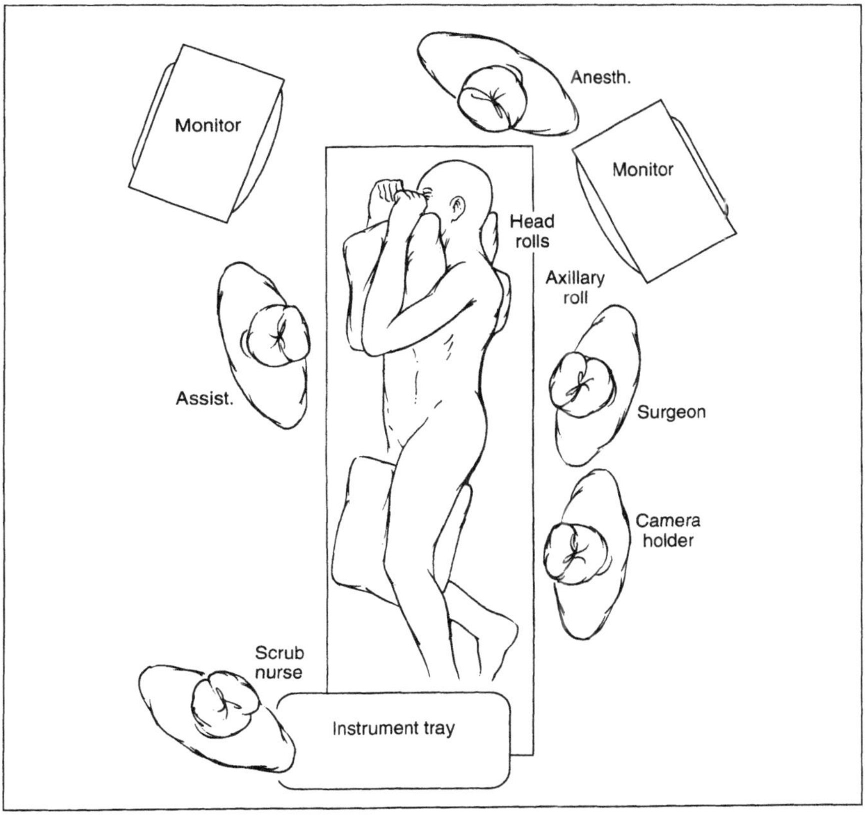

Fig. 2. Operating room setup for laparoscopic retroperitoneal nephrectomy. Two videc monitors are used to provide an unobstructed view of the operation to the surgeon and assistants

Access and Trocar Placement

Three trocars are positioned in the anterior, mid, and posterior axillary lines (Fig. 3). Retroperitoneal access is initially obtained via the open Hassan technique. A 1.5-cm transverse incision is made just anterior and inferior to the tip of the 12th rib. The incision is carried down sharply through the posterior thoracolumbar fascia, flank muscles, and anterior thoracolumbar fascia. Upon entering the retroperitoneal space, the index finger is used to sweep the peritoneum anteriorly and develop a space between the psoas muscle anteriorly and Gerota's fascia posteriorly (Fig. 4).

When performing a nephrectomy, the surgeon's finger can be used to initially develop the space. With simple nephrectomy, the index finger is placed cephalad to palpate the lower pole of the kidney, enter Gerota's fascia, and develop the space within Gerota's fascia. When performing a radical nephrectomy, the index finger is used to develop the space between the psoas muscle and Gerota's fascia. The working space is then created by balloon dissection (Fig. 5). This expands the

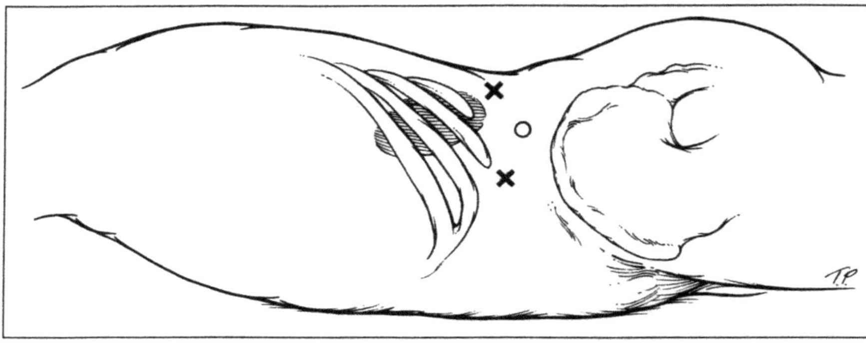

Fig. 3. Trocar placement. The laparoscope is positioned in the mid-axillary line. A 12-mm port is placed in the posterior axillary line. A 5-mm port is placed in the anterior axillary line

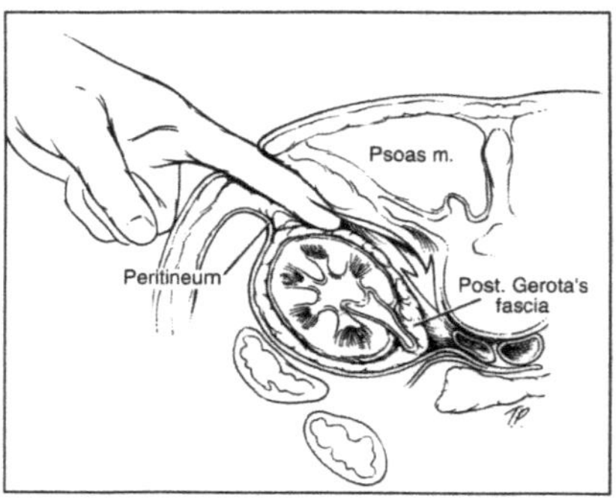

Fig. 4. The surgeon's finger is used to start the retroperitoneal dissection. A space behind the kidney is created to place the balloon dissector

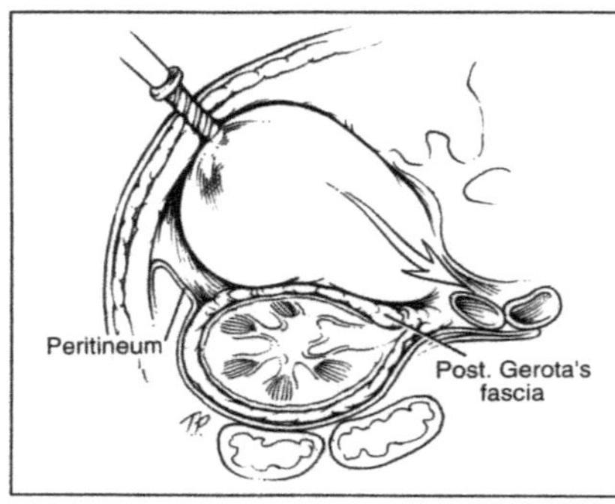

Fig. 5. The working space is created by balloon dissection. The kidney and peritoneum are displaced anteriorly exposing the renal hilum

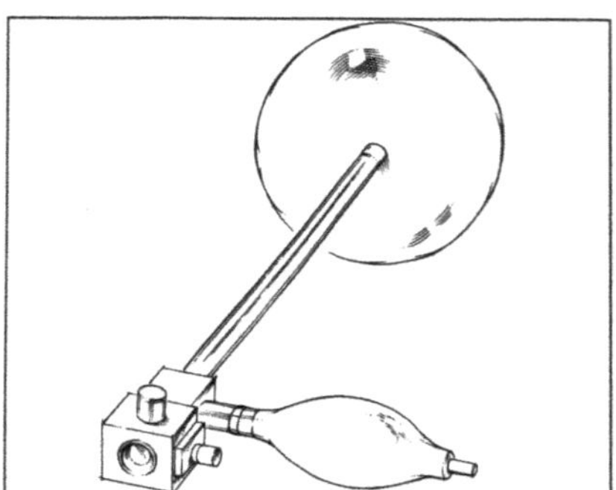

Fig. 6. The trocar-mounted balloon, which accommodates the laparoscope, allows the surgeon to visually inspect the retroperitoneum while the balloon is expanding

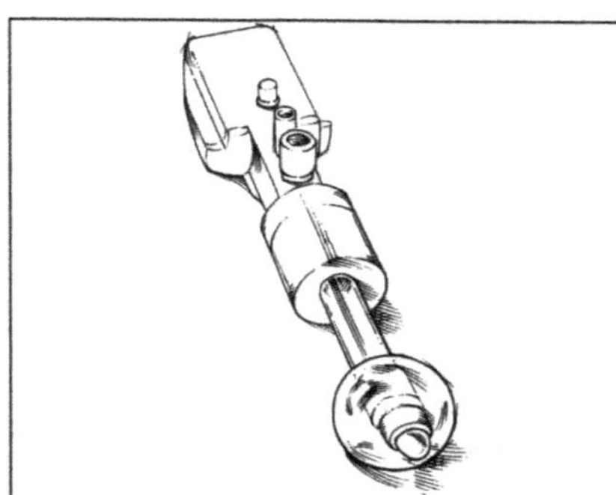

Fig. 7. Blunt-tipped trocar. The collar on the port slides down against the balloon tip to prevent loss of pneumoretroperitoneum

retroperitoneal space to between 800 and 1,000 ml. Trocar-mounted balloons are available, allowing direct visualization while the space is developed (Fig. 6). Alternatively, Clayman et. al and Micali et. al described the technique of entering the retroperitoneum under laparoscopic control using a visualizing port [4, 5].
After the space has been developed, a 10-mm blunt-tipped trocar is inserted (Fig. 7). The trocar has a balloon on its distal end and a cushion proximally which helps maintain a tight seal. The pneumoretroperitoneum is established with CO_2 to a pressure of 15-20 mmHg and the working space is inspected. The entry sites for the two remaining ports are viewed laparoscopically to aid in their placement. If the peritoneal reflection still lies too far posteriorly, preventing placement of the anterior port, it can be swept anteriorly with the laparoscope itself.

Surgical Technique

Maintaining orientation is important throughout the procedure. This helps in identifying landmarks such as the psoas muscle, peritoneal reflection, ureter, gonadal vein, and pulsations of the renal artery. Initial dissection is carried out inferiorly and posteriorly to isolate the ureter and mobilize the lower pole (Fig. 8).

The peritoneal attachments anterior to the kidney are not divided in order to prevent the kidney from falling into the working space. Blunt dissection along the ureter reveals the gonadal vein. The ureter is traced cephalad to the renal hilum. Bipolar cautery can be used to clear off the hilum and isolate the renal vessels. The renal artery is encountered first as it lies posterior to the vein (Fig. 9). The artery can be ligated with vascular clips or stapled with a stapling device using an endovascular load. The renal vein, which lies anteriorly and caudally, is then isolated. Figure 10 shows the stump of the ligated renal artery with the renal vein behind it.

The size of the renal vein usually does not allow safe ligation with clips. The endovascular stapler is used to ligate and transect the vein. Figure 11 demonstrates the staple line on the stump of the renal vein after division with a vas-

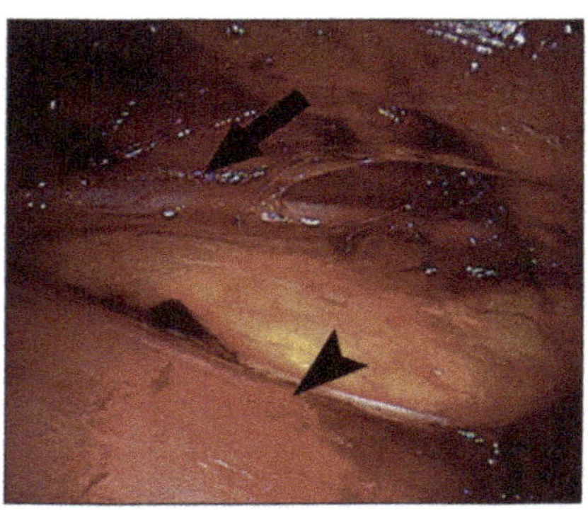

Fig. 8. Retroperitoneal working space after balloon dissection. The ureter (*arrow*) and psoas muscle (*arrowhead*) are seen

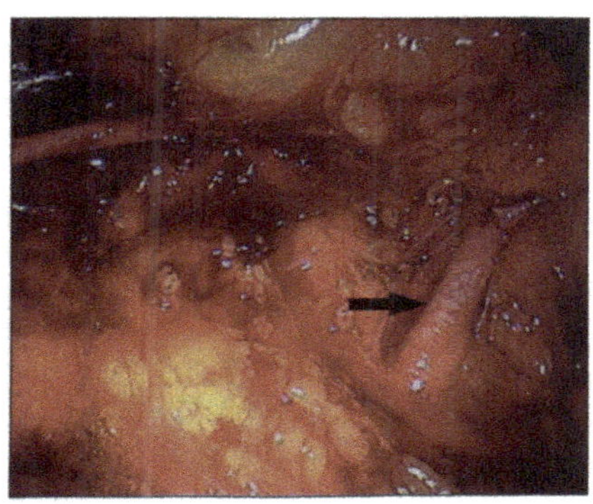

Fig. 9. The renal artery (*arrow*) is encountered first during the hilar dissection

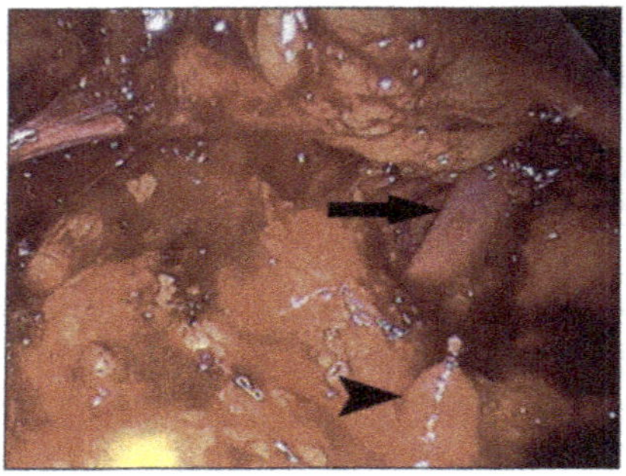

Fig. 10. The renal vein (*arrow*) is revealed after division of the renal artery. The stump of the renal artery (*arrowhead*) is seen in the foreground

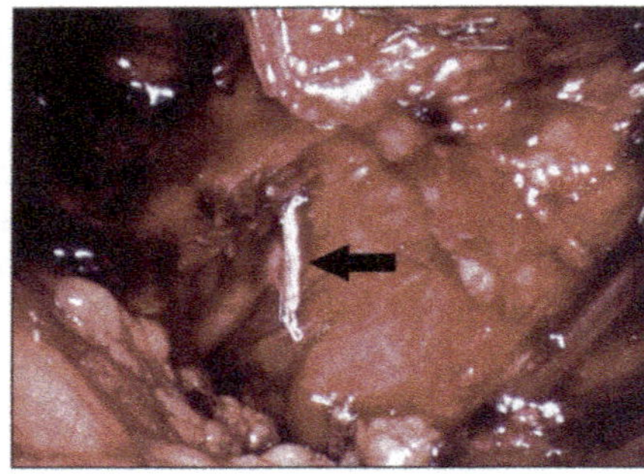

Fig. 11. After ligation with a linear stapling device, the stump of the renal vein is seen (*arrow*)

cular load of Endo-GIA stapler. When performing a left nephrectomy, dissection reveals the entry of the adrenal vein superiorly (Fig. 12). The Endo-GIA vascular stapler can be placed distal to the adrenal vein when performing a simple nephrectomy. When performing a radical nephrectomy, the renal vein is divided proximal to the adrenal branch in order to allow removal of the adrenal gland with the specimen.

Once the vessels have been controlled, the anterior surface of the kidney is mobilized from its peritoneal attachments. Care is taken not to enter the peritoneum and injure the adjacent bowel and mesentery.

The ureter remains attached to keep the kidney from retracting cephalad. The kidney is then mobilized superiorly, thus freeing it completely. After ligating and dividing the ureter, the kidney is inspected to confirm that all the attachments have been divided. Finally, the specimen is entrapped in a sac and extracted (Fig. 13).

This is done by placing the laparoscope in the lateral port and inserting the 15-mm endocatch through the trocar at the tip of the 12th rib. The specimen can be morcellated or extracted whole by extending the incision. In cases where the working space in the retroperitoneum limits entrapment, the peritoneum can be opened to help place the specimen in the bag.

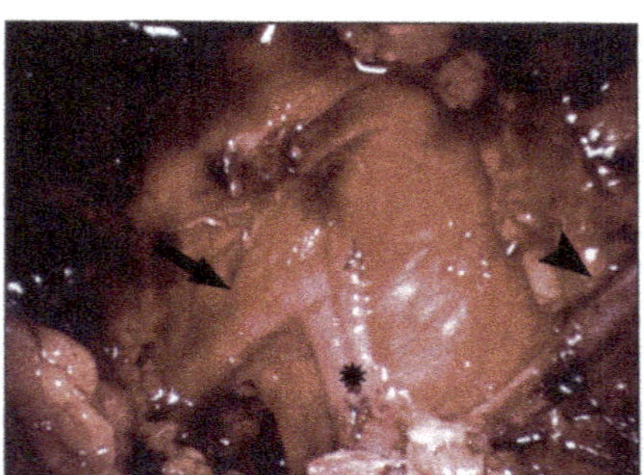

Fig. 12. Dissection during a left nephrectomy reveals the adrenal vein (*arrow*) entering the renal vein (*asterisk*). The gonadal vein (*arrowhead*) is also seen draining into the renal vein

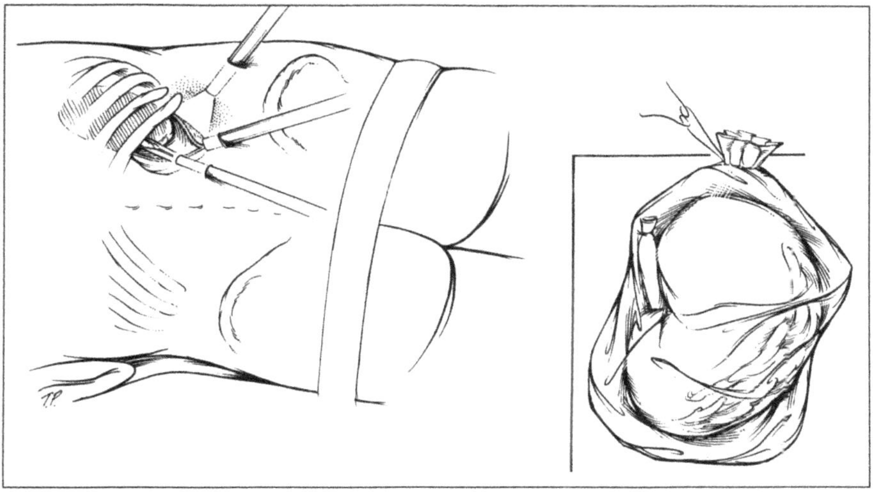

Fig. 13. Specimen entrapment

Nephroureterectomy

Indications

Nephroureterectomy is the gold standard treatment for transitional cell carcinoma of the kidney or ureter. In cases where endoscopic management is not appropriate, i.e., high-grade or multifocal disease, laparoscopic nephroureterectomy is a minimally invasive alternative. The first reported cases described a transperitoneal approach [6]. Subsequently, Gill and associates popularized the retroperitoneal approach [7].

Technique

Setup and Patient Position

The patient is initially placed in the dorsal lithotomy position for management of the distal ureter and bladder cuff. This will be described later in the chapter. The patient is then repositioned in true flank position as described previously.

Access and Trocar Placement

Trocar positioning is the same as for standard nephrectomy. The development of the working space, however, is slightly different. Since access to the distal ureter and bladder is necessary, a double balloon dilation is required. It is first placed behind the kidney as is done for standard nephrectomy. After this space is developed, it is passed a second time more caudal, toward the bladder (Fig. 14).

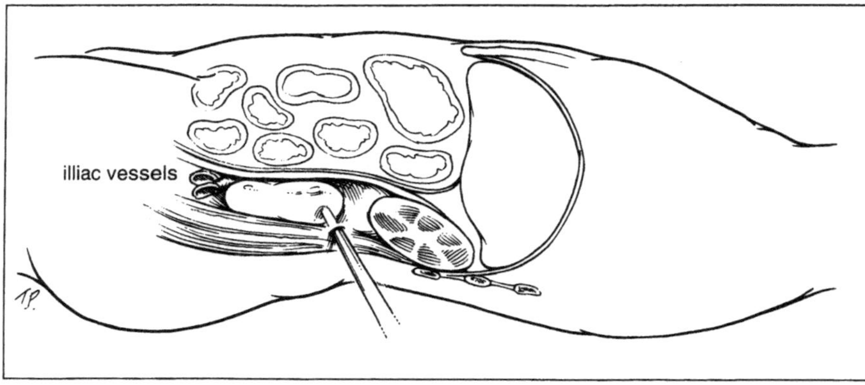

Fig. 14. A second, caudal balloon dissection is carried out after creating the working space posterior to the kidney

Surgical Technique

With the patient in the dorsal lithotomy position, cystoscopy is performed. After ruling out concomitant bladder tumors, two 3-mm trocars are placed into the bladder one finger-breadth above the symphysis pubis. They are placed with the bladder distended and under cystoscopic guidance (Fig. 15). An endoloop tie is passed through the ipsilateral trocar and around the ureteral orifice. An open-ended ureteral catheter is passed into the ureter and the entire intramural segment is mobilized with a resectoscope and Collin's knife (Fig. 16). A laparoscopic grasper passed through the contralateral trocar aids in this dissection. When com-

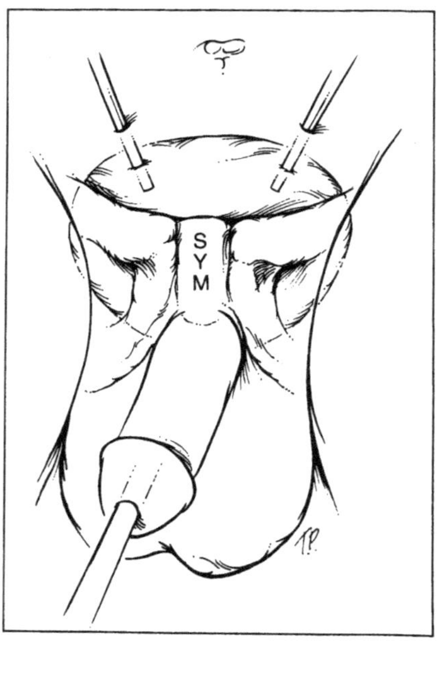

Fig. 15. Once the bladder is filled, cystoscopy guides the insertion of the 3-mm ports

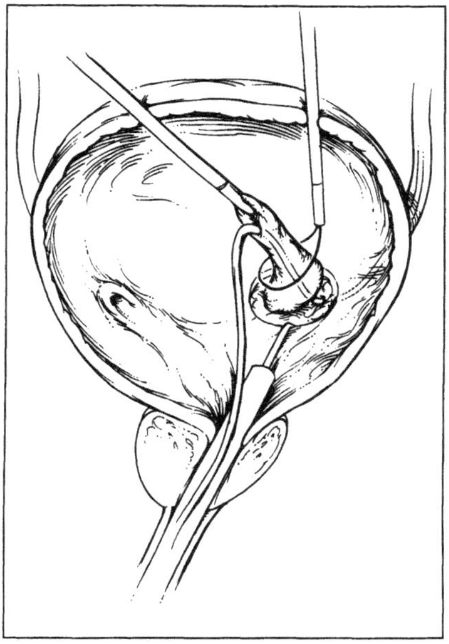

Fig. 16. The distal ureter is mobilized and secured with an endoloop

pletely mobilized, the ureteral catheter is removed and the endoloop cinched down around the mobilized ureter. Bleeding points are fulgurated and a large-caliber Foley catheter is placed for drainage.

After repositioning the patient, the nephrectomy is carried out as previously described. The ureter is then traced distally to its entry into the bladder. It is important to remember that the ureteral blood supply changes from medial in its mid-portion to lateral at its distal end. Sharp and blunt dissection, along with gentle traction on the ureter, delivers the distal segment. The endoloop around the orifice confirms that the ureter, in its entirety, has been removed. Specimen retrieval is carried out as previously described.

There are alternative methods to managing the distal ureter and bladder cuff. Instead of the previously described cystoscopic method, the entire ureter and bladder cuff can be removed laparoscopically. The opening in the bladder can then be sutured or the distal ureter can be resected and stapled with the Endo-GIA stapler. A perivesical drain is then placed.

Partial Nephrectomy

Indications

Although initially indicated for tumors involving a solitary kidney or bilateral disease, nephron-sparing surgery is now performed for tumors smaller than 4 cm in the presence of a normal contralateral kidney. Indications have been extended due to the favorable results reported in multiple series [8-11]. As recommended for open surgery, laparoscopic partial nephrectomy is limited to tumors less than or equal to 4 cm in size.

Technique

Setup and Patient Position

The operating room staff and equipment are positioned as described in the section on radical nephrectomy. Additional materials that should be made available are laparoscopic vascular clamps, an argon beam coagulator, Surgicel pledgets, fibrin glue, indigo carmine or methylene blue, an ultrasound with laparoscopic transducer, a cystoscope, and a ureteral catheter. The patient is initially placed supine on the operating table for insertion of an open-ended ureteral catheter. This is followed by repositioning to the true flank position as was previously described.

Access and Trocar Placement

Trocar positioning and development of the working space is carried out as for standard nephrectomy.

Surgical Technique

With the patient supine, flexible cystoscopy is performed and an open-ended ureteral catheter is placed on the relevant side. A syringe filled with methylene blue or indigo carmine is attached to the ureteral catheter which is secured to the Foley catheter with a silk tie. The patient is then repositioned.

As in the approach to standard nephrectomy, landmarks such as the psoas and ureter are first established. The renal hilum is isolated, exposing the renal artery and vein for possible temporary occlusion. Gerota's fascia is then entered and dissected off the renal capsule with endoshears. Care is taken to leave a cap of fat over the tumor. Visual inspection of the kidney along with intraoperative sonography is used to rule out the presence of other lesions and determine the extent of the tumor.

Exophytic masses attached by a narrow base can be excised without the need for vascular occlusion. The capsule around the tumor is scored with cautery, and the mass is removed with the aid of laparoscopic scissors or an ultrasonic scalpel. Alternatively, we have used a laparoscopic scalpel to cut into the parenchyma. This is created by fixing a urethrotome to the end of the laparoscopic suction/irrigator wand or laparoscopic kitner (Fig. 17).

Large, more broad-based tumors often require interruption of renal blood flow. An osmotic diuretic is administered to initiate a brisk diuresis. The capsule around the mass is scored, and a laparoscopic bulldog clamp is placed on the renal artery. Alternatively, a laparoscopic Satinsky vascular clamp can be used, but this requires the placement of an additional 12-mm trocar. The tumor is excised ensuring a rim of normal parenchyma around it. It is entrapped in a sac, and left temporarily in the wound. Biopsy specimens are taken from the base and sent for

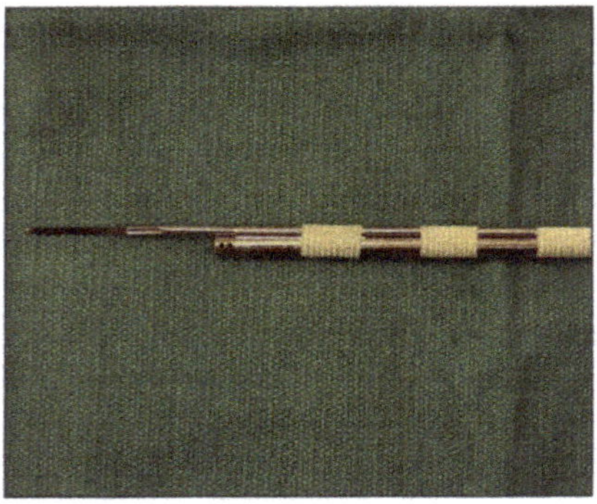

Fig. 17. Laparoscopic scalpel fashioned from an urethrotome and laparoscopic suction/ irrigator wand

frozen section to determine margin status. Methylene blue is injected through the ureteral catheter to check for any openings in the collecting system. If one is found, it is sewn laparoscopically with 4-0 absorbable suture. Smaller defects can be handled with fibrin glue alone. The resected base is then sealed. First, bleeding points are controlled with the argon beam coagulator. Next, fibrin glue is applied to the entire raw surface. The vascular clamp is removed and the pneumoretroperitoneum is lowered to 5 mmHg to ensure adequate hemostasis.

Mid-pole lesions are excised by wedge resection. In these cases, Surgicel pledgets are created on the bench before starting the procedure (Fig. 18).

After excision, hemostasis is obtained as previously described. But in addition, the Surgicel pledgets are placed in the defect. The capsule is sutured over them to reapproximate and compress the defect in the parenchyma.

Cold ischemia is technically feasible laparoscopically, but not practical. Therefore, when operating under the time constraints of warm ischemia, it is important to be expeditious in your approach to resection and reconstruction of the kidney.

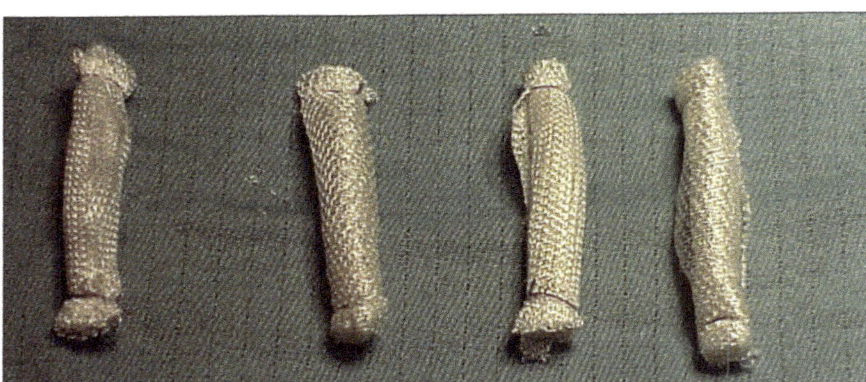

Fig. 18. Surgicel pledgets, approximately 1 cm wide and 4 cm long, are prepared prior to wedge resection

Decortication of Renal Cysts

Indications

Renal cysts, whether inherited or acquired, are often without symptoms and are found incidentally. Yet simple cysts or cysts associated with autosomal dominant polycystic kidney disease (ADPKD) can become symptomatic. When pain cannot be managed with analgesics or infection becomes refractory to antibiotics, intervention may be necessary. Aspiration and sclerosing of cysts may be considered first-line therapy, but recurrent cysts often require more definitive therapy [12]. Laparoscopic decortication or marsupialization is a minimally invasive alternative to the standard open flank approach.

Technique

Setup and Patient Position

The patient position and operating room setup is the same as for nephrectomy. In addition, the argon beam coagulator should be available to control parenchymal bleeding if encountered. Other instruments that should be made available include an ultrasound with laparoscopic transducer, indigo carmine or methylene blue, a cystoscope, and a ureteral catheter.

Access and Trocar Placement

Trocar positioning and development of the working space is carried out as for standard nephrectomy.

Surgical Technique

As was described for partial nephrectomy, cystoscopy and placement of a ureteral catheter is performed with the patient supine. Although the risk of entering the collecting system is low for peripheral and simple cysts, central and peripelvic cysts may abut the collecting system. Injection of methylene blue at the end of the procedure will identify a collecting system injury, which can then be repaired laparoscopically. The laparoscopic part of the procedure is carried out in the flank position.

Gerota's fascia is opened longitudinally near the psoas muscle. The renal hilum and entire kidney are exposed. Gerota's fascia is dissected off the renal capsule, exposing the cysts. It is necessary to mobilize the kidney completely when multiple cysts are present. Subcapsular cysts can be identified with the aid of intraoperative ultrasound. The extrarenal cyst wall is then grasped and excised with laparoscopic scissors or ultrasonic shears. It is sent for pathological examination. The base of the cyst is inspected for any irregularities. If suspicious areas are found, they are biopsied with a laparoscopic cup biopsy forceps. The edge of the cyst wall is cauterized with electrocoagulating scissors or the argon beam coagulator. The cyst base is not fulgurated to prevent collecting system injury [13]. If the renal cyst is too large to mobilize, it can be first drained with a spinal needle. In an attempt to prevent cyst recurrence, Gerota's fascia or perirenal fat can be laid onto the cyst base and tacked in place with absorbable sutures. A closed suction drain is left in place if a single large cyst or multiple cysts are unroofed.

Peripelvic cysts require complete mobilization of the renal hilum. In addition to intraoperative sonography, injecting methylene blue into the collecting system can help differentiate the cyst from the pelvis.

For indeterminate cysts, the cyst is decorticated and the base biopsied for analysis by frozen section. If malignant tissue is found, radical or partial nephrectomy can be performed in the same setting.

References

1. Clayman RV, Kavoussi LR, Soper NJ, et al (1991) Laparoscopic nephrectomy: initial case report. J Urol 146:278-282
2. Gaur DD (1992) Laparoscopic operative retroperitoneoscopy. J Urol 148:1137-1139
3. Gill IS, Schweizer D, Hobart MG, et al (2000) Retroperitoneal laparoscopic radical nephrectomy: the Cleveland clinic experience. J Urol 163:1665-1670
4. Clayman RV, McDougall EM, Kerbl K, et al (1993) Laparoscopic nephrectomy: transabdominal vs. retroperitoneal. J Edourol 7:S139
5. Micali S, Caione P, Virgili G, et al (2001) Retroperitoneal laparoscopic access in children using a direct vision technique. J Urol 165:1229-1232
6. Clayman RV, Kavoussi LR, Figenshau RS (1991) Laparoscopic nephroureterectomy: initial Case Report. J Laparoendosc Surg 16:343-349
7. Gill IS, Sung GT, Hobart MG, et al (2000) Laparoscopic radical nephroureterectomy for upper tract transitional cell carcinoma: the Cleveland Clinic experience. J Urol 164:1513-1522
8. Licht MR, Novick, AC (1993) Nephron sparing surgery for renal cell carcinoma. J Urol 149:1-7
9. Steinbach F, Stöckle M, Müller SC, et al (1992) Conservative surgery of renal tumors in 140 patients: 21 years of experience. J Urol 148:24
10. Provet J, Tessler A, Brown J, et al (1991) Partial nephrectomy for renal cell carcinoma: indications, results and implications. J Urol 145:472-476
11. Hafez KS, Fergany AF, Novick AC (1999) Nephron sparing surgery for localized renal cell carcinoma: impact of tumor size on patient survival, tumor recurrence and TNM staging. J Urol 162:1930
12. Lang EK (1987) Renal cyst puncture studies. Urol Clin N Amer 14:91
13. Hoenig DM, McDougall EM, Shalhav AL, et al (1997) Laparoscopic ablation of peripelvic renal cysts. J Urol 158:1345-1348

Chapter 14

Laparoscopic Urologic Surgery in Malignancies

G. Breda, A. Caruso, N. Piazza

Introduction

The last decade has witnessed major shifts in the popularity of laparoscopic procedures for therapy of urologic pathology.

The pioneering work of Ralph Clayman in 1990 prompted an explosion in the interest in such techniques, which, however, was soon tempered by the realization that the benefit gained (vs. open procedures) was offset by the disproportionate time and financial investment needed to acquire the technical skills and to maintain and improve them.

A second change in the winds occurred in the last few years after it was demonstrated that such techniques could be safely used in the therapy of neoplastic diseases of the kidney and prostate.

At the present time laparoscopic surgery for the therapy of various urologic tumors can be roughly divided in three main categories: widely accepted, controversial, and experimental (Table 1) [1].

Table 1. Indications for laparoscopic surgery in urology for malignancies

WIDESPREAD INDICATIONS:
• Radical nephrectomy for renal carcinoma (T1)
• Pelvic lymphadenectomy for carcinoma of prostate
• Radical prostatectomy for prostate cancer
CONTROVERSIAL INDICATIONS:
• Partial nephrectomy for renal cancer
• Nephrouretectomy for trasnitional cell carcinoma (Ta/T1)
• Retroperitoneal lymph node dissection for testicular cancer
• Pelvic lymphadenectomy for bladder cancer
EXPERIMENTAL INDICATIONS:
• Radical cystectomy and urinary reconstruction for bladder cancer

Widespread Indications

Laparoscopic Pelvic Lymphadenectomy for Carcinoma of the Prostate

Lymph node dissection for prostatic tumors was one of the first laparoscopic procedures to be done and one of the most commonly used and best evaluated applications of laparoscopy in urologic practice [2]. An estimation of the risk of the lymph node metastases can be made on the basis of algorithms such as the table of Partin. Nowadays, however, because of increased public awareness and screening, a substantial number of prostate cancer patients present with prostate-specific antigen (PSA) levels < 10 ng/ml and, subsequently, it is to be expected that the number of men qualifying for lymph node dissection will decrease dramatically. The indications for laparoscopic pelvic lymphadenectomy for prostatic carcinoma are high risk of positive nodes (PSA > 10 ng/ml; Gleason score > 7; >2 positive biopsies), prior to perineal prostatectomy, radiotherapy, or brachytherapy. The technique is performed in many centers; the length of the procedure is less than 2 h and patients can usually be discharged within 48 h after surgery. Fornara et al. in 1999 reviewed a total of 1,847 cases in 19 centers in Europe and the United States [3].

Laparoscopic Radical Prostatectomy

Laparoscopic radical prostatectomy was first performed in 1991 by Schuessler and colleagues and an initial series of nine cases was published in 1997 [4]. Laparoscopic radical prostatectomy is now performed routinely in several centers where the feasibility and reproducibility of this technique have been established. The indications are the same as for open surgery (T1-T2 N0); it is not advisable in prostates < 20 g or > 80 g, or in patients who have previously undergone Transureteral Resection of the Prostate (TURP) or adenomectomy. The improvement in the quality of intraoperative vision related to magnification of the image and selective illumination allows for a more precise procedure with the potential of better preserving the viability of neurovascular and muscular structures. Therefore, laparoscopic prostatectomy can achieve excellent functional results in connection with atraumatic dissection.

Table 2. Multicenter European experience of laparoscopic radical prostatectomy (Zurich, Paris, Bordeaux, Berlin, Creteil, Brussels, Schaffhausenn)

Period	January 1998 - November 2000
No. Pts	1228
Catheter time (mean, days)	7
Hospitalization (mean, days)	7.8
Conversion open	2%
Operative time (mean-min)	262
Blood loss (ml)	488
Complications	Rectal injuries 2% Ureteral injuries 1%
Stage:	4 pT0, 883 pT2; 298 pT3, 13 pt4, 6 pTxN1
Positive surgical margins	17.8% (219 Pts)

Guillonneau and Vallancien reported full continence rates of 83 % after 12 months of follow-up and 73.9% of spontaneous erections in bilateral nerve-sparing and 51.8% in unilateral nerve-sparing procedures [5].
At the most recent AUA meeting in Anaheim 2001, a European multicenter study revealed the following data in 1,228 cases: mean operative time of 262 min, mean blood loss of 488 ml, mean hospitalization of 7.8 days, mean catheter time of 7.5 days, and intraoperative complications in 2.2% of the patients. The positive surgical margin rate was for all operative specimens 17.8% (Table 2) [6].
Despite a short-term follow-up, laparoscopic radical prostatectomy confers pathologic tumor control in patients with favorable preoperative tumor profiles. The excellent vision provided by laparoscopic surgery allows meticulous dissection of the anatomic structures and thus low morbidity and overall complication rates. Further investigations should focus on the oncologic and functional results in the long-term follow-up of this procedure.

Laparoscopic Radical Nephrectomy

After the first laparoscopic radical nephrectomy performed by Clayman in 1990 [7], laparoscopic nephrectomy now has gained in popularity as an alternative to open surgery for localized renal cell carcinoma [8].
The technique can be performed either by transperitoneal or retroperitoneal approach and the widespread indications for this procedure are medium-sized renal tumors > 4 cm (4-10 cm) - T1/T2 N0M0. A general contraindication is severe cardiopulmonary comorbidity.
The procedure is technically more demanding. The retroperitoneal space is limited in a smaller working space and it is more difficult to perceive surgical landmarks, but there is no violation of the peritoneum and no need for mobilizing the colon. Removal is possible through specially manufactured endobags made of impermeable material in which the kidney can be entrapped. The only disadvantages are the steep learning curve and longer operating times, although the latter does decrease with experience.
Over 500 laparoscopic radical nephrectomies have been published in the literature and worldwide experience shows good oncologic results with decreased postoperative morbidity and analgesic requirements, improved cosmetic results, and more rapid convalescence and return to normal activity than in open surgery (Table 3) [9]. The drawback to the laparoscopic approach continues to be the costs. To date, there have been only two reports of port site seeding, but only with morcellation [10, 11]. Laparoscopic radical nephrectomy confers long-term oncologic effectiveness that is equivalent to traditional surgery [12].

Table 3. Laparoscopic radical nephrectomy worldwide experience: (Janetschek, Ono, Barret, Clatman, Kavoussi, Gill)

Follow-up (mean, months)	20
No. Pts	345
Hospitalization (mean, days)	3.1
Operative time (mean-hours)	3.8
Blood loss (ml)	195
Mortality	0.3%
Stage:	pT1/pT3b

AUA Atlanta 2000

Controversial Indications

Laparoscopic Partial Nephrectomy

Traditionally, partial nephrectomy for renal cell carcinoma was initially reserved only for tumors occurring in a solitary kidney or when the patient presented with bilateral disease. Several series have shown partial open nephrectomy to be equivalent to open radical nephrectomy in terms of long-term cancer-free survival in cases of unilateral renal involvement, unifocal disease, and tumor size less than 4 cm [13, 14]. Nephron-sparing surgery is becoming the standard of care for most small renal cancers.

The indications for nephron-sparing surgery were also extended in laparoscopy to include patients with small tumors and a normal contralateral kidney (solid lesion <4 cm). Tissue is removed under direct vision and ultrasound is used to assess multifocality and margins intraoperatively. The advantages of this procedure are a reduction in the postoperative morbidity, a "small incision for small tumors," and favorable results in terms of patient survival and tumor control.

More than 100 partial nephrectomies have been published and the cumulative overall disease-free survival rate after 3 years of follow-up is 100%; the operating time is 90-320 min and the mean postoperative hospital stay is shorter than with traditional surgery (Table 4). The limitations of this procedure are the very difficult learning curve, the time of the hemostasis and consequent renal ischemia, and the hypothetical risk of tumor cell spillage [16-18].

Table 4. Laparoscopic partial nephrectomy

	Cleveland	Austria
Patients	40	52
Tumor Size (cm)	3.0	2.1
Warm ischemia (min)	23	-
Blood loss	270	275
Operative time (min)	146	148
Complications	-	9.6%
Surgical margins pos	-	-

Margerber M, Klinger C, et al: Panel Session "Update on renal cell carcinoma", AUA, 2001

Laparoscopic Radical Nephroureterectomy

Laparoscopic radical nephroureterectomy has evolved more slowly than nephrectomy for benign or malignant renal disease because of the rarity of upper tract transitional cell cancer (TCC) and the overall difficulty of the procedure. This technique is an effective minimally invasive treatment for selected patients with upper tract TCC, but longer follow-up is needed before laparoscopy can be considered standard treatment. At this time the efficacy of laparoscopic nephroureterectomy appears to be similar to that of open surgery in regard to bladder recurrence, metastatic disease, and crude and cancer-specific survival [18].

At the most recent AUA meeting in Anaheim 2001, an American-European multicenter study showed in 100 patients an acceptable operating time (4 h), significantly less postoperative discomfort, fewer pulmonary complications, quicker return to resuming oral intake of food,, and a shorter hospital stay compared to open surgery [19]. Major drawbacks are the longer operating time and the risk of tumor spillage.

Further data on efficacy and cost-effectiveness will determine the practical future of the laparoscopic approach to upper urinary TCC (Table 5).

Table 5. Nephroureterectomy for TCC worldwide experience

	Keely (1998)	Shalhav (1999)	Cleveland Clinic (2000)
N. pts.	22	25	42
Approach	TP	TP	RP
T.op.m. (h)	2.6	7.7	3.9
Hosp. stay (days)	5.5	3.6	2.3
Tumor recurrance:			
- Bladder	-	7	8
- Local		1	3 0
- Metastases	1	3	3

Gill IS, Office of Education, Radical nephroureterctomy in upper tract transitional cell carcinoma, AUA, 2001

Laparoscopic Retroperitoneal Lymph Node Dissection

More controversy exists about laparoscopic retroperitoneal lymph node dissection for testis cancer (LRPLND) and about lymphadenectomy for bladder cancer. The former is still considered experimental by the AUA and the German Society of Urology.

The discussion of the treatment of clinically stage I testicular cancer is ongoing; some urologists advocate a "wait and see" policy while others tend to perform LRPLND in patients who have a high risk for retroperitoneal lymph node metastasis. Laparoscopy may offer a way out of this dilemma because it substantially reduces the morbidity, with a shorter hospital stay than after open surgery, provided that the efficacy of laparoscopy is comparable with that of traditional surgery.

The procedure was first performed in 1992 by Hulbert and Fraley and, to date, more than 100 patients who underwent a LRPLND have been reviewed worldwide. As yet, only insufficient data have been collected for defining the value of LRPLND [2, 20, 21].

Pelvic lymphadenectomy for bladder cancer may be considered in patients who refuse radical cystectomy and desire definitive alternative treatments (radiotherapy, chemotherapy, combined).

With this procedure, lymph node dissection can be performed with the same results as open surgery; the advantage is lower morbidity and a shorter hospital stay in these selected patients [2].

Experimental Indications

Further experimental treatments have been performed, such as radical cystectomy with ileum-conduit, ileal neobladder, and Mainz-Pouch at the Cleveland Clinic and the Charité in Berlin. The results are very stimulating; with more experience and improvement in the surgical technique, LAP radical cystectomy may become an attractive alternative in the surgical treatment of selected patients with localized muscle-invasive bladder cancer [22, 23].

References

1. Breda G, Nakade SY, Rassweiler JJ (2001) Future developments and perspectives in laparoscopy. Eur Urol 40 : 84-91
2. Schuessler WW, Vancaille TG Reich H, Griffith DP (1991) Transperitoneal endosurgical lymphadenectomy in patients with localized prostate cancer. J Urol 145: 988-991
3. Fornara P, Doehn C, Jocham D (1999) Role of laparoscopy in the lymph node staging of urological malignancies. Min Invas Ther Allied Technol 8: 271-279
4. Schuessler WW, Schulan P, Clayman R, Kavoussi L (1997) Laparoscopic radical prostatectomy: initial short term experience. Urology 50:854-857
5. Guillonneau B, Vallancien G (2000) Laparoscopic radical prostatectomy: the Montsouris experience. J Urol 163:418-422
6. Sulser T, Guillonneau B, Vallancien G (2001) Complications and initial experience with 1228 laparoscopic radical prostatectomy at 6 European Centers. J Urol 165 (abstract 615)
7. Clayman RV, Kavoussi LR, Sopen NY et al (1991) Laparoscopic nephrectomy: initial case report. J Urol. 146: 278
8. Jarrett TW (2001) Editorial: the present and future of laparoscopic renal and adrenal surgery. J Urol 165:1882-1883
9. Ono Y, Kinukawa T, Hattori R et al (1999) Long-term outcome of laparoscopic radical nephrectomy. J Urol 161 (abstract 73)
10. Castilho LN, Fugita O, et al (2001) Port site tumor recurrence of renal cell carcinoma after videolaparoscopy radical nephrectomy. J Urol 165:519-520
11. Fentie D, Barrett PH, Taranger LA et al. (2000) Metastatic renal cell cancer after laparoscopic radical nehrectomy long term follow up. J Endourol 14:407-411

12. Gill IS, Hobart M, Soble J et al (1999) Retroperitoneal laparoscopic radical nephrectomy: comparison with open surgery. J Urol 161 (abstract 637)
13. Hafez KS, Fergany AF, Novick AC (1999) Nephron sparing surgery for localized renal cell carcinoma: impact of tumor size on patient survival, tumor recurrence and TNM staging. J Urol 162:1930
14. Butler BP, Novick AC, Miller DP, Campbell SA, Light ME (1995) Management of small unilateral renal cell carcinomas: radical versus nephron sparing surgery. Urology 45: 34
15. Rassweiler JJ, Abbou C, Janetschek G, Jeschke K (2000) Laparoscopic partial nephrectomy. The European experience. Urol Clin North Am :27(4):721-736
16. Kozlowsky PM, Winfield HN (2001) Laparoscopic partial nephrectomy and wedge resection for malignancy. J Endourol 15(4):369-374
17. Marberger M, Klingler C, Janetscheck G, Jeschke K (2001) Panel session "Update on Renal Cell Carcer." AUA, Anaheim
18. Abou HI, Gill I, Jarrett T, Kavoussi L et al (2001) Laparoscopic radical nephroureterectomy multicenter study-intermediate-term follow-up. J. Urol 165 (abstract 9)
19. Gill IS (2001) Postgraduate Course: radical nephroureterectomy in upper tract transitional cell carcinoma. AUA, Anaheim
20. Janetschek G, Hobsch A, Höltl L, Bartsch G (1996) Retroperitoneal lymphadenectomy for clinical stage I non seminomatous testicular tumor. Laparoscopy vs. open surgery and impact of learning curve. J Urol 156:89-94
21. Rassweiler JJ, Seeman O, Henkel C et al (1996) Laparoscopic retroperitoneal lymphnode dissection for non seminomatous germ cell tumors; indications and limitations. J Urol 156: 1108-1113
22. Gill I, Sung GT, Mereney AM et al (2001) Laparoscopic radical cystectomy with urinary diversion-completely intracorporeal technique in the male and female. J Urol 165 (abstract V374)
23. Tuerk I, Loening SA, Deger S, Ninkelmann B et al (2001) Laparoscopic radical cystectomy with continent urinary diversion (rectum-sigma-pouch) performed completely intracorporeally. J Urol 165 (abstract 362)

Chapter 15

Retroperitoneoscopic Varicocelectomy in Children and Adolescents

J.S. Valla

Introduction

Varicocele is an abnormal dilatation of the veins of the pampiniform plexus. It typically develops during adolescence and is present in 10%-15% of the male adult population. Varicocele is usually located on the left side for anatomical reasons. There are still many preliminary questions about this condition that remain unanswered: for example, the etiology, particularly anatomical factors that may contribute to the formation of varicocele; the pathophysiology; the relationships between varicocele and infertility, and varicocele and testicular volume loss; techniques for clinical classification and preoperative setup (venography, scrotal thermography, Doppler ultrasound?); and finally when and how to manage varicocele. Because varicocele is associated with a progressive duration-dependent decline in testicular function, the importance of early treatment in childhood and adolescence so as to prevent testicular damage is widely accepted, especially in boys with significant ipsilateral testicular growth failure [1, 2]. However, proper management of adolescent varicocele is controversial.

To date, common treatment options include: spermatic vein sclerotherapy or embolization; classic surgical treatment via the scrotal, inguinal or high retroperitoneal approach in order to ligate only the veins (Ivanissevitch technique) or the vein and artery (Palomo technique); microsurgery for the artery and lymphatic-sparing surgery or venous bypass.

In the last 10 years, many urologists have adopted the laparoscopic technique for treating varicocele, particularly the intraperitoneal approach [3-12], which is never used with classic open surgery. Therefore, after the report by Gaur in 1994 [13], and in order to reproduce, with a minimally invasive technique, the same procedure as in open surgery, we have tried to develop the retroperitoneal minimally invasive approach for treatment of varicocele in adolescents. To get the most minimally invasive technique, it seems logical — in cases of simple surgical procedures like varicocelectomy — to use only one port instead of two or three. Furthermore, an operating channel telescope is widely used in pediatric urology and is also used for appendectomy in our department [14]; thus, we have naturally chosen the monotrocar retroperitoneal approach for varicocele management. Our purpose is to describe this new approach, whose usage has not spread; however, until new prospective randomized studies are published, the question of the ideal technique for repair of varicocele remains open [15-20].

Operative Technique for One-Puncture Retroperitoneoscopic Varicocelectomy

Our technique for one-puncture retroperitoneoscopic varicocelectomy has been described in a previous publication [21].

Preparation

Patients

No special preparation is needed (no gastric tube, no ureteral catheter, no antibiotic).

Materials

We use a short (27 cm), 0° telescope with a 5.5-mm operating channel (external diameter of telescope, 10 mm), specially developed by the Karl Storz Company (Tuttlinglen, Germany) for pediatric surgery. This short telescope allows the use of all the usual 5-mm instruments, especially bipolar forceps, ultrasonic coagulators, or clip appliers. For the open approach, narrow and deep Farabeuf retractors are useful and a trocar with a specific system to avoid its extraction (balloon or umbrella).

Technique

Under general anesthesia, the patient is placed in the lateral decubitus position, monitored with an oximeter and a capnometer. A soft bolster is applied underneath the patient. The surgeon and assistant stand at the patient's back, the video stands on the other side, and the cables are fixed to the inferior part of the operative field at the level of the thigh. The left scrotum can be left in the operative field (see Fig. 1).

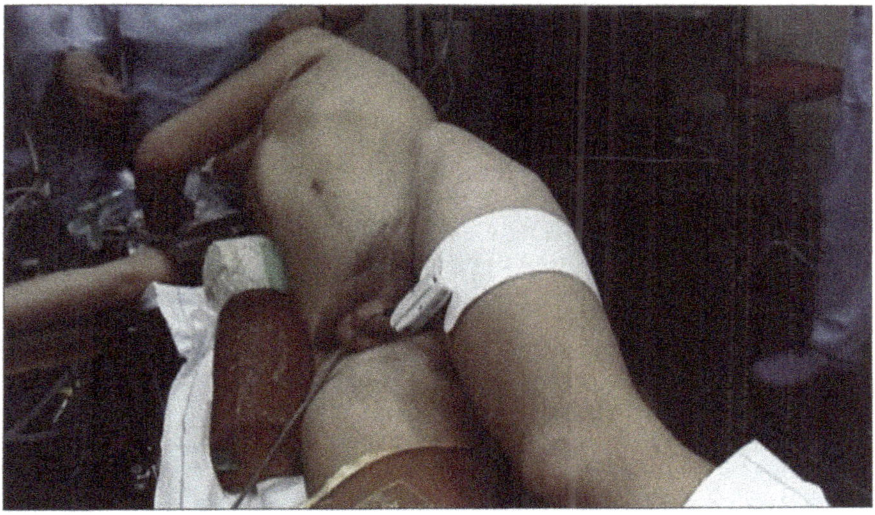

A

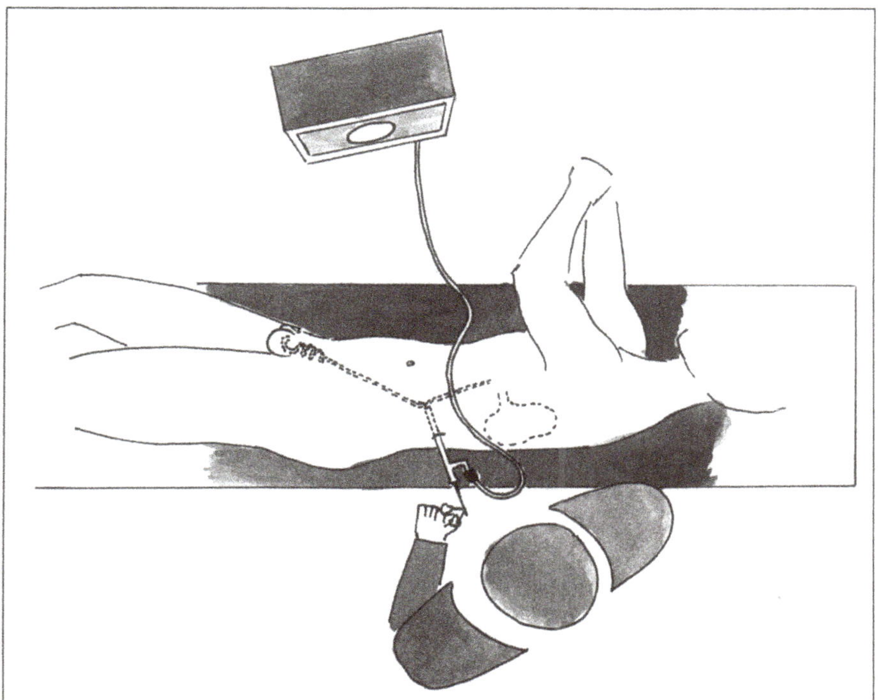

B

Fig. 1A, B. Positioning of the patient and equipment. The surgeon stays in the back

Retroperitonal Approach

A 15-mm-long skin incision is made at the tip of the 11th rib in the midaxillary line. This incision is deepened by blunt dissection down to the retroperitoneal space. Dissecting forceps, Farabeuf retractors, and Metzenbaum scissors are usually sufficient. In children and adolescents, the cutaneous incision is too small to enable finger dissection of the retroperitoneal space but large enough to visualize the retroperitoneal fat; at this point, two strong stitches must be made on each side of the muscular layers to facilitate the two next steps.

Creation of the Working Space

The working space is first created by using gauze to dissect the retroperitoneal space: the surgeon must keep this dissection in close contact with the posterior muscular wall to avoid peritoneal perforation.

The next step involves introduction of the 10-mm trocar and insufflation of the retroperitoneal space with a 12- to 15-mmHg pressure, 1 l/min. The operating channel telescope is introduced in the retroperitoneal space; the first landmark is the anterior part of the psoas muscle. The working space continues to be progressively created by moving the tip of the telescope and using a palpator or peanut. The second landmark is the ureter, located on the psoas and presenting typical peristaltic movements. The spermatic vessels are then identified as they cross the ureter (uretero-venous angle) from the anterolateral to the medial side; these vessels are sticked to the posterior part of the peritoneum. Manual traction on the testicle may aid in the identification of the vessels to ensure that they are indeed the spermatic vessels and not the inferior mesenteric vessels. The testicular artery and one or two veins are dissected using a 5-mm hook or curved forceps (see Fig. 2), and completely freed. Hemostasis is achieved by coagulation (mono- or bipolar), or by using a clip or an ultrasonic coagulator, and then the vessels are divided.

The retroperitoneal space is exsufflated; muscles and skin are closed with absorbable sutures. No drainage is necessary. Wound closure is performed using local anesthetic.

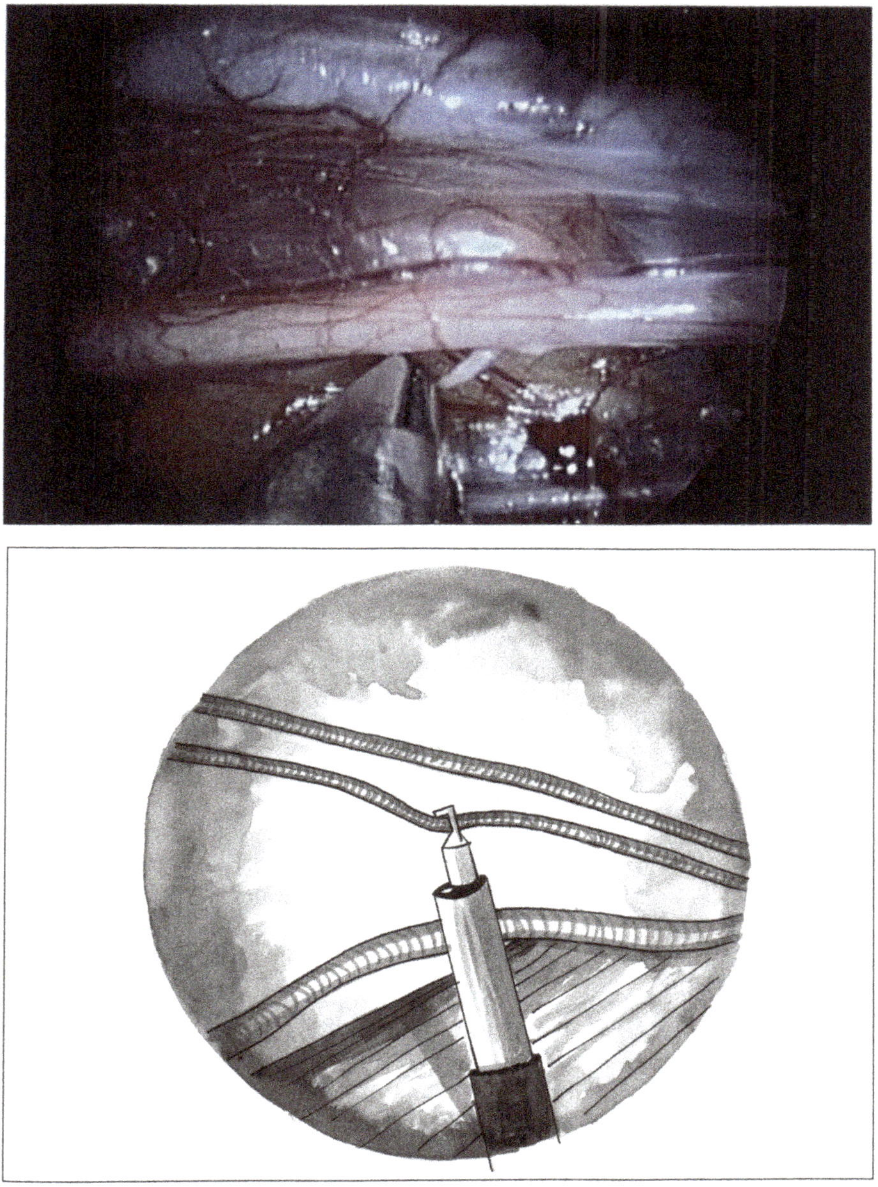

A

B

Fig. 2 A, B. Dissection of the retroperitoneal space (left side) and visualization of the psoas muscle, ureter, and spermatic vessels; —>, uretero-venous angle

Results of Personal Experience

From 1995 to 2000, 42 boys underwent monotrocar retroperitoneoscopic varicocele management. All cases were left-sided varicocele, mean age 14 years (range 11-18 years). All patients were evaluated clinically and with a Doppler ultrasound probe (28 palpable grade 2; 14 palpable grade 3). Testicular hypotrophy (difference of at least 25%) was recorded in 28 patients (67%).

The testicular artery was identified in 42 cases (100%) at surgery. The artery and vein were divided in 39 cases; because of the parental preference, three arteries were preserved.

Hemostasis was achieved by monopolar coagulation (22 cases), bipolar coagulation (17 cases), clip (2 cases), or ultrasonic scalpel (1 case). Two peritoneal perforations occurred in our first ten cases, which needed two (4.8%) conversions (one patient was treated by classic surgery, one was treated by introduction of two additional operating 3-mm trocars). There were no other intraoperative incidents.

The average operation time was 35 min (range 14-70 min) and hospital stay was 1 day.

All but two patients who underwent retroperitoneoscopic varicocelectomy were seen at follow-up, at least 6 months postoperatively. There were no wound complications. One severe postoperative complication was recorded: a ureteral burn injury (case no. 22) due to monopolar coagulation, which required a repair 8 days after surgery with good final results. At an average follow-up of 24 months (range 6-60), 38 of the 42 boys were monitored (90%): there were three recurrences (8%), one complete recurrence which needed reoperation and two mild recurrences still under supervision, and four hydroceles (10%), of which one needed reoperation. There were no cases of atrophy: on the contrary, 22 testes of 28 patients (79%) had an increased volume.

Discussion

Choosing a Method of Varicocele Repair

Our experience shows that our recurrence rate and complication rate are comparable to those of the open or intraperitoneal laparoscopic approach. What exactly are the criteria with which to judge the results?

One of the criteria to judge a method of varicocele repair is the quality of sperm and pregnancy rate: this criterion is always missing in studies concerning adolescents and is also missing in our data. At this age, only the volume of the testis has been considered, and our results are good concerning this particular point. However, the main criterion is the overall success rate: 92% in our data. Concerning the persistence/recurrence rate of varicoceles, the problem is not how to approach the vessels — classically or laparoscopically — but what procedure to use on the vessels: vein only or vein and artery? In many reports [10-15], the recurrence rate is at its lowest level after ligature of the whole pedicle, vein, and artery. Interestingly, the only relapse needing reoperation in our series occurred after artery-sparing surgery (1/3 cases). However, because the lymphatic vessels are also ligated, this last technique gives the highest rate of postoperative hydrocele: 28% for Glassberg [22], 3% for Kass [15], and 10% in our experience. In order to avoid this complication, recent reports [22, 23] emphasize lymphatic-sparing surgery; magnification is essential for success and could be provided by a telescope [24] as well as a microscope [25]. The future of retroperitoneoscopic management of varicocele could be a true microdissection with two additional 3-mm-diameter operating devices.

The final criterion for choosing a method of varicocele repair is the complication rate [5]. Minimally invasive techniques may offer some advantages in reducing the morbidity, but a significant disadvantage of laparoscopy is that there are some specific risks: bowel or vascular injury with the intraperitoneal technique, ureteral injury with the retroperitoneal technique. These risks must be eliminated by a faultless and well-mastered technique. Great care must be taken in the choice of devices for hemostasis. The monopolar hook is very effective and cost effective but also very dangerous for the surrounding structures: the ureteral burn injury which occurred in one of our patients was located 3 cm above the area of coagulation and was probably due to a transmitted electric current. Since this incident, we use only bipolar or ultrasound coagulation and have had no further accidents.

Why Choose the Laparoscopic Technique?

What are the possible advantages of laparoscopy? One of the main arguments is that there is less scarring, less pain, and faster recovery. But classic surgery — especially microdissection by an inguinal or subinguinal incision [26] — can also achieve the same results (3-cm-long incision and 1-day hospital stay). However, after 9 years' practice of inguinal incision with a loupe or a microscope, I find that dissection at that level is tedious and time-consuming if all the veins, the artery, and the lymphatic vessels are to be dissected free. Sometimes the testicular artery cannot be identified: e.g., 7.6% of cases for Abdulmaaboud [19]. Because the numerous vascular plexuses progressively disappear from the testis area to the renal area, the dissection is easier in the retroperitoneal space just above the internal ring and even easier some centimeters above that. In my experience, there are fewer hematomas, fewer scrotal edemas, and less pain if the vascular pedicle is divided in its high retroperitoneal part than in its inguinal part. Thus, if you compare high division of spermatic vessels by classic surgery or laparoscopy, it becomes evident that the retroperitoneoscopic approach involves less scarring and less pain.

Intraperitoneal Versus Retroperitoneal Laparoscopic Technique

Between the two laparoscopic techniques — intra- and retroperitoneal — which is the better choice? It is difficult to answer this question because no comparative data have been published. However, the intraperitoneal approach is obviously the favorite: about 10 publications and 500 cases versus only 3 publications [13, 21, 27] and 70 cases for the retroperitoneal approach.

The following arguments help assess the pros and cons. The intraperitoneal laparoscopic approach provides access just above the internal inguinal ring, and permits dissection of the spermatic vessels and the deferential vessels on both sides. The anatomical landmarks are obvious and well known. The working space is large and there is no learning curve in this approach, for example, no conversion in the 161 cases published by Esposito [10]. It allows treatment of other intra-abdominal pathological conditions such as inguinal hernia [10]. It has the following disadvantages: It is difficult to reach a retroperitoneal structure with the intraperitoneal approach; it has never been used in classic surgery; there is a risk of intra-abdominal organ injury, especially in case of previous abdominal surgery; there is also a risk of postoperative shoulder pain, omental evisceration, or intestinal adhesions. At least three trocars are needed to open the peritoneum and dissect the vessels. In case of abdominal adhesion of the sigmoid colon, the dissection of spermatic vessels can be difficult, if not impossible: two cases of conversion for that reason in the data of Belloli [9]. Jarrow noted [5] that, "There was a significant learning curve in our ability to spare the testicular artery," and they remained unable to identify the artery in 11% of cases even with the help of a Doppler probe. In the same manner, the artery was not identified in 4.6% of cases for Abdulmaaboud [19], in 7% of cases for Donovan [7], and in 20% of cases for Ralph [6].

The retroperitoneal approach gives a much better access than the intraperitoneal approach, in an area where one encounters only one or two major veins coursing parallel to the testicular artery. At this level, the testicular artery is usually readily identified and easily dissected; the artery was identified and dissected free in 100% of our 42 cases without the help of a Doppler probe, which is recommended with the intraperitoneal technique [28]. Some fine retroperitoneal venules could be seen, but not the deferential vein and, with the lateral approach, only one side could be reached. However, a bilateral retroperitoneal approach has been described by Ourpinar [27]. The retroperitoneoscopic approach is logical, anatomical, direct, and fast; varicocelectomy is possible with only one trocar. Moreover, one of the great advantages of the retroperitoneoscopic approach is, once training is gained with this technique, it is helpful for many others indications in pediatric urology [21]. The first disadvantage of the retroperitoneal approach is the lack of a natural cavity: the working space needs to be created and this step brings some difficulties at the beginning of the learning curve. This point is illustrated by our conversion rate: as for Gaur [13], there were 2 cases due to peritoneal perforation in our 10 first cases, but 0 perforations during the next 32 cases. The second disadvantage of the retroperitoneal approach is that the working space is smaller than with the intraperitoneal approach; however, with the operating channel telescope and only one instrument, this reduced working space is not a handicap as it is when performing a more complex procedure with three or four trocars.

Finally, in obese patients, thick retroperitoneal fat could hinder the dissection; however, I have never encountered such a situation because varicoceles are more common in tall, thin boys.

To conclude, personal preferences aside (the intraperitoneal technique for general surgeons, retroperitoneal technique for urologists), the intraperitoneal approach is indicated in case of contraindication of the retroperitoneal approach: bilateral varicocele, obese patient, and retroperitoneal fibrosis.

Conclusion

A conclusion cannot be reached on the choice of the ideal management of varicocele in adolescents, because we do not have current evidence-based studies. A few comparative studies have been published [15, -17-20] mainly in adults: apart from the Sayfan study [16], all these studies are retrospective and limited to two or three techniques. No comparative study has included the retroperitoneoscopic approach. Randomized prospective studies are needed to determine which method is the best and fulfills the following criteria: preservation of optimal testicular function, elimination of the varicocele, minimal current and future morbidity, and cost effectiveness [1]. However, in selected cases such as unilateral left varicocele in a nonobese adolescent — which is the usual situation in our practice — the retroperitoneoscopic approach, after a short but necessary learning period, allows the spermatic vessels to be quickly reached and the artery, veins, and lymphatic vessels to be easily separated.

References

1. Golstein M (1995) Editorial: adolescent varicocele. J Urol 153:484-485
2. Sayfan J, Sillovich L, Kiltun L, Benyamin N (1997) Varicocele treatment in pubertal boys prevents testicular growth arrest. J Urol 157:1456-1457
3. Matusda T, Horii Y, Higashi S, et al (1992) Laparoscopic varicocelectomy: a simple technique for clip ligation of the spermatic vessels. J Urol 147:636-638
4. Hagood PG, Mehan DJ, Worischeck JH, et al (1992) Laparoscopic varicocelectomy: preleminary reports of a new technique. J Urol 147:73-76
5. Jarrow JP, Assimos DG, Pittaway DE (1993) Effectiveness of laparoscopic varicocelectomy. Urology 42:544-546
6. Ralph DJ, Timoney AG, Parker O, Pryor JP (1993) Laparoscopic varicocele ligation. Br J Urol 72:230-233
7. Donovan JF, Winfield HN (1992) Laparoscopic varix ligation. J Urol 147:77-81
8. Humphrey GME, Najmaldin AS (1997) Laparoscopic in the management of pediatric varicoceles. J Pediatr Surg 32:1470-1472
9. Belloli G, Mussi L, D'Agostino S (1996) Laparoscopic surgery for adolescent varicocele: preliminary report on 80 patients. J Pediatr Surg 31:1488-1490
10. Esposito C, Monguzzi GL, Gonzalez Sabin MA, Rubino R, Montinaro L, Papparella A, Amici G (2000) Laparoscopic treatment of pediatric varicocele: a multicenter study of the Italian society of video surgery in infancy. J Urol 163:1944-1946
11. Darzi A, Carey P, Menzies-Cow N, Monson JTR (1994) Laparoscopic varicolectomy. Surg Lap Endosc 4:210-212
12. MacKinlay GA (1999) Laparoscopic varicocele. In: Bax NMA, Georgeson KE, Najmaldin A, Valla JS (eds) Endoscopic surgery in children. Springer, Heidelberg Berlin New York, pp 408-414

13. Gaur DD, Agarwal DK, Purohit KC (1994) Retroperitoneal laparoscopic varicocelectomy. J Urol 151:895-897
14. Valla JS, Ordorica Flores RM, Steyaert H, Merrot T, Bartels AM, Breaud J, Ginier C, Cheli M (1999) Umbilical one puncture laparoscopic assisted appendectomy in children. Surg Endosc 13:83-85
15. Kass EJ, Marcol B (1992) Results of varicocele surgery in adolescents: a comparison of techniques. J Urol 148:694-696
16. Sayfan J, Soffer Y, Orda R (1992) Varicocele treatment: prospective randomized trial of 3 methods. J Urol 148:1447-1449
17. Mandressi A, Buizza C, Antonelli D, et al (1996) Is laparoscopy a worthy method to treat varicocele ? Comparison between 160 cases of two-port laparoscopic and 120 cases of open inguinal spermatic vein ligation. J Endourol 10:935
18. Atassi O, Kass EJ, Steneirt BW (1995) Testicular growth after successful varicocele correction in adolescents; comparison of artery sparing technique with Palomo procedure. J Urol 153:482-483
19. Abdulmaaboud MR, Shokeir A, Farage Y, et al (1998) Treatment of varicocele: a comparative study of conventional open surgery, percutaneous retrograde sclerotherapy and laparoscopy. Urology 52:294-300
20. Lynch WJ, Badenoch DF, McAnena OJ (1993) Comparison of laparoscopic and open ligation of the testicular vein. Brit J Urol 72:796-798
21. Valla JS (1999) Videosurgery of the retroperitoneal space in children. In: Bax NMA, Georgeson KE, Najmaldin A, Valla JS (eds) Endoscopic surgery in children. Springer, Heidelberg Berlin New York, pp 379-392
22. Glassberg KI, Gershbein A, Horowith M (2000) Hydrocele formation after varicocelectomy in adolescents: a long term follow up. Br J Urol 85[Suppl 4]:36 Abstract 63
23. Oswald J, Koerner I, Riccabona M (2000) The use of isosulfan blue to identify lymphatic vessels in the high retroperitoneal ligation of adolescent varicocele to avoid post operative hydrocele. Brit J Urol 85[Suppl 4]:34 Abstract 64
24. Kocvara R, Koi J, Dite Z, Novak K, Dvoracek J (2001) Lymphatic sparing varicocele repair in children and adolescents. A laparoscopic modification. Br J Urol 87[Suppl 1]:35 Abstract E.59
25. Golstein M, Gilvert BR, Dicker AP, Dwosh J, Gnecco C (1992) Microsurgical inguinal varicolectomy with delivery of the testis: an artery and lymphatic sparing technique. J Urol 148:1808-1811
26. Lemack GE, Uzzo RG, Schlegel PN, Golstein M (1998) Microsurgical repair of the adolescent varicocele. J Urol 166:179-181
27. Ourpinar T, Sariyuce O, Balbay MD, Ozkan S, Gurel M (1995) Retroperitoneoscopic bilateral spermatic vein ligation. J Urol 153:127-128
28. Loughlin KR, Brooks DC (1992) The use of Doppler probe to facilitate varicocele ligation. Surg Gyn Obst 174:326-328

Chapter 16

Laparoscopic Bladder Surgery

Kenneth Ogan and Jeffrey A. Cadeddu

Introduction

Laparoscopy has been established as a minimally invasive alternative to open surgery for many procedures. Disciplines such as general surgery and gynecology have been quick to implement laparoscopy as the procedure of choice for operations such as cholecystectomy and tubal ligation. In the late 1980s, urologists entered the laparoscopic arena with laparoscopic pelvic lymph node dissections in patients with biopsy-proven prostate cancer. However, with the advent of prostate-specific antigen (PSA) testing and early detection, the indications for laparoscopic lymph node dissection markedly decreased. Thereafter, the enthusiasm for laparoscopic urological surgery decreased. It was not until Clayman and others developed laparoscopic nephrectomy that laparoscopy made a resurgence in the field of urology.

Laparoscopic surgery on the bladder has been applied sparingly but ranges from relatively simple procedures such as closure of a cystotomy, to the extremely challenging radical cystectomy and orthotopic urinary diversion. As experience increases and instrumentation improves, such procedures will become more common. The task for the physician is to assess whether laparoscopic bladder surgery is equally effective as its open counterparts with decreased morbidity.

Cystectomy

Parra and colleagues first described simple cystectomy in 1992 [1]. In their report, laparoscopic cystectomy was first performed on a 27-year-old paraplegic female who had previously undergone supravesical diversion and then subsequently developed recurrent pyocystis. In general, laparoscopic bladder procedures are usually arranged with four ports configured in a "diamond" (Fig. 1a), or five ports in a "fan" (Fig. 1b) configuration. Using three ports, the peritoneal reflection was incised bilaterally from the bifurcation of the iliac vessels to the pubic symphysis (Fig. 2). The prevesical space between the lateral walls of the bladder and pelvic sidewall were developed with a combination of sharp and blunt dissection. Then with cephaled traction on the bladder, a plane was created between the posterior vesical wall and the vagina, thus defining the lateral pedicles of the bladder. The pedicles were divided using serial endo-GIA (US Surgical, Norwalk, CT) staplers.

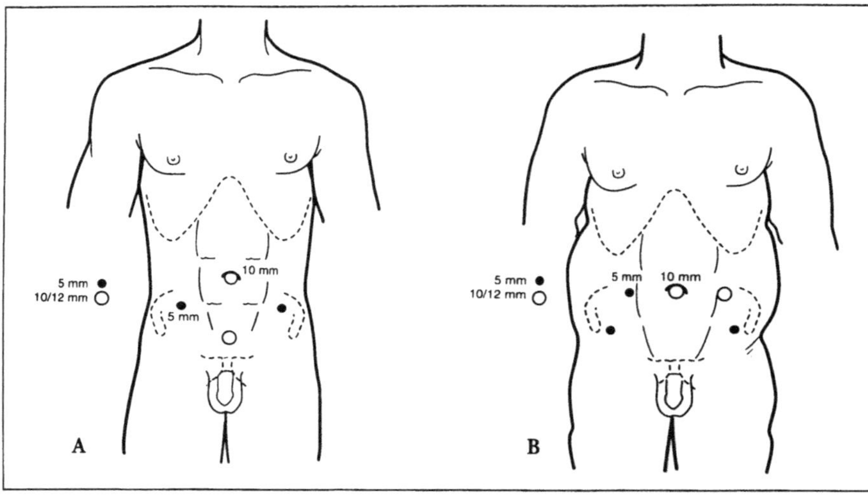

Fig. 1A, B. Two variations of port placement are commonly used, the "diamond" and the "fan". **A** In the diamond configuration, two 10-mm trocars are used, one at the umbililus and the other approximately 4-6 cm above the symphysis pubis in the midline. Two 5-mm trocars are also used, near McBurney's point in the midclavicular line on each side. **B** In the fan configuration, five trocars are used. A 10-mm trocar is placed at the umbilicus for the laparoscope. A second 10-mm trocar is placed on the left side and a 5-mm trocar on the right side at the level of the umbilicus, lateral to the inferior epigastric vessels and in line with the anterosuperior iliac crest. Two 5-mm trocars are placed laterally midway between the umbilicus and the symphysis pubis. (From [42])

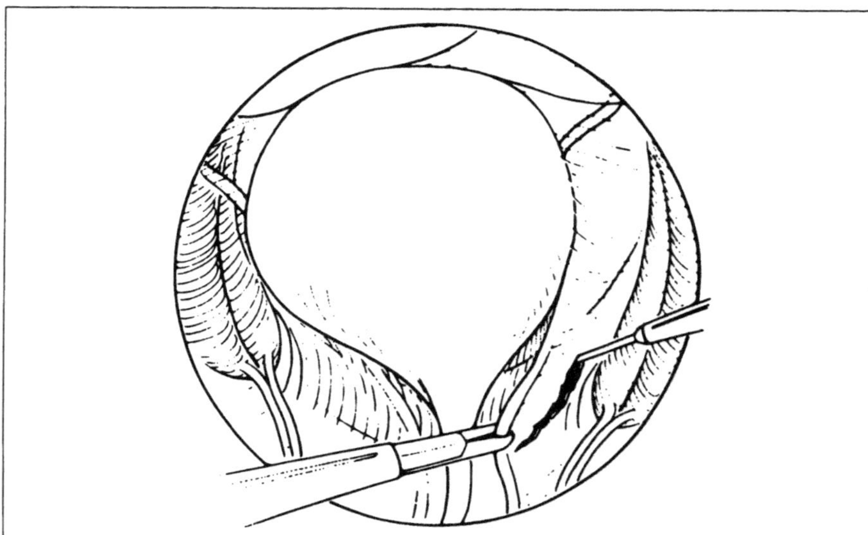

Fig. 2. Initial step of laparoscopic cystectomy, incision of the peritoneal reflection from the bifurcation of the common iliac artery to the pubic ramus. (From[43])

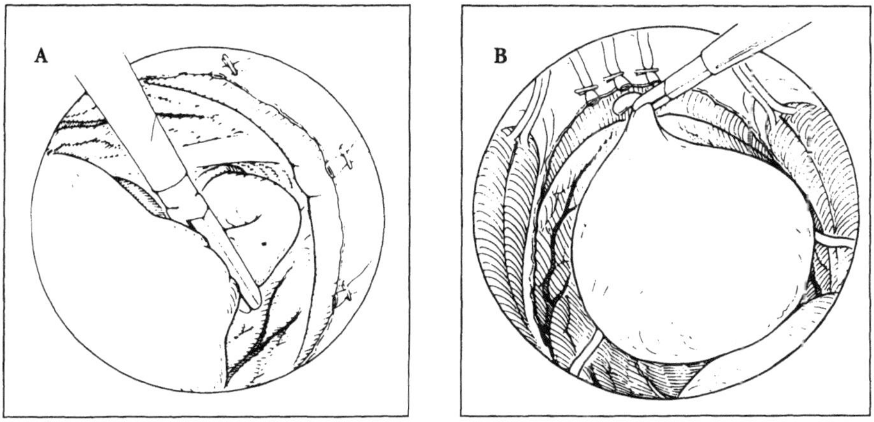

Fig. 3A, B. A Division of the urethra in a female patient with Endo-GIA-30 stapler. B Divided urethra in a female patient. (From [43])

With posterior traction on the bladder, the urethrovesical junction was defined and divided with an Endo-GIA stapler (Fig. 3). Intact specimen removal was accomplished through one of the 12-Fr trocar sites.

Over the past few years laparoscopic radical cystectomy and urinary diversion has been demonstrated to be a feasible procedure in the management of invasive bladder cancer. Initial reports [2-4] on laparoscopic urinary diversion describe a combined intracorporeal/extracorporeal approach in which the creation of the ileal conduit and ureterointestinal anastomosis were performed extracorporeally through a small abdominal incision. Gill and colleagues were the first to perform laparoscopic radical cystectomy with creation of an ileal conduit urinary diversion [5] completely intracorporeally in the porcine model. Using a five-port transperitoneal technique, they were able to perform cystoprostatectomy and ileal conduit urinary diversion in ten male pigs. Cystectomy, isolation of the ileal conduit, restoration of bowel continuity, and creation of precise ureterointestinal anastomosis were all accomplished utilizing intracorporeal techniques. There were no intraoperative or immediate postoperative complications, and the average operative time was only 200 min. Subsequently, their group has applied this technique to two human patients with muscle invasive bladder cancer [6]. The operative time was 11.5 and 10 h, respectively, for each case. There were no major complications and the hospital stay was 6 days for both.

The creation of an orthotopic neobladder, which is the preferred method of urinary diversion status post cystectomy, remains a more technically demanding endeavor. Gill and colleagues performed this procedure entirely intracorporeally in the porcine model [7]. Laparoscopic cystectomy with preservation of the urethral sphincter was initially performed. An ileal segment was then isolated and bowel continuity was reestablished with a stapled anastomosis. Ileal detubularization, urethroileal anastomosis, and bilateral stented ileoureteral anastomosis to a tubular Studer limb extension were all created intracorporeally using only laparoscopic free-hand suturing and knot-tying. As with the ileal conduit, there were no intraoperative or immediate postoperative complications, and the mean operating time was 5.4 h. Their conclusion was that the application of these techniques to clinical practice was imminent.

Turk and colleagues were the first to report on their experience with laparoscopic cystectomy and continent urinary diversion in clinical practice [8]. They performed a radical cystectomy with bilateral pelvic lymphadenectomy and creation of a rectal sigmoid pouch in five patients with organ-confined muscle invasive bladder cancer. As with the initial porcine experiments described by Gill, the procedure was performed intracorporeally with free-hand laparoscopic suturing and in situ knot-tying. Median operating time was 7.4 h, with no intraoperative or immediate postoperative complications.

Bladder Augmentation

Bladder augmentation has been used in patients with high pressure contracted bladders refractory to conservative management. The dysfunctional bladder is typically secondary to neurological deficits, such as meningomyeloceles, traumatic spinal cord injuries, and demyelinating disorders. However, nonneurogenic conditions may result in a contracted bladder, including interstitial cystitis, radiated bladders, postintravesical chemotherapy, and other, idiopathic causes.

The objectives of bladder augmentation are to increase bladder capacity, decrease intravesical pressure, and thereby increase compliance. As a result, the upper tracts are protected, and hopefully social continence is attained.

Classically, various intestinal segments from the stomach to the rectum have been utilized for augmentation cystoplasty. However, this technique is associated with numerous problems: excessive mucous production, stone formation, recurrent infection, metabolic disorders, spontaneous perforation, and potential malignancy [9, 10]. Therefore, numerous biodegradable grafts have been investigated in the animal model to avoid the inherent complications of incorporating segments of the gastrointestinal tract into the bladder [11]. As another alternative, Cartwright and Snow devised the concept of the "auto-augment"; this technique creates a large bladder diverticulum by partially excising the bladder detrussor while leaving the bladder mucosa intact [12].

Numerous investigators have described laparoscopic enterocystoplasty in the animal model as well as sporadically in humans [13-15]. Lifshitz and colleagues recently described laparoscopic transverse hemicystectomy and ileocystoplasty in a porcine model [14]. The procedure was begun laparoscopically with the use of four ports. The segment of ileum to be used for the augmentation was first grasped with endoscopic bowel clamps and positioned just beneath the umbilical port. The umbilical port was then removed and the port site incision was extended to 3 cm to exteriorize the ileum. A 12-cm segment was separated from the bowel and bowel continuity was reestablished using gastrointestinal staplers. The isolated segment was then opened on its antimesenteric border and configured into a U-shaped patch, as in standard open augmentation cystoplasty. Pneumoperitoneum was reestablished and the patch was transferred back into the intraperitoneal cavity where the remainder of the procedure was performed laparoscopically. The hemicystectomy was accomplished using laparoscopic scissors and the enterovesical anastomosis was performed in a running single layer of 3-0 Vicryl, utilizing an Endostitch laparoscopic suturing device (US Surgical Corporation, Norwalk, CT). Meraney et al. [13] describe the first series of enterocystoplasty in humans using ileum, cecum, or sigmoid. As above, the procedure was performed laparoscopically except for the isolation of the bowel segment and reestablishment of bowel continuity, which were performed through a small incision.

As for gastrocystoplasty, Docimo et al. describe the first laparoscopic case in a 17-year-old girl with sacral agenesis [16]. This procedure was completed solely laparoscopically, but no bowel anastomosis was done. Instead, a 20-cm wedge of stomach body was removed using serial firings of the Endo-GIA stapler. The bladder was then opened in the standard "clam shell" pattern and the stomach patch was sutured to the bladder laparoscopically.

In order to avoid the difficulties of a laparoscopic bowel anastomosis and intracorporeal suturing, other investigators have performed auto-augmentation. McDougall et al. describe an extraperitoneal laparoscopic auto-augmentation in a 26-year-old woman with bladder hyperreflexia following a spinal cord injury [17]. Prior to beginning the procedure, a 5-F angiographic catheter was passed through the end of an 18-F Council catheter. To the end of this angiographic catheter the small finger of a sterile glove was attached to create an intravesical dilating balloon once inserted into the bladder. Once all ports were placed, the bladder was completely mobilized at the anterior, lateral, and posterior aspects. The balloon on the end of the angiographic catheter was then inflated with 60 cc of normal saline to aid in the subsequent bladder dissection. Using electrocautery, the bladder detrussor was incised in the midline, starting at the bladder neck and continuing posteriorly toward the trigone. The bladder mucosa was not incised (Fig. 4A). Bladder flaps were then developed bilaterally between the detrussor and the mucosa and reflected laterally to the pelvic sidewall where they were sutured to Cooper's ligament (Fig. 4B). The balloon catheter was left in place for 2 weeks postoperatively in order to prevent subsequent fibrosis and scarring.

Another technique described to avoid using bowel segments is the use of biodegradable grafts for augmentation cystoplasty. These materials provide scaffolding on which normal bladder epithelium can migrate and grow. Porcine small intestine submucosa (SIS) has been used successfully to augment the bladder in the animal model [18]. Portis et al. laparoscopically excised a portion of a porcine bladder and replaced the segment with a biodegradable patch twice the size of the resected specimen [11]. The biodegradable materials utilized were porcine bowel acellular tissue matrix, bovine pericardium, human placental membranes, or porcine small intestinal submucosa.

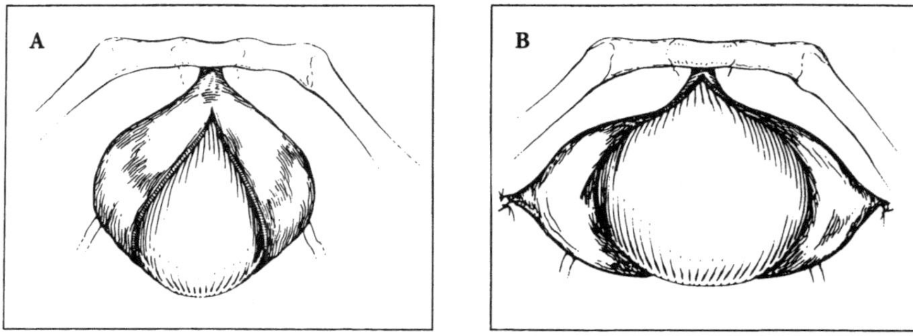

Fig. 4A, B. A Detrussor muscle was incised down to but not through mucosa in midline. **B** Detrussor flaps were dissected from bladder mucosa and sutured back to respective side wall of pelvis. (From [44])

Repair of Cystotomy

Bladder lacerations are classified as being intraperitoneal versus extraperitoneal. Whereas extraperitoneal lacerations may be managed conservatively with Foley catheter drainage, intraperitoneal injuries warrant laparotomy and surgical repair. The most common cause of intraperitoneal bladder injury is trauma, often associated with fractures of the pelvis [19]. These cases would, for the most part, preclude laparoscopic repair due to hemorrhage, bone fragments, and associated injuries. With the advent of more complex transurethral and laparoscopic procedures, iatrogenic bladder injuries have become more prevalent. In contrast to trauma-induced injuries, these iatrogenic injuries are better suited for laparoscopic repair, thus avoiding laparotomy to manage the complication

Complex gynecological laparoscopic procedures have been associated with injuries to the urinary tract. In a review by Said, serious urinary complications were found in 15 (1.6%) of 953 major laparoscopic cases [20]. Bladder lacerations accounted for eight cases, of which seven were identified intraoperatively. These lacerations were successfully closed laparoscopically prior to the conclusion of the procedure, thus avoiding laparotomy and open surgical closure. Intraperitoneal bladder lacerations incurred during transurethral surgery have also been shown to be amenable to laparoscopic repair [21].

Bladder Neck Suspension

Laparoscopic bladder neck suspension was initially developed as a minimally invasive alternative to transabdominal or transvaginal treatment of anatomic stress urinary incontinence. The procedure is usually performed extraperitoneally, utilizing balloon distension to expose the retropubic space. There are two main techniques described to suspend the bladder neck. The first performs the suspension similar to the open Burch procedure. Once the urethrovesical junction is visualized, the endopelvic fascia is incised and then secured to Cooper's ligament bilaterally. Initial results were encouraging, revealing short-term success rates of 90.6% at a follow-up of 24 months [22]. However, a review by McDougall that compared the long-term results of this technique in 58 patients followed over a mean of 45 months to a matched group of patients undergoing transvaginal Raz bladder neck suspension revealed that, while the laparoscopic group had a decreased time of surgery, required less pain medication, and returned to normal activities faster, the long-term success rates were unacceptable [23]. At a mean of 45 months, only 30% of the laparoscopic group was completely continent, with a mean time to failure of 18 months.

The second technique uses a synthetic mesh sling for bladder neck suspension. The mesh is placed suburethrally and either sutured [24] or stapled [25] to Cooper's ligament to provide support and prevent bladder neck hypermobility. In the series of Hanah et al., of 300 patients with sutured mesh, the long-term cure rate was 67% at 3.28 years [24]. Ou and Rowbotham [26] had a cure rate of 88% at 5 years with stapled mesh. While these reports seem to favor the use of synthetic slings in laparoscopic bladder neck suspensions, one must consider the inherent risks of placing synthetic materials intracorporeally.

Excision of Urachal Remnants

Urachal remnants may take the form of urachal cysts, sinuses, or diverticula [23]. Traditionally, the removal of these remnants has been managed with infraumbilical incision. Numerous investigators have described reports of laparoscopic approaches for these anomalies that appear to decrease surgical morbidity compared to the open approach [27-29]. Some investigators have even reported the laparoscopic resection of urachal adenoma [30].

Cadeddu et al. reported on a series of four adults who underwent laparoscopic removal of a urachal remnant [31]. Transperitoneal access was obtained using four ports. The urachus was divided near the umbilicus, taking care to leave a large resection margin cephaled to the urachal sinus. Dissection was then continued in a caudal direction towards the dome of the bladder, excising the anterior wall attachments to the urachus. The medial umbilical ligaments were included as part of the resected specimen. When the bladder was reached, the urachal cyst was sharply dissected off the dome of the bladder and the specimen was removed in a laparoscopic sac via a port site. In three of the four cases a segment of bladder cuff was excised due to significant fibrosis around the urachal cyst at the dome of the bladder.

Bladder Diverticulectomy

Treatment of bladder diverticula has classically been described as an open surgical procedure necessitating laparotomy. However, treatment of small bladder diverticula (<5 cm) with transurethral incision of the diverticulum neck and mu-

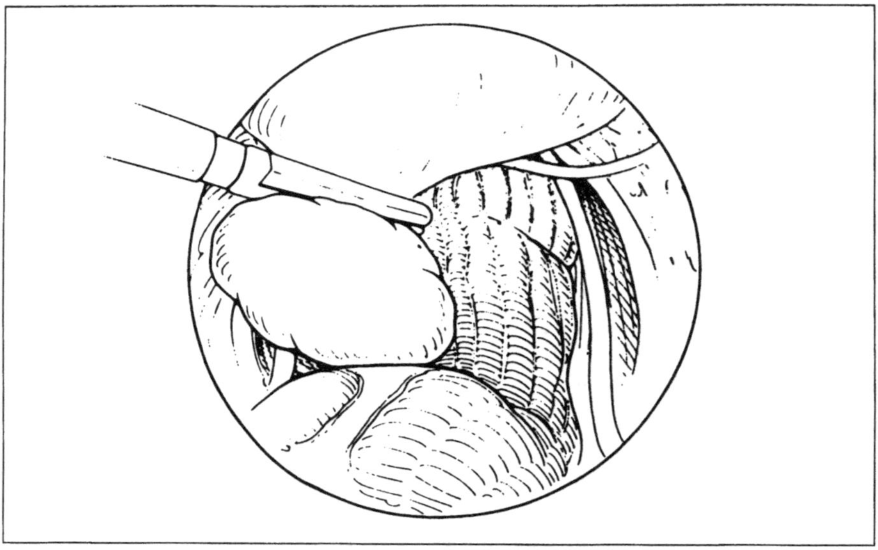

Fig. 5. Dissection of diverticular neck with Endo-GIA-30 stapler. (From [43])

cosal fulguration has been shown to be successful [32]. In an effort to treat larger bladder diverticula in a minimally invasive fashion, combined transurethral and laparoscopic techniques have been developed. Okumura and colleagues describe an endoscopic transvesico-transurethral approach in two patients [33]. Under direct transurethal cystoscopic visualization, the mouth of the diverticulum is closed laparoscopically using two percutaneous ports placed into the bladder. Transperitoneal laparoscopic diverticulectomy has also been advocated. The extravesical visualization of the bladder with transperitoneal laparoscopy allows for superior visualization of the diverticulum and surrounding vital structures such as the ureters. Excision of the bladder diverticulum (Fig. 5) is then safely performed with an Endo-GIA stapler (US Surgical, Norwalk, CT). If the ureter is involved with the diverticulum, it may be laparoscopically reimplanted [34]. Of course, with all of these techniques, if there is any evidence of bladder outlet obstruction this must be treated as well. Iselin and colleagues describe performing transurethral resection of the prostate followed by immediate laparoscopic diverticulectomy at the same sitting [35].

Bladder Endometriosis

Endometriosis is a common problem encountered in gynecology. The most frequent locations are the pouch of Douglas, the ureterosacral ligaments, the rectovaginal septum, and the vesicouterine space [36]. In addition, the bladder has been reported to be involved in 1%-2% of patients with endometriosis [37].

Patients with endometriosis of the bladder may undergo hormonal treatment with either gonadotropic-releasing hormone (GnRH) and/or progestational hormones. Transurethral resection of bladder lesions can also be performed. However, both hormonal and transurethral surgical treatments are associated with high recurrence and failure rates. Therefore, most patients proceed to laparotomy for definitive resection of their bladder endometriosis.

Chapron and Dubuisson performed laparoscopic partial cytectomy on eight patients with deep bladder endometriosis [38]. Following transperitoneal laparoscopic inspection of the abdomen, the first step involves dissection of the vesicouterine space in order to render the endometriotic lesion fully accessible. The uterus is mobilized by cannulating it as during laparoscopic hysterectomy [39]. Once exposed, a partial cystectomy is performed by excising the entire nodule with a margin of normal bladder tissue. To avoid injury, ureteral catheters are placed initially to help in the identification of the ureters. The bladder is then reconstructed with a single-layer closure with appropriate postoperative bladder drainage.

Conclusion

Laparoscopic surgery when compared to open surgery has generally proven to result in a quicker recovery time, shorter hospitalization, decreased need for pain medication, and a superior cosmetic result [41]. While these advantages have been shown to be true for laparoscopic nephrectomy [41], they have not yet been analyzed for laparoscopic bladder surgery. All indications are that bladder procedures will yield similar results but the data are still too premature to make any meaningful assessments. As the results of larger series on bladder laparoscopy become available, we will be better able to determine whether the laparoscopic approach has similar efficacy as open surgery, with the aforementioned advantages.

References

1. Parra RO, Andrus CH, Jones JP, Boullier JA (1992) Laparoscopic cystectomy: initial report on a new treatment for the retained bladder. J Urol 148: 1140-1144
2. Denewer A, Kotb S, Hussein O, El-Maadawy M (1999) Laparoscopic assisted cystectomy and lymphadenectomy for bladder cancer: initial experience. World J Surg 23: 608-611
3. Sanchez de Badajoz E, Gallego Perales JL, Reche Rosado A, Gutierrez de la Cruz JM, Jimenez Garrido A (1995) Laparoscopic cystectomy and ileal conduit: case report. J Endourol 9: 59-62
4. Zayyan KS, See WA (2000) Their initial experience with laparoscopy-assisted cystectomy. World J Surg 24: 1282-1283
5. Fergany AF, Gill IS, Kaouk JH, Meraney AM, Hafez KS, Sung GT (2001) Laparoscopic intracorporeally constructed ileal conduit after porcine cystoprostatectomy. J Urol 166: 285-288
6. Gill IS, Fergany A, Klein EA, Kaouk JH, Sung GT, Meraney AM, Savage SJ, Ulchaker JC, Novick AC (2000) Laparoscopic radical cystoprostatectomy with ileal conduit performed completely intracorporeally: the initial 2 cases. Urology 56: 26-29; discussion 29-30

7. Kaouk JH, Gill IS, Desai MM, Meraney AM, Fergany AF, Abdelsamea A, Carvalhal EF, Skacel M, Sung GT (2001) Laparoscopic orthotopic ileal neobladder. J Endourol 15: 131-142
8. Turk I, Deger S, Winkelmann B, Schonberger B, Loening SA (2001) Laparoscopic radical cystectomy with continent urinary diversion (rectal sigmoid pouch) performed completely intracorporeally: the initial 5 cases. J Urol 165: 1863-1866
9. McDougal WS (1992) Metabolic complications of urinary intestinal diversion. J Urol 147: 1199-1208
10. Filmer RB, Spencer JR (1990) Malignancies in bladder augmentations and intestinal conduits. J Urol 143: 671-678
11. Portis AJ, Elbahnasy AM, Shalhav AL, Brewer A, Humphrey P, McDougall EM, Clayman RV (2000) Laparoscopic augmentation cystoplasty with different biodegradable grafts in an animal model. J Urol 164: 1405-1411
12. Cartwright PC, Snow BW (1989) Bladder autoaugmentation: partial detrusor excision to augment the bladder without use of bowel. J Urol 142: 1050-1053
13. Gill IS, Rackley RR, Meraney AM, Marcello PW, Sung GT (2000) Laparoscopic enterocystoplasty. Urology 55: 178-181
14. Lifshitz DA, Beck SD, Barret E, Simmons G, Chang L, Lingeman JE, Shalhav AL (2001) Laparoscopic transverse hemicystectomy with ileocystoplasty in a porcine model. J Endourol 15: 199-203
15. Cadeddu JA, Docimo SG (1999) Laparoscopic-assisted continent stoma procedures: our new standard. Urology 54: 909-912
16. Docimo SG, Moore RG, Adams J, Kavoussi LR (1995) Laparoscopic bladder augmentation using stomach. Urology 46: 565-569
17. McDougall EM, Clayman RV, Figenshau RS, Pearle MS (1995) Laparoscopic retropubic auto-augmentation of the bladder. J Urol 153: 123-126
18. Xie H, Shaffer BS, Wadia Y, Gregory KW (2000) Use of reconstructed small intestine submucosa for urinary tract replacement. ASAIO J 46: 268-272
19. Parra RO, Worischeck JH, Hagood PG (1995) Laparoscopic simple cystectomy in a man. Surg Laparosc Endosc 5: 161-164
20. Saidi MH, Vancaillie TG, White AJ, Sadler RK, Akright BD, Farhart SA (1996) Complications of major operative laparoscopy. A review of 452 cases. J Reprod Med 41: 471-476
21. Parra RO (1994) Laparoscopic repair of intraperitoneal bladder perforation. J Urol 151: 1003-1005
22. Papasakelariou C, Papasakelariou B (1997) Laparoscopic bladder neck suspension. J Am Assoc Gynecol Laparosc 4: 185-189
23. McDougall EM, Heidorn CA, Portis AJ, Klutke CG (1999) Laparoscopic bladder neck suspension fails the test of time. J Urol 162: 2078-2081
24. Hannah SL, Roland B, Gengenbacher PM (2001) Extraperitoneal retropubic laparoscopic urethropexy. J Am Assoc Gynecol Laparosc 8: 107-110
25. Soygur T, Safak M, Yesilli C, Arikan N, Gogus O (2000) Extraperitoneal laparoscopic bladder neck suspension using hernia mesh and tacker. Urology 56: 121-124
26. Ou CS, Rowbotham R (1999) Five-year fallow-up of laparoscopic bladder neck suspension using synthetic mesh and surgical staples. J Laparoscopic Adv Surg Tech A 9(3):249-252
27. Linos D, Mitropoulos F, Patoulis J, Psomas M, Parasyris V (1997) Laparoscopic removal of urachal sinus. J Laparoendosc Adv Surg Tech A 7: 135-138
28. Redmond HP, Ahmed SM, Watson RG, Hegarty J (1994) Laparoscopic excision of a patent urachus. Surg Laparosc Endosc 4: 384-385
29. Trondsen E, Reiertsen O, Rosseland AR (1993) Laparoscopic excision of urachal sinus. Eur J Surg 159: 127-128
30. Hubens G, De Vries D, Hauben E, Van Marck E, Corthouts B, Michielsen P, Vaneerdeweg W, Eyskens E (1995) Laparoscopic resection of an adenoma of the urachus in combination with a laparoscopic cholecystectomy. Surg Endosc 9: 914-916

31. Cadeddu JA, Boyle KE, Fabrizio MD, Schulam PG, Kavoussi LR (2000) Laparoscopic management of urachal cysts in adulthood. J Urol 164: 1526-1528
32. Errando Smet C, Laguna Pes P, Salvador Bayarri J, Vicente Rodriguez J (1996) Endoscopic surgery of bladder diverticulum. Actas Urol Esp 20: 783-785
33. Okamura K, Watanabe H, Iwasaki A, Tsuji Y, Ohshima S (1999) Closure of mouth of bladder diverticulum via endoscopic transvesico- transurethral approach. J Endourol 13: 123-126
34. McDougall EM, Urban DA, Kerbl K, Clayman RV, Fadden P, Royal HD, Chandhoke PS, Stone AM (1995) Laparoscopic repair of vesicoureteral reflux utilizing the Lich-Gregoir technique in the pig model. J Urol 153: 497-500
35. Iselin CE, Winfield HN, Rohner S, Graber P (1996) Sequential laparoscopic bladder diverticulectomy and transurethral resection of the prostate. J Endourol 10: 545-549
36. Cornillie FJ, Oosterlynck D, Lauweryns JM, Koninckx PR (1990) Deeply infiltrating pelvic endometriosis: histology and clinical significance. Fertil Steril 53: 978-983
37. Aldridge KW, Burns JR, Singh B (1985) Vesical endometriosis: a review and 2 case reports. J Urol 134: 539-541
38. Chapron C, Dubuisson JB (1999) Laparoscopic management of bladder endometriosis. Acta Obstet Gynecol Scand 78: 887-890
39. Chapron C, Dubuisson JB, Aubert V, Morice P, Garnier P, Aubriot FX, Foulot H (1994) Total laparoscopic hysterectomy: preliminary results. Hum Reprod 9: 2084-2089
40. Richards W, Watson D, Lynch G, Reed GW, Olsen D, Spaw A, Holcomb W, Frexes-Steed M, Goldstein R, Sharp K (1993) A review of the results of laparoscopic versus open appendectomy. Surg Gynecol Obstet 177: 473-480
41. Dunn MD, Portis AJ, Shalhav AL, Elbahnasy AM, Heidorn C, McDougall EM, Clayman RV (2000) Laparoscopic versus open radical nephrectomy: a 9-year experience. J Urol 164: 1153-1159
42. West, DA (2000) Laparoscopic pelvic lymphadenectomy. In: Bishoff JT, Kavoussi LR (eds) Atlas of laparoscopic retroperitoneal surgery. Saunders Philadelphia, p 228
43. Parra RO, Boullier JA (1996) n. Semin Surg Oncol 12: 147
44. McDougall EM, Clayman, RV (1995) n. J Urol 153: 124

Chapter 17

Extraperitoneal Laparoscopic Radical Prostatectomy: Results After 50 Cases

R. Bollens, M. Vanden Bossche, T. Roumeguere, A. Damoun, S. Ekane, P. Hoffmann, A.R. Zlotta, C.C. Schulman

Introduction

After the first description of laparoscopic radical prostatectomy in 1992 [1], the interest for this approach remained limited due to multiple technical difficulties [2]. Following the technical modifications of Gaston with initial transperitoneal dissection of the seminal vesicles, Guillonneau and Vallancien developed this procedure further based on the same principle [3]. In 1997, Raboy reported two cases of extraperitoneal radical prostatectomy but did not pursue this approach [4]. After initial experience with transperitoneal laparoscopic radical prostatectomy, we have shifted to a purely extraperitoneal approach, since it seems more comparable to the open technique and avoids the potential disadvantages of a transperitoneal dissection.

We describe in this chapter the different steps of the extraperitoneal approach and report the early oncological results after 50 laparoscopic procedures. We also analyze the preliminary results in terms of continence and potency.

Material and Method

Patient Characteristics

Between September 1999 and September 2000, four surgeons operated on 50 patients for localized prostate cancer by a laparoscopic approach. Only chronic respiratory diseases were considered as a relative contraindication for laparoscopic surgery. There was no patient selection and indications were similar to open prostatectomy in our institution. Twelve patients had a history of previous surgery, including Transuretral Resection of Prostate (TURP) (n=2), open retropubic prostate adenomectomy (n=1), appendectomy (n=4), herniorrhaphy (n=2), hepatic graft (n=1), anterior nephrectomy (n=1), or hemicolectomy (n=1). The surgical preparation included an enema the day before the operation but antibiotic prophylaxis was not given systematically.

On average, patients were 63 years old (47-71), had mean prostate-specific antigen (PSA) values of 9.1 ng/ml (1.1-23), a median Gleason score of 6 (4-8), 2.5 positive biopsies (1-6) and ultrasound prostate volumes of 40 cc (17.5-95). The clinical stages were: T1 in 46.3%, T2a in 41.5%, T2b in 9.8%, and T3 in 2.4%.

Surgical Technique

The patient is placed in lithotomy position with Trendelenburg. The creation of the extraperitoneal space starts by an incision of the rectus abdominalis muscle aponeurosis just below the umbilicus. The optical trocar is introduced in the prevesical space and used to dissect the space between the epigastric vessels on both sides and the pubic arch anteriorly. First, one 5-mm port is introduced 5 cm above the pubic arch on the midline. A bipolar forceps is introduced in this port and is used to dissect the working space more laterally. Two 10-mm ports are placed just medial to the anterior iliac crests and, finally, a 5-mm port is placed in the right flank. The fatty tissue is removed to define the prostate landmarks.

Dissection requires reusable monopolar scissors and bipolar forceps (R/Microfrance) only. The first step in our approach is dissection of the bladder neck. We begin with this step to avoid possible uncontrolled bleeding from the apex during seminal vesicle dissection. After careful bladder neck-sparing dissection, the bladder catheter is removed and the urethra sectioned. We then replace the catheter by a 20-Fr metal bougie. This device enables us to further mobilize the prostate during the next steps. The posterior part of the bladder neck is incised to expose and dissect the vas deferens and seminal vesicles. The endopelvic fascia is then incised on both sides, followed by ligation of the dorsal vein complex with a 15-cm-long Vicryl 0 MH endosuture. The neurovascular bundles are dissected from the lateral surface of the prostate before sectioning the main prostatic pedicles. Denonvillier's fascia is incised to free the posterior prostate wall. The prostatic apex is carefully and gradually divided. Laparoscopic vision improves visualization of the urethra and dissection of the neurovascular bundles. The urethra is sectioned and the prostate freed after dissection of the last attachments. We use a laparoscopic bag (R/Endocatch) to catch the prostate, which is placed laterally from the operative field. Hemostasis is controlled before performing the anastomosis, using six to eight separate stitches (15-cm 2/0 vicryl SH+) starting at 5 o'clock. An 18-Fr catheter is placed on a metallic guide in the bladder and 200 cc of saline are injected to check that the bladder is water-tight. A suction drain is placed for 24-48 h. The prostate is removed through an enlarged, 10-mm port site and the largest aponeurosis openings are closed with vicryl 0 sutures.

Results

Among our first 50 cases, a transperitoneal approach was used in eleven patients (two initial operations, three due to previous prevesical surgery, one open adenomectomy, one hemicolectomy, one herniorrhaphy, and three due to incidental peritoneal opening). Among those eight transperitoneal procedures, nine were performed according to the Heilbronn technique [7] and two according to the Montsouris experience [8]. Only one conversion was performed for technical difficulties during dissection of the neurovascular bundles in a patient previously under hormone therapy.

Operative Data

Operative Time

Mean operative time ("skin to skin") was 317 min [293 without pelvic length node dissection (PLND) and 373 min with PLND]. Taking into account the learning curve, the development of the technique and separating our population in groups of ten patients, the mean operative time was 367 min for the first ten patients and 242 min for the last ten patients. Noteworthy, four different urologists took part in these operations, each with individual skill and an individual learning curve (Table 1).

Table 1. Evolution of mean operative time and blood loss per group of ten patients

Patients	Operative time (min)	Blood loss (cc)
1-10	367.7	1350
11-20	316/5	520
21-30	296	530
31-40	345	405
41-50	235	492

Blood Loss and Transfusion Rate

Blood loss is not easy to evaluate since the volume aspirated is a mixture of blood and urine (increased by high perfusion). The blood loss decreased progressively from 1350 cc for the first ten patients to 492 cc for the last ten patients. The transfusion rate was 13% in all patients (the majority in the twenty first patients). We observed an important decrease in blood loss after the first ten patients using a more efficient bipolar forceps (Table 1).

Postoperative Course

Postoperative Analgesia

In our initial experience, patients received classical analgesics for pain control (intravenous paracetamol, morphine, or nonsteroidal anti-inflammatory drugs). After re-evaluation we chose to give intramuscular morphine only if it was necessary according to a validated pain scale during the first 24 h.

Catheterization Time and Hospital Stay

Catheterization time was 10.1 days for the first ten patients and decreased to 5.5 days for the last ten patients. Two patients had longer duration of catheterization. The first one (patient 9) developed acute transient renal failure due to a tubular necrosis (the bladder catheter was left in to monitor diuresis) and the second one (patient 22) had incorrect repositioning of the catheter with a large defect of the anastomosis. The hospital stay evolution was related to the catheter duration, adding 24 h (Table 2).

Table 2. Evolution of mean catheterization time and hospital stay per group of ten patients

Patients	Catheterization time (days)	Hospital stay (days)
1-10	10.1	13.5
11-20	6.5	9.3
21-30	7.8	8.9
31-40	6.6	7.5
41-50	5.5	7.5

Complications

Only two of 50 patients suffered from a major complication. One immediately developed postoperative transient acute renal failure due to a tubular necrosis on a solitary kidney. This patient underwent hemodialysis for 10 days and recovered normal renal function. The second patient had a urethrorectal fistula on day 20, probably due to a rectal wall necrosis after coagulation. The fistula was closed by a perineal surgical approach.

The minor complications included three epigastric vessel injuries treated laparoscopically during the procedure, two urinary tract infections, one prolonged ileus (transperitoneal approach), two cases of urinary leakage (treated by an additional 10 days of catheterization), four transient urinary retentions probably due to early removal of the catheter and treated by 2 further days of catheterization, one laparoscopic drain removal (transperitoneal approach), one case of thrombophlebitis, and one late hernia on a 10-mm port site (before we began systematically closing 10-mm port sites). No death or intraperitoneal organ injury occurred.

Oncological Results

Pathological Analysis

According to the 1997 UICC classification, the stage distribution was: pT1a in 2.2%, pT2a in 8.5%, pT2b in 42.5%, pT2c in 2.2%, pT3a in 34%, and pT3b in 10.6%. Lymph node dissection was performed in 12 patients (PSA>10 ng/ml) and was positive in two cases. Mean Gleason score was 6.5 [4-10]. The rate of positive

Table 3. Pathological findings

	Pathological stage		(%) Patients with positive surgical margins (*n*)
	pT1a	2.5	
	pT2a	10	2
	pT2b	42.5	
	pT2c	2.5	8
	pT3a	30	
	pT3b	12.50	1
	N1	16	2
TOTAL			(22%)

surgical margins was 22% (five lateral margins, four apical margins, and two bladder neck margins) occurring in two pT2b, eight pT3a, and one pT3b specimen. The average prostate weight was 51 g (17-116 g) (Table 3).

Follow-up: PSA

Out of 35 patients with at least 3 months of follow-up at the time of writing the manuscript, only two had postoperatively detectable levels of serum PSA. One was a patient with a pT3a specimen and positive surgical margins and the other was a pT2b tumor with negative surgical margins (probably incomplete removal of the prostate gland in our initial experience in a gland over 100 cc).

Functional Results: Continence and Potency

For many patients follow-up is too short and data have only been reported for a limited number of them. At 3 months 39% (n= 23) and at 6 months 85% (n=14) were perfectly continent and did not use any pad.

We used an international classification (IIEF) to evaluate postoperative potency. (Q1: complete impotence; Q2: tumescence; Q3: insufficient erection; Q4: sufficient erection for sexual activity; and Q5: perfect erection). We offered medical treatment (sildenafil or PGE1) 1 month postoperatively to help recover potency. We evaluated the results obtained for patients with previously normal sexual activity and in whom a bilateral nerve-sparing procedure was performed (seven patients evaluable at 3 months and six at 6 months). In this group, spontaneous sexual activity was observed in three of seven 7 patients at 3 months and in four of six patients at 6 months. In the same group, sexual activity with addition of sildenafil or PGE1 was observed in five of seven and in five of six patients at 3 and 6 months, respectively. In our experience, when a patient presents a Q1 quality erection, sildenafil does not give satisfaction and we prefer the use of intracavernous PGE1. Results after unilateral nerve sparing are poor and the majority of the patients have not reported a spontaneous erection so far at 6 months.

Discussion

After a short initial experience with the transperitoneal approach as described by Guillonneau and Vallancien [3], we shifted to a purely extraperitoneal radical prostatectomy technique. This approach seems more comparable to the classical open retropubic radical prostatectomy. The mean operative time for our first 50 patients is similar to other series at the same stage of the learning curve [5-7] and is actually decreasing progressively. As mentioned, four surgeons with an individual learning curve operated on those patients. We observed an important decrease in blood loss by using bipolar forceps after our initial experience with the harmonic scalpel (three cases: patients 2-4). As we work in a closed space, the volume aspirated is accurate but represents a mixture of blood and urine loss. In the transperitoneal series, the blood loss is probably less accurate and the transfusion rates seems higher than at our institution, which is 13% [3]. The optimal catheterization time is unknown and probably depends on several parameters and surgeons' preferences. Progressive reduction of the catheterization time was due to the improvement in the water-tightness of the urethrovesical anastomosis. It is important to consider that patients in most European countries with a social health care system will not accept returning home with a catheter. Early continence rates at 6 months seem comparable to other series [6, 8]. This also probably depends on several parameters, such as the quality of the anastomosis and the traction on the suture. Shorter catheterization times may eventually increase the delay in recovering perfect continence. The potency rate is equally encouraging but the analysis concerns a limited number of patients only. Thus, these early results should be interpreted with great care.

Regarding cancer control in a short-term evaluation, positive surgical margins were observed in 22% of cases. This is comparable to several other initial reports [5, 6], but could be improved by patient selection (we have a high percentage of pT3a in our population) and increasing experience as shown by the Montsouris group [8, 9].

We did not have any intraperitoneal injury, which was observed using a transperitoneal approach in initial studies [3, 6]. Previous abdominal surgery is not a contraindication, but may render a purely extraperitoneal approach more difficult.

The potential advantages of a purely extraperitoneal laparoscopic radical prostatectomy combine the usual advantages of a laparoscopic approach (less painful, reducing morbidity, earlier recovery, etc.) and the advantages of the retropubic open approach (avoids intraperitoneal organ injuries, potential risk of cancer spillage in the peritoneal cavity, and intraperitoneal bleeding or urine leakage, and also allows possible later adjuvant radiotherapy). The disadvantages of the extraperitoneal approach include the slightly reduced working space and the potential increase in traction on the anastomosis due to a slightly more limited bladder mobilization. For this reason, we avoid running sutures when performing urethrovesical anastomosis.

Conclusions

We have developed a reproducible extraperitoneal laparoscopic radical prostatectomy technique. Cancer control results seem comparable to an open or transperitoneal laparoscopic approach. Preliminary results in terms of potency and continence seem equal to those of other techniques. At the present time, the criteria for choosing between an extraperitoneal and a transperitoneal laparoscopic approach have not been investigated and remain open to further evaluation and preference. Only long-term follow-up of large series and comparative studies of the different approaches will define the advantages, disadvantages, and limitations of these new techniques.

References

1. Schluesser WW, Kavoussi LR, Clayman RV, Vancaille TH (1992) Laparoscopic radical prostatectomy: initial case report. J Urol 147: 246A (abstract 130)
2. Schluesser WW, Schulan PG, Clayman RV, Kavoussi LR (1997) Laparoscopic radical prostatectomy: initial short-term experience. Urology 50: 854-857
3. Guillonneau B, Cathelineau X, Barre E, Rozet F, Vallancien G (1999) Laparoscopic radical prostatectomy: technical and early oncological assessment of 40 operations. Eur Urol 36: 14-20
4. Raboy A, Ferzli G, Albert P (1997) Initial experience with extraperitoneal endoscopic radical retropubic prostatectomy. Urology 50: 849-853
5. Guillonneau B, Cathelineau X, Barret E, Vallancien G (2000) Short term oncological results of laparoscopic radical prostatectomy, statement after 135 first procedures. Eur Urol 37 [Suppl 2]: 1-175 (Abstract 386)
6. Jacob F, Salomon L, Hoznek A, Bellot J, Antiphon P, Chopin DK, Abbou CC (2000) Laparoscopic radical prostatectomy : preliminary results. Eur Urol 37: 615-620
7. Rassweiler J, Sentker L, Seeman O, Hatzinger M, Stock C, Frede T, (2001) Heilbronn laparoscopic radical prostatectomy. Technique and results after 100 cases. Eur Urol 40(1):1-96
8. Guillonneau B, Vallancien G (2000) Laparoscopic radical prostatectomy: the Montsouris experience. J Urol 163: 418-422
9. Guillonneau B, Vallancien G (2000) Laparoscopic radical prostatectomy: the Montsouris technique. J Urol 163: 1643-1649

Chapter 18

Laparoscopic Access for Female Urinary Incontinence

Errico Zupi, Daniela Marconi, Carlo Romanini †

Introduction

Urinary incontinence is the demonstrable involuntary loss of urine that is socially or hygienically unacceptable or detrimental to the patient.

The problem of urinary incontinence — which affects 20%-40% of elderly women [1] — is becoming more and more frequent due to the increase in the average age of the population. The three most common types of incontinence are genuine stress incontinence (27%), detrusor instability (12%), and mixed incontinence (56%). These three types reflect the three most common mechanisms of incontinence [2-4].

More than 160 different types of surgical techniques to correct urinary incontinence have been described, but the best approach to this problem has not yet been established [5]. Retropubic colposuspension following the Marshall-Marchetti-Kranz technique or Burch's technique has the best prognosis and the least incidence of complications [6, 7]. All the urinary incontinence correction procedures that require the vaginal route need only a short operative time; however, the long-term results cannot be favorably compared with those of patients treated according to Burch's intervention [8-13].

With advancements in laparoscopic technology, surgeons' increased proficiency in laparoscopic suturing techniques, and a less morbid postoperative course for the patient [31, 32], the laparoscopic approach to management of genuine stress incontinence has increased in popularity [14].

The endoscopic approach for treatment of urinary stress incontinence dates to around 1990. The techniques were perceived as demanding, and laparoscopic knots were considered to be difficult to master. After a few years of work on the subject, a number of authors have demonstrated that this approach has considerable advantages, including improved visibility of Retzius's cavity, better understanding of the anatomy, improved assessment of defects in this area, and better treatment.

Vancaille and Nezhat were the first to describe the technique in which retropubic colposuspension was executed laparoscopically [15-17]. This technique offers the advantage of out-patient surgery along with the possibility of a long-term solution to the problem of stress urinary incontinence [18-20]. In addition, when executed laparoscopically, the exposure of the retropubic area is excellent; the magnification obtained by the videolaparoscope increases the surgeon's ability to suture in the best possible place.

Preoperative Evaluation

The preoperative evaluation includes the patient's clinical history, an accurate gynecologic, urologic, and neurologic assessment, a stress test, a Q-tip test, a urine analysis, and a urine culture [21, 22]. Each patient undergoes urodynamic examination with particular attention paid to the volume of the bladder and time needed for it to be emptied, and the consequential residual volume [23-28].

Technique

For mild-to-moderate stress urinary incontinence, nonsurgical treatment options can be tried. Patients with severe stress incontinence and those who fail conservative management may benefit from surgery. Because stress incontinence is a non-life-threatening condition and symptom severity is subjective, the decision to undergo surgery should be made by the patient. The objectives of surgery with its attendant risks and complications should be clearly outlined to the patient. The principal goal of surgery is to correct stress incontinence and improve quality of life. Risks include the de novo development of detrusor incontinence in 5%-18% of patients undergoing surgery for isolated stress incontinence and the possibility of voiding dysfunction.

The goals of surgery for hypermobility stress incontinence are as follows:

1. To support and stabilize the suburethral fascia (pubocervical fascia) so as to prevent excessive displacement of the urethra during periods of increased intra-abdominal pressure.
2. To allow posterior rotational descent of the bladder base.
3. To preserve the pliability and compressibility of the urethra.
4. To avoid compromising the urethral sphincteric mechanism.

Using general anesthesia and endotracheal intubation, the patient is placed in the dorsolithotomy position with both legs supported in stirrups. An 18-F Foley catheter with a 30-ml balloon tip is then inserted into the bladder. A 10-mm laparoscope is inserted through an intraumbilical incision and three 5-mm puncture sites are made in the lower abdomen. The lower pair of puncture sites is made lateral to the deep inferior epigastric vessels and the upper pair lateral to the abdominal rectus muscle near the umbilical level. The patient is then placed in a 20-degree Trendelenburg position, the bowels are displaced back toward the upper abdomen, and the pelvic organs are then meticulously examined. All visible signs of pathology, such as adhesions and endometriosis, are excised laparoscopically. Additional procedures, such as adnexectomy, hysterectomy, vaginal vault suspension, and repair of enterocele, are performed if indicated. The cul-de-sac is obliterated with permanent suture using a modified Moschowitz technique through the laparoscope. A transverse incision is made using laparoscope scissors on the parietal peritoneum about 1 in above the symphysis pubis between the two lateral umbilical ligaments (Fig. 1). The

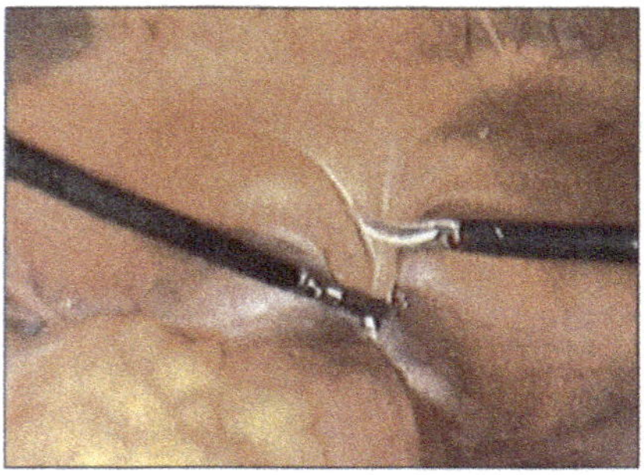

Fig. 1. Peritoneal incision with monopolar scissors

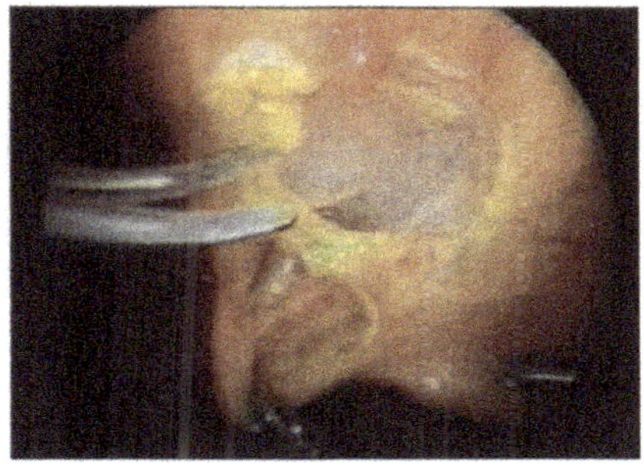

Fig. 2. Dissection of the preperitoneal space

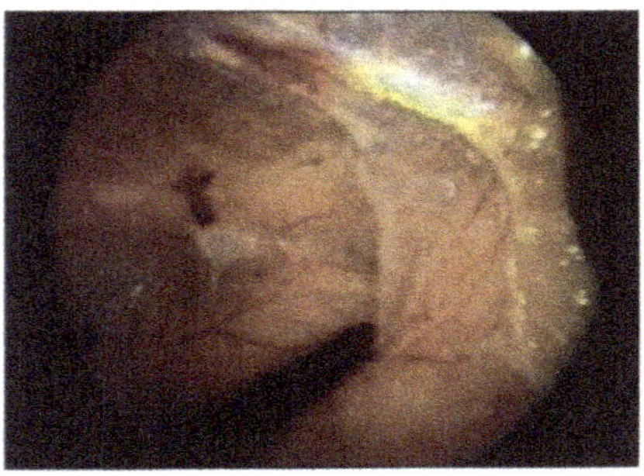

Fig. 3. The retropubic space is dissected

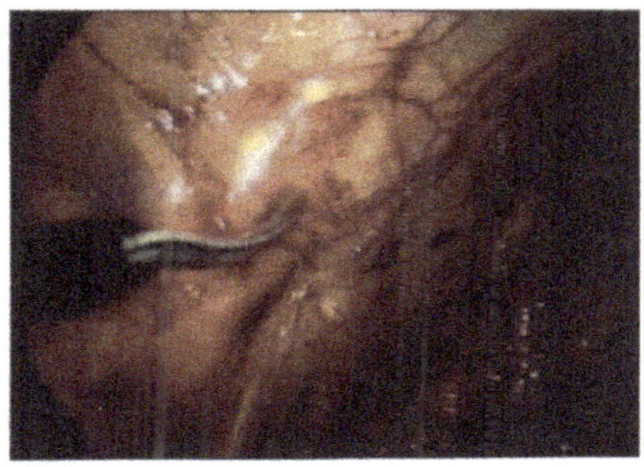

Fig. 4. The symphysis pubis, obturator neurovascular bundles, Cooper's ligaments, arcus tendineus fascia of pelvis, and levator ani are exposed

anterior peritoneum is dissected away from the anterior abdominal wall toward the pubic bone and the retropubic space entered (Fig. 2). The retropubic space is dissected (Fig. 3), and important anatomic landmarks such as the symphysis pubis, obturator neurovascular bundles, Cooper's ligaments, arcus tendineus fascia of pelvis, and levator ani are exposed (Fig. 4). No dissection is made within 2-2.5 cm of the urethra and urethrovesical junction. The paravaginal fat is removed to promote fibrosis and scar formation in the paravaginal area. The bladder is mobilized medially, and the pubocervical fascia is identified on both sides of the urethra. Retropubic dissection and bladder mobilization can damage the paraurethral vascular plexus, causing troublesome bleeding, but effective hemostasis can always be achieved by bipolar electrocoagulation with or without suture.

Two nonabsorbable sutures are placed (Fig. 5) on each side at the level of the midurethra and also at the urethrovesical junction at least 2 cm lateral to these structures. A double bite of the whole thickness of the anterior vaginal wall, avoiding the vaginal canal, is taken and is then passed through Cooper's ligament of the ipsilateral side at a level immediately above the anterior vaginal wall suture

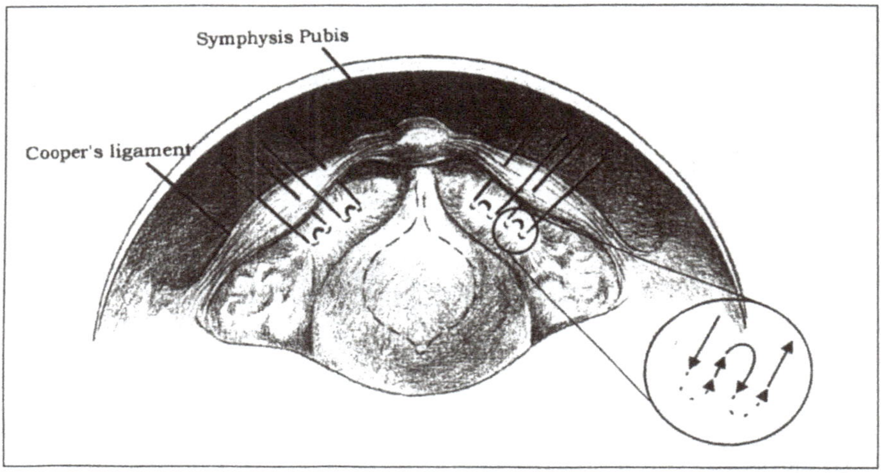

Fig. 5. Two nonabsorbable sutures are placed

(Fig. 6). During the placement of sutures, the assistant, or preferably the operating surgeon, places the middle and index fingers at the level of the urethrovesical junction identified by the balloon and the drainage tube of the Foley catheter. Tenting of the anterior wall in this manner facilitates the correct placement of sutures. The sutures are tied using an extracorporeal knot-tying technique with the Clark-Reich knot pusher while elevating the vagina up toward Cooper's ligament. Adequate support will be obtained if the sutures are tied without undue tension. Excessive tension will compress or kink the urethra, increasing the risk of voiding

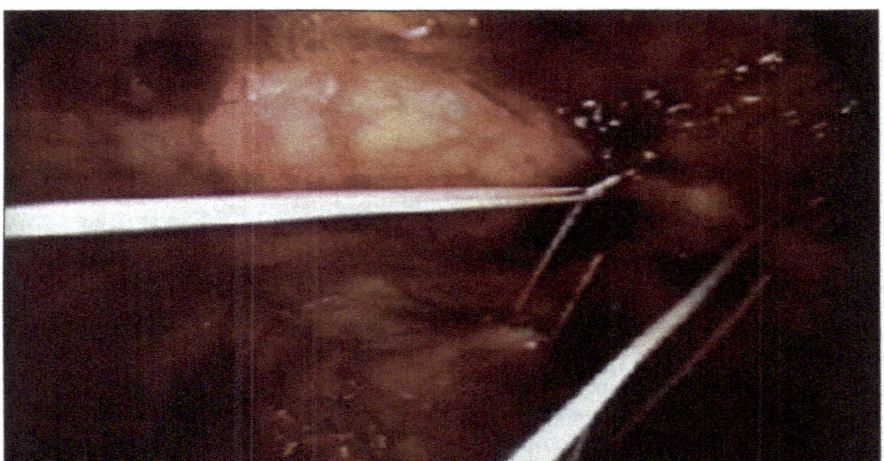

Fig. 6. Cooper's ligament of the ipsilateral side at a level immediately above the anterior vaginal wall suture

dysfunction and of necrosis at the suture sites, resulting in suture release and surgical failure. The retropubic space is then irrigated with copious amounts of Ringer's lactate solution. Hemostasis is achieved using bipolar diathermy forceps or sutures. A suprapubic catheter is inserted into the bladder under direct laparoscopic vision, and the peritoneal defect is closed with absorbable sutures. Transurethral or suprapubic cystoscopic examination is performed to ensure that no suture material has penetrated the bladder wall. A total of 5 ml of indigo-carmine dye and 10 mg of furosemide (Lasix) may then be injected intravenously to confirm the integrity of the ureters. Peristalsis and ejection of dye from ureteral orifices can be clearly observed cystoscopically [21, 29].

Postoperative Care

Postoperative care is similar to that provided in any major laparoscopic surgery. Most patients can be discharged from the hospital within 24 h of surgery while receiving mild analgesic medication. Some patients must return home with an indwelling suprapubic catheter that can be removed when residual urine amounts are less than 50 ml in three consecutive voids.

All patients are allowed to drive and return to work within 2 weeks of surgery provided that their jobs do not require much physical exertion. Detailed instructions are given regarding postoperative physical activities and the importance of consuming a high-fiber diet to avoid constipation. Patients are instructed to limit activities for at least 3 months after surgery to promote strong fibrosis and scar tissue formation in the retropubic area, which will ensure improved long-term results [30-33].

The studies undertaken to evaluate the effectiveness of a laparoscopic retropubic colposuspension demonstrate that this technique is efficient in selected women who undergo operative laparoscopy for stress urinary incontinence. The exposure of the tissue is better than in a laparotomy, the endoscopic approach is both less traumatic and less invasive in relation to operative time, and has less risk of complications, to which we can add a shorter period of hospitalization. The blood vessels can be identified and respected, due to the laparoscopic magnification, thus obtaining a wider operative vision and eliminating the need for drainage and the formation of postoperative hematoma.

The preliminary results obtained from different authors are promising, with a success rate of more than 90%. Long-term studies including follow-up are needed in order to determine whether the laparoscopic urethral suspension gives similar results to those obtained using the laparotomic route [34-37].

Paravaginal Suspension

Paravaginal repair or paravaginal suspension is based on the concept that the urethral cystocele and stress urinary incontinence may be the consequence of a break in the pubocervical fascia from its peripheral attachments or a break inside the pubocervical fascia itself [29, 38, 39]. In 1902, White described a transvaginal reattachment of the anterior vaginal fornix to the arcus tendineus fascia of the pelvis as a treatment for cystocele.

Successively in the 1970s, Richardson, Walker, and Baden took up the concepts expressed by White and described repair of paravaginal defects to restore normal anatomic integrity for the treatment of cystocele.

Richardson emphasized that the cystocele is not caused by stretching or attenuation of the pubocervical fascia but is the result of a break. The pubocervical fascia supports the bladder and the urethra, forming a shelf and allowing the bladder neck and proximal urethra to be compressed in an anteroposterior fashion during periods of stress.

When this supportive structure is debilitated due to childbirth, chronic obstructive pulmonary disease, or chronic constipation, the stability of the pubocervical fascia is reduced and may fail. This leads to cystocele formation and the development of germine stress incontinence (GSI) if the defect involves the regions of the bladder neck and the proximal urethra. Cadaver dissections and observations during numerous surgical cases led Richardson to identify four different pubocervical fascial defects that can cause cystocele and associated stress urinary incontinence.

1. The paravaginal defect is a result of detachment of the pubocervical fascia from its lateral attachment to the fascia of the obturator internus muscle at the level of the arcus tendineus fascia of the pelvis (white line). It can be unilateral or bilateral and accounts for approximately 80% of all urethrocystoceles.
2. The transverse defect is the next most common defect, resulting from transverse separation of the pubocervical fascia from the pericervical ring onto which the cardinal and uterosacral ligaments insert. The base of the bladder herniates into the anterior vaginal fornix and forms a pure cystocele without displacing the urethra or urethrovesical junction.
3. The midline defect is caused by a break in the central portion of the hammock-like sling of the pubocervical fascia on which the bladder rests. There may be concomitant stress urinary incontinence if the area under the bladder neck is involved in the break. A midline defect is a rare occurrence for which the traditional anterior colporrhaphy works well. One must identify the edges of the fascial defects during the repair by dissecting the vaginal mucosa off the underlying pubocervical fascia and reapproximating the edges of the defect.
4. The distal defect is the result of avulsion of the urethral attachment to the urogenital diaphragm as it passes under the symphysis pubis. It is a rare defect and can be seen in patients who have had surgical amputation of the distal urethra as part of a radical vulvectomy.

Technique

The patient lies in the laparoscopic position (Fig. 7); the preparation of the Retzius space is as for colposuspension described above, except that the dissection is carried cephalad on the pelvic side wall to the ischial spine. The bladder is then

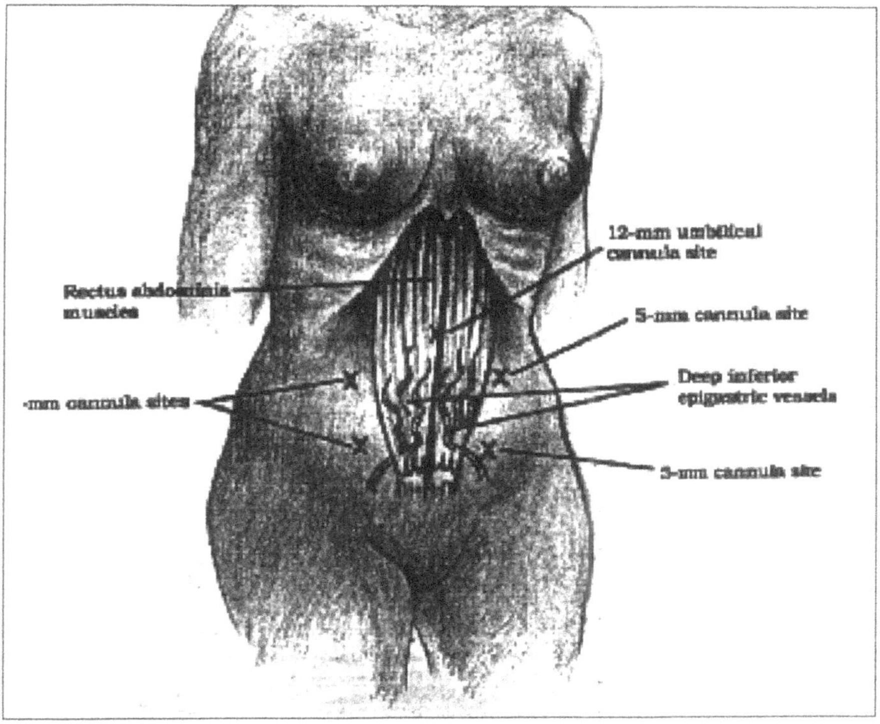

Fig. 7. Trocar placement. (From [37])

mobilized medially, facilitated by the surgeon's fingers in the vagina and an atraumatic laparoscopic instrument in the retropubic space. The pubocervical fascia should be well exposed, especially around the level of the ischial spine where the ureters run medially and anteriorly to it. The location of the ischial spine can be identified and confirmed by vaginal digital palpation and simultaneous visualization with the laparoscope. The pelvic floor defects are repaired using permanent sutures: the superior lateral sulcus of the vagina is reattached to the arcus tendineus fascia of the pelvis (white line) (Fig. 8).

Richardson and coworkers reported more than 95% patient satisfaction with paravaginal repair of cystoceles and cystourethrocele; the same results are reported laparoscopically.

We can conclude that when a patient has paravaginal defects associated with stress urinary incontinence, a combination of paravaginal and Burch colposuspension is required.

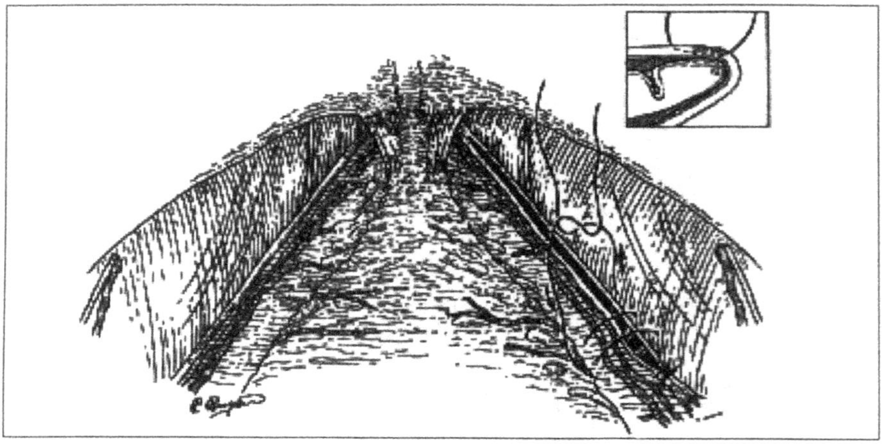

Fig. 8. Repair of paravaginal defects. (From [37])

Extraperitoneal Access for Female Urinary Incontinence

The retroperitoneal route presents the most advantages in cases of urinary stress incontinence on its own. The steps involving opening the peritoneum and peritonization are eliminated. There are several techniques for access to the retroperitoneal, of which the earliest is probably that described by Dargent and Salvat.

After carefully locating the midline, a suprapubic midline incision about 2 cm long is made. The subcutaneous space is dissected, and the aponeurosis located and incised. The subaponeurotic space is opened, after which the surgeon introduces a finger into the suprapubic space to search for Cooper's ligaments.

The surgeon then penetrates the Retzius cavity, and moves the finger sideways and upward to detach the lateral preperitoneal space and prepare it for the operating trocars.

Once the two operating trocars have been inserted, the optics trocar is positioned. This may be a normal trocar or one specially designed for open laparoscopy. The air seal is provided by a purse of skin or aponeurosis.

The gas is insufflated directly via the trocar once it is confirmed that the instrument is located correctly.

The disadvantage of this method is the restricted field of vision because of the lens being in the suprapubic position. This problem can be solved by reaching the Retzius cavity via the subumbilical retroperitoneal access in order to carry out retropubic colposuspension.

The operator stands on the left of the patient; the first assistant who manipulates the laparoscope and the attached camera stands on the right. A 1-mm operative laparoscope is inserted through a Hasson's cannula placed 1 cm infraumbilically in the preperitoneal space. The abdominal fascia is fixed by two sutures inserted through the sheath of the blunt trocar. The Retzius cavity is dissected using CO_2; an insufflation pressure of 12-15 mmHg can be used to help with the dissection. The dissection can be continued easily and without difficulty by blunt dissection of the preperitoneal space, using monopolar scissors or a bipolar needle when necessary to coagulate the preperitoneal vessels. The dissection can be carried down to the lower part of the retropubic space until the anterior bladder wall, the vaginal wall, and the urethra are visualized.

Duluc insufflates directly into the retroperitoneal space. He pierces the abdominal wall level with the pubis using a Veress needle, and when he feels he has gone through the fascia transversalis, he insufflates the preperitoneal space, enabling him to introduce the trocar into this space in the same way as for ordinary laparoscopy, except that his incision is made 10 mm below the umbilicus and not in the umbilicus itself.

An alternative trocar with dissecting balloon can be used. This is introduced via a cutaneous incision and positioned under the aponeurosis. The balloon is insufflated once the endoscope is in position. Dissection then proceeds by distension under visual control. The anatomic structures are easy to identify and there is no risk of hypercapnia.

References

1. Thomas TM, Plymat DR, Blannin J, et al (1980) Prevalence of urinary incontinence. Br Med J 281:1243-zzzz
2. Diokno AC, Brock BM, Brown MD, et al (1986) Prevalence of urinary incontinence and other urological symptoms in the noninstitutionalized elderly. J Urol 136:1022
3. Yarnell JW, St Leger AS (1979) The prevalence, severity and factors associated with urinary incontinence in a random sample of the elderly. Age Aging 8:81
4. Holst K, Wilson PD (1988) The prevalence of female urinary incontinence and reasons for not seeking treatment. N Z Med J 101:756
5. Rosenzweig BA, Hischke MD, Thomas S, et al (1991) Stress incontinence in women: Psychological status before and after treatment. J Reprod Med 36:835
6. Horbach NS (1992) Genuine SUI: best surgical approach. Contemp Obstet Gynecol 37:53
7. Marshall VF, Marchetti AA, Krantz KE (1941) The correction of stress incontinence by simple vesicourethral suspention. Surg Gynecol Obstet 88:509-518
8. Burch JC (1968) Cooper's ligament urethrovesical suspension for stress incontinence. Am J Obstet Gynecol 100:764-772
9. Stanton SL (1986) Colposuspension. In: Stanton SL, Tanagho E (eds) Surgery of female incontinence, 2nd ed. Springer, Berlin Heidelberg New York, pp 95-103
10. McGuire EJ, Layton B (1973) Pubovaginal sling procedure for stress incontinence. Surg Gynecol Obstet 136:547
11. Pereyra AJ, Lebherz TB (1976) Combined urethrovesical suspension and vaginouretheroplasty for correction of urinary stress incontinence. Obstet Gynecol 30:537
12. Raz S (1981) Modified bladder neck suspension for female stress incontinence. Urology 17:82
13. Hohnfellner R, Petrie E (1986) Sling procedures in surgery. In: Stanton SL, Tanagho E (eds) Surgery of female incontinence, 2nd edn. Springer Berlin Heidelberg, New York, pp 105-113
14. Gittes RF, Loughlin KR (1987) No incision pubovaginal suspension for stress incontinence. J Urol 138:568
15. Bhatia NN, Bergman A (1980) A modified Burch versus Pereyra retropubic urethropexy for stress urinary incontinence. Obstet Gynecol 66:255
16. Mundy AR (1983) A trial comparing the Stamey bladder neck suspension procedure with colposuspension for the treatment of stress incontinence. Br J Urol 33:687-690

17. Green DF, McGuire EJ, Lytton B (1986) A comparison of endoscopic suspension of vesical neck versus anterior urethropexy for the treatment of stress urinary incontinence. J Urol 136:1205-1207
18. Tanagho EA (1976) Colpocystourthropexy: the way we do it. J Urol 116:751-753
19. Bergman A, Ballard C, Koonings P (1989) Primary stress urinary incontinence and pelvic relaxation: prospective randomized comparison of three different operations. Am J Obstet Gynecol 161:97-101
20. Bergman A, Ballard C, Koonings P (1989) Comparison of three different surgical procedures for genuine stress incontinence: prospective randomized study. Am J Obstet Gynecol z:1102-1106
21. Wall LL, Wank K, Robson I, Stanton SL (1990) The Pyridium pad test for diagnosing urinary incontinence. A Comparative study of asymptomatic and incontinent women. J Reprod Med 1:3-6
22. Walters MD, Dombrosky RA, Prihoda TJ (1990) Perineal Pad testing in the quantation of urinary incontinence. Int Urogynecol J 1:3-6
23. Karram MM, Bhatia NN (1989) Transvaginal needle bladder neck suspension procedure for stress urinary incontinence: a comprehensive review. Obstet Gynecol 73:906-914
24. Penttinen J, Lindholm EL, Kaar K, Kauppila A (1989) Successful colposuspension in stress urinary incontinence reduces bladder neck mobility and increases pressure transmission to the urethra. Acta Gynecol Obstet 244:233-238
25. Van Geelen JM, Theeuwes AGM, Eskes TKAB, Martin CB (1989) The clinical and urodynamic effects of anterior vaginal repair and Burch colposuspension. Am J Obstet Gynecol 159:137-144
26. Hilton P, Stanton SL (1983) A Clinical and urodynamic assessment of the Burch colposuspension for genuine stress incontinence. Br J Obstet Gynaecol 90:934-939
27. Bahatia NN, Bergman A (1986) Use of preoperative uroflowmetry and simultaneous urethrocystometry for predicting risk of prolonged post-operative bladder drainage. Urology 28:440
28. Bergman A, Bhatia NN (1985) Uroflowmetry for predicting postoperative voiding difficulties in women with SUI. Br J Obstet Gynaecol 92:835-838
29. Griffiths DJ, McCraken PN, Harrison GM (1991) Incontinence in the elderly: objective demonstration and quantitative assessment. Br J Urol 67:467-471
30. Nezhat C, Nezhat F, Nezhat CH (1992) Operative laparoscopy (minimally invasive surgery): state of the art. J Gynecol Surg 8:111-141
31. Vancaille TG, Schessler W (1991) Laparoscopic bladder neck suspension. J Laproendsc Surg 1:169
32. Nezhat CH, Nezhat F, Nezhat C, Rottenberg H (1994) Laparoscopic retropubic cystourethropexy. J Am Assoc Gynecol Laparosc
33. Walters M, Shields L (1988) The diagnostic value of history, physical examination and the Q-tip cotton swab test in women with urinary incontinence. Am J Obstet Gynecol 159:145-149
34. Wiskind AK, Creighton SM, Stanton SL (1992) The incidence of genital prolapse after Burch colposuspension. Am J Obstet Gynecol 176:399-405
35. Cordozo LD, Stanton SL, William JE (1979) Detrusor instability following surgery for genuine stress urinary incontinence. Br J Urol 51:204
36. Zupi E, Marconi D, Romanini C (1997) Preperitoneal laparoscopic colposuspension for genuine stress urinary incontinence: a modified Burch procedure. J Gynecol Surg 13:65
37. Hulka JF, Reich H (1997) Textbook of laparoscopy, 2nd edn. Saunders, Philadelphia
38. Burch JC (1961) Urethrovaginal fixation to Cooper's ligament for correction of stress incontinence, cystocele, and prolapse. Am J Obstet Gynecol 81:281-290
39. Stanton SL (1984) The Burch colposuspension procedure. Acta Urol Belg 52:280-282

Chapter 19

Complications of Retroperitoneal Laparoscopy in Pediatric Urology: Prevention, Recognition, and Management

CRAIG A. PETERS

Introduction

Retroperitoneal laparoscopic or retroperitoneoscopic procedures introduce a new range of potential complications to the arena of laparoendoscopic surgery. The principle organ of interest is the kidney and this can be affected by a variety of surgical complications in any type of laparoendoscopic surgery. When a retroperitoneal access technique is performed, however, there are specific issues that need to be addressed.

The majority of complications deal with access techniques and the development of a working field. It is critical to recognize these potential sources of problems, acknowledge their presence, and deal with the important issues. Prevention is the most important element of this discussion in that it can eliminate the need for the other two elements. This is not always possible, but should be striven for. Recognition is the second critical element and is almost as important, since the lack of recognition of a developing complication will usually lead to more complex problems. Finally, efficient management of complications during a surgical procedure is the best assurance of an adequate outcome and a healthy patient.

Complications of Access

The principle complications of access are shown in Table 1. The most important of these is inadequate development of a surgical field. This limits all subsequent work.

Table 1. Complications of retroperitoneal access

Complication	Signs	Management
Parietal hematoma	Bleeding, loss of field	Localize bleeder, control
Visceral injury	Inadequate field, hemorrhage, absent normal landmarks	Control bleeding, localize injury, convert to open procedure
Peritoneal insufflation	Loss of working field, bulging peritoneum	Vent peritoneal cavity, window peritoneum, convert to transperitoneal procedure

The types of complications are a product of the type of access elected. The options are usually direct access, balloon insufflation to create a working space, or formal blunt dissection from a working port using a camera. Blunt dissection may be started using the Visiport system for direct vision placement of the port into the retroperitoneal space [10]. There are two basic approaches to retroperitoneal access, the lateral and the prone approaches. Each has advantages and disadvantages with specific best uses. The lateral approach seems to be associated with a higher incidence of peritoneal violation, but offers a somewhat larger working space. No other significant difference between the two approaches was noted in a recently published comparison [4].

The first essential element is appropriately functioning equipment, including the balloon, cannulae, and endoscopes. We have used a dissecting balloon, made from the finger of a surgical glove tied securely to the end of a 12-Fr straight catheter [3]. Double ties maintain an adequate seal. These may be slowly insufflated with 150-200 cc of saline. They are left in position, deflated and removed, with placement of the scope quickly thereafter. While waiting, a box stitch is placed in the muscle and fascia to secure the cannula, maintain a gas seal, and ultimately close the port site. Leakage will limit the working space and compromise the operation. Accurate placement and avoidance of over-filling can prevent problems of dissecting within muscle layers or balloon rupture with fragments left in the wound [1]. Adequate visualization is critical. With the initial field started, this is developed under direct vision with blunt dissection by the camera. The aim is to identify the peritoneal reflection and make sure that subsequent port placement is accurate and avoids the peritoneum.

The placement of secondary ports in retroperitoneal procedures may not be able to be viewed directly, but the line of movement of the introducing trocar/needle should be anticipated and observed. These cannulae need to be secured. Dislodgment of a working port is frustrating and may create problems, especially if it occurs during a critical maneuver. If this happens, one of the best ways to deal with it is to pass a blunt instrument through the cannula and watch for its movements through the tissues of the retroperitoneum, then guide it into the operative field, following it with the cannula.

After development of the retroperitoneal space, identification of the kidney is not always easy. It is possible that the kidney has been displaced upward (posteriorly) by the blunt dissection, and will be found along the posterior retroperitoneum.

During development of the retroperitoneal space, the peritoneum may be torn, particularly in smaller children where it is thinner and less layered with fat [4]. This will immediately insufflate the peritoneum, which will limit the working space in the retroperitoneum. This might not create a significant problem, but usually will. It can occur at any time during the procedure. There are several potential solutions. The peritoneum may become preferentially insufflated almost like a tension pneumothorax, in which there is preferential insufflation of the lower pressure intraperitoneal space. Venting the peritoneum with an 18-g angiocatheter can effectively reduce the impact of that insufflation and provide an adequate working space. Alternatively, the peritoneum may be windowed widely to equilibrate the pressures and insufflation. If these measures do not improve the working space, the peritoneum is opened widely and the procedure is performed in a retro- and intraperitoneal manner. There is generally no need to convert to an open procedure solely on the basis of intraperitoneal insufflation, as long as the basic requirements of safe endoscopic surgery are provided: exposure, ready vascular control, and working space for the procedure.

Complications Specific to Retroperitoneal Procedures

There are particular complications associated with the specific operation being performed retroperitoneally, which are similar to when the procedure is performed transperitoneally, with distinct features. There are also general complications associated with insufflation that may be different in retroperitoneal access than in transperitoneal access. There are very few reports in the pediatric literature, however, and most information can only be gained from adult retroperitoneal procedures. These include the potential for CO_2 absorption through the retroperitoneal working area or through a vascular injury. Hypercarbia does not appear to be more severe with retroperitoneal insufflation in adults [12].There is one case report of fatal CO_2 embolism without major vascular injury evident [2]. Major vascular injuries are possible, most likely due to inadequate visualization.

Nephrectomy

The essence of nephrectomy is vascular control. From the retroperitoneal approach, this is facilitated by posterior access to the hilum, which provides initial exposure of the renal artery. Once controlled, the vein may be more safely dissected and ligated. There is a tendency to isolate the artery near the renal hilum, which may require taking several branches for complete control. It is better to isolate the artery more medially to permit control of a single vessel. This also provides better access to the renal vein. These vessels do not need to be taken at their origin with the aorta and vena cava, but a sufficiently wide area of exposure to permit placement of clips with adequate space in between for ligation is important. When taking the vein, careful identification of the anatomy is essential. In the posterior approach, it is possible for the vena cava to be mistakenly isolated instead of the renal vein, particularly on the right side. A slight misorientation of the camera and the direction of the cava may appear to be that of the renal vein. Attention needs to be paid to the size of the vessels as well. Double-checking the direction and orientation is necessary prior to clip placement. One case report of aortic occlusion from a gastrointestinal staple line placed to control bleeding illustrates this potential problem [13]. Some have advocated use of electrocautery for controlling the vessels in small dysplastic renal units [7], but this author continues to use clips in all situations.

Control of serious bleeding is an essential skill for the laparoendoscopic surgeon. This may occur at almost any part of the procedure. When it develops during mobilization and control of the renal hilum, rapid recognition and management are critical. As with all renal surgery, careful attention needs to be paid to avoiding inadvertent injury to the adrenal and lumbar vessels.

Because of the small working area in retroperitoneal laparoendoscopic surgery, it may not be apparent that all vessels have not been controlled, so it is essential to check the entire surface of the kidney before starting to remove it. Small polar vessels may not have been controlled and avulsion will cause bleeding that may be difficult to control. With each maneuver, including dissection, clip placement, or transection, the surgeon should be thinking about what structures are nearby and where they will move with the planned maneuver. This allows a mental view of the origin of the bleeding. The initial action with the onset of bleeding is to attempt to slow the bleeding by pressure with an instrument on the area of presumed origin. If one instrument is maintaining exposure, that is not the instrument to use. Loss of exposure will waste valuable time. An efficient suction-irrigating device is necessary and should be readily available. The origin of bleeding may be pinpointed by looking for the source of a swirl or jet of blood. If a delicate dissecting instrument can be quickly brought into play, it can be used to stop bleeding by grasping and cautery. It is risky to cauterize blindly in a field of blood. Traction may also facilitate control and identification of the bleeding point. At all times, an endoscopic clip applier must be available. It is our practice to always have two appliers in the room in case of misfire. The judgment as to when bleeding cannot be safely controlled endoscopically, and conversion to open surgery is needed, is difficult. Some bleeding can appear to be significant only because of the magnification of the endoscope. If, however, real control cannot be obtained within 10-15 min and there is continued welling up of blood, conversion may be the best option.

Partial Nephrectomy

The basic principles of nephrectomy obviously apply in partial nephrectomy, but this procedure also requires specific attention to controlled transection of the renal parenchyma between the poles. The goals are to remove as much of the nonfunctioning dysplastic tissue as possible without injury to the remnant pole, or to enter the collecting system of the remnant pole, and do so with adequate vascular control. In most cases this is relatively straightforward after vascular control, but in the setting of a pole with prior infection, it may be difficult. The harmonic scalpel is particularly useful in this task. The curve blade is probably more useful than the scissor blade. It is important to keep in mind that the harmonic scalpel works best with tension on the tissues and with slow incision. We have not routinely checked the integrity of the collecting system with laparoscopic partial nephrectomy, but have seen one persistent collection of fluid (urine) following upper pole removal. Alternatively, a drain could be considered, which has not been part of the routine.

The most serious complication of partial nephrectomy is injury to the remnant pole vessels and loss of the remnant pole. This is due to excessive manipulation of the remnant pole or misidentification of the remnant pole vessels. With identification of the problem acutely, as manifest by duskiness of the remnant pole, clear vascular transection, or vasospasm, can be treated. Vasospasm is best handled by irrigation of the vessel with papaverine [8]. Transection would mandate conversion to an open procedure with reconstruction of the artery. Delayed identification may be noted with clinical symptoms of pain, fever, and hematuria; but may also only be noted with an ultrasound showing atrophy or absence of flow on Doppler ultrasound interrogation. There is little to be done at that time, except to monitor for hypertension.

Pyeloplasty

The close working space of retroperitoneal laparoendoscopic surgery is the primary limitation in performing an efficient pyeloplasty. This limitation will largely be reflected in less accurate anastomoses and possible failure of the repair. It may also be more likely to injure the renal vessels during mobilization and manipulation to perform the pyeloplasty.

Complications of Completion

There are few complications of completion of the retroperitoneal laparoendoscopic surgery. These involve bleeding in the operative area, which was masked by the insufflation pressure, and at the cannula sites, which need to be recognized prior to loss of the pneumoretroperitoneum. After completion of the operative procedure and removal of the specimen (if applicable), the operative area, particularly near the hilum, is inspected. If the insufflation has been lost with specimen removal, it can be inspected immediately for new bleeding, or the retroperitoneal pressure can be reduced to below 5 mmHg by stopping inflow and venting off the insufflating gas. Venous bleeding can be completely masked due to the insufflating pressures and will only become evident when those pressures are reduced. The cannulae are best removed under direct vision. This may be difficult to do, owing to the angle and close placement of the ports. A 30° lens can permit viewing of the port sites. Alternatively, watching for blood dripping after removal of the cannula can indicate the need for hemostasis.

The need to close port sites is unclear. In the retroperitoneum, we close all 5- and 3.5-mm sites that are not near the iliac crest. Placing a musculofascial stitch just before placing the cannula provides this closure. This stitch is also useful for preventing cannula dislodgment. A single simple stitch can be used after the cannula is removed for small ports where the fascial stitch was not previously placed.

Postoperative Complications

The complications that arise postoperatively are generally manifestations of complications that should be recognized intraoperatively. This is primarily hemorrhage, intraperitoneal injury, or urine leak. Hemorrhage may be in the operative site or in the body wall. Prevention is as indicated above. Recognition is based on clinical parameters such as pain, decreased hematocrit, or bleeding from a port site. Management is usually supportive, unless there is indication of severe blood loss, which would probably necessitate open exploration for control.

Intraperitoneal injury is likely to present as intraperitoneal sepsis due to bowel injury. This may be difficult to note intraoperatively and is best prevented by careful attention to anatomic landmarks, notice of possible violations of the peritoneum, and a careful final check of the operative field. After a laparoendoscopic procedure, the finding of free air on an abdominal film may not be able to be accurately interpreted, but the clinical scenario should guide further evaluation. Management is directed by the nature of the injury and the clinical scenario.

Urine leak may be evident as leakage from a port site, pain, fever, infection, or incidentally noted at routine follow-up. Prevention is directed toward maintaining the integrity of the remnant collecting system. During partial nephrectomy, retrograde injection of methylene blue dye through a previously placed ureteral catheter permits identification of an opening in the collecting system. This would permit direct closure. Alternatively, drainage of the retroperitoneum would prevent urinoma formation. Internal drainage of the remnant pole does not seem to be advisable. The natural history of a contained, asymptomatic urinoma is unclear.

Conclusions

The complications associated with retroperitoneoscopic surgery in children are qualitatively similar to those in adults, but appear to be quantitatively less similar (Table 2). This may simply reflect the early series and in all likelihood will increase as more surgeons undertake retroperitoneoscopic procedures. These complications are predictable and preventable with appropriate recognition and vigilance. Avoidance of over-aggressive development of the retroperitoneal space, caution with development of the working field, constant attention to the anatomy, and a methodical approach to the renal hilum will go a long way in preventing complications that might necessitate conversion to open surgery or create a significant problem. It is essential to be open to recognition of these complications should they occur, so that they may be dealt with expeditiously. Denial of the possibility of a complication is not effective management of that complication. Retroperitoneoscopic surgery is effective and safe in children and offers a unique and exceptional surgical exposure. When performed carefully, it is able to offer a low incidence of significant complications.

Table 2. Reported complication rates in pediatric retroperitoneal surgery

Author	Conversion to open	Hemorrhage	Peritoneal violation	Comment
Valla et al. 1996 [15]	1/18	0/18		
El-Ghoneimi et al. 1998 [7]	3/42	2/42	12/42	1 Duodenal perforation; 1 lower pole loss
Shanberg 1998 [14]	1/20	1/20	3/20	Venacaval laceration
Borer et al. 1999 [3]	0/14	0/14	0/14	2-mm Instruments
El-Ghoneimi et al. 2000 [6]	0/9	1/9	3/9	High-risk patients
Caione et al. 2000 [5]	1/20	1/20	1/20	Renal biopsy
Yeung et al. 2001 [16]	1/12	1/12	0/12	Pyeloplasty
Borzi 2001 [4]	2/55	0/55	6/55	
Micali et al. 2001 [10]	0/31	0/31	1/31	Visiport use
Mirallie et al. 2001 [11]	1/2			Adrenal
Pediatric %	4.5	2.7	12.8	Kumar et al.
Adult %	11.7	2.2	5.4	2001 [9]

References

1. Adams JB 2nd, Micali S, Moore RG, Babayan RK, Kavoussi LR (1996) Complications of extraperitoneal balloon dilation. J Endourol 10:375-378
2. Blaser A, Rosset P (1999) Fatal carbon dioxide embolism as an unreported complication of retroperitoneoscopy. Surg Endosc 13:713-714
3. Borer JG, Cisek LJ, Atala A, Diamond DA, Retik AB, Peters CA (1999) Pediatric retroperitoneoscopic nephrectomy using 2 mm instrumentation. J Urol 162:1725-1730
4. Borzi PA (2001) A comparison of the lateral and posterior retroperitoneoscopic approach for complete and partial nephroureterectomy in children. BJU Int 87:517-520
5. Caione P, Micali S, Rinaldi S, Capozza N, Lais A, Matarazzo E, et al (2000) Retroperitoneal laparoscopy for renal biopsy in children. J Urol 164:1080-1083
6. El-Ghoneimi A, Sauty L, Maintenant J, Macher MA, Lottmann H, Aigrain Y (2000) Laparoscopic retroperitoneal nephrectomy in high risk children. J Urol 164:1076-1079
7. El-Ghoneimi A, Valla JS, Steyaert H, Aigrain Y (1998) Laparoscopic renal surgery via a retroperitoneal approach in children. J Urol 160:1138-1141
8. Gearhart JP, Jeffs RD (1985) The use of topical vasodilators as an adjunct in infant renal surgery. J Urol 134:298-300
9. Kumar M, Kumar R, Hemal AK, Gupta NP (2001) Complications of retroperitoneoscopic surgery at one centre. BJU Int 87:607-12

10. Micali S, Caione P, Virgili G, Capozza N, Scarfini M, Micali F (2001) Retroperitoneal laparoscopic access in children using a direct vision technique. J Urol 165:1229-1232
11. Mirallie E, Leclair MD, de Lagausie P, Weil D, Plattner V, Duverne C, et al (2001) Laparoscopic adrenalectomy in children. Surg Endosc 15:156-160
12. Ng CS, Gill IS, Sung GT, Whalley DG, Graham R, Schweizer D (1999) Retroperitoneoscopic surgery is not associated with increased carbon dioxide absorption. J Urol 162:1268-1672
13. Sautter T, Haueisen H, Stierli P, Kwiatkowski M, Recker F (2001) A severe complication of retroperitoneoscopic nephrectomy. J Urol 165:515-516
14. Kobashi KC, Chamberlin DA, Rainpoot O, Shanberg AM (1998) Retroperitoneal laparoscopic nephrectomy in children. J Urol 160:1142-1144
15. Valla JS, Guilloneau B, Montupet P, Geiss S, Steyaert H, El Ghoneimi A, et al (1996) Retroperitoneal laparoscopic nephrectomy in children. Preliminary report of 18 cases. Eur Urol 30:490-493
16. Yeung CK, Tam YH, Sihoe JD, Lee KH, Liu KW (2001) Retroperitoneoscopic dismembered pyeloplasty for pelvi-ureteric junction obstruction in infants and children. BJU Int 87:509-513

Chapter 20

Advantages and Future Perspectives

Eduardo F. Carvalhal, Inderbir S. Gill

Introduction

During the last two decades, urology has benefited tremendously from advancements in technology. In the same vein as other minimally invasive treatment modalities, such as extracorporeal shock-wave lithotripsy and advanced endourological procedures, laparoscopy has recently been established as an effective minimally invasive treatment alternative for a variety of urological disorders. Retroperitoneoscopy and extraperitoneal laparoscopy reflect the continued search for less invasive approaches and have been increasingly utilized as an important approach in the urologic laparoscopic armamentarium [1].

We review the advantages and potential drawbacks of this method and critically discuss the current status and future applications of this approach. Detailed descriptions of the surgical techniques are presented in other sections of this book and are beyond the scope of this chapter. However, a brief overview of specific procedures is outlined when indicated to highlight distinct characteristics of the retroperitoneal/extraperitoneal approach.

Retroperitoneoscopy: Historical Aspects

Since the description of retroperitoneoscopy by Bartel in 1969 [2], initial attempts of retroperitoneoscopic procedures were limited by the suboptimal pneumoretroperitoneum and visualization. [3, 4] The first retroperitoneoscopic nephrectomy was reported by Clayman's group, in St. Louis [4]. After Gaur's seminal description of a balloon technique for atraumatic retroperitoneal dissection [5], a resurgence of interest in retroperitoneoscopy and pelvic extraperitoneal laparoscopy occurred. Expanding the capability of the method and providing a more adequate working space, this concept allowed a larger number of procedures to be performed extraperitoneally [6]. Although it is possible to perform major operations without the use of balloon dissection [7, 8], the commercial availability of balloon dilators has increased the effectiveness and popularity of this approach. The use of some type of balloon dilator has recently been reported by 36 institutions included in a survey about worldwide urologic extraperitoneal laparoscopy [1]. At the Cleveland Clinic, we routinely employ atraumatic balloon dilation as the primary step in establishing retroperitoneoscopic access.

Advantages of Retroperitoneal/Extraperitoneal Laparoscopy

Retroperitoneoscopy is mainly characterized by avoiding violation of the peritoneal cavity (Fig. 1). This concept constitutes the main advantage of the method compared to the transperitoneal approach and explains many of its benefits [9] (Table 1). Since no bowel segments are directly manipulated during the procedure and the need to mobilize the colon is obviated, the risk of an intraperitoneal organ injury is reduced, although not eliminated. Also, in the case of a postoperative hematoma or urinoma, these fluid collections remain restricted to the retroperitoneal space, which decreases the morbidity of these complications and facilitates its management. As such, intra-abdominal seeding is minimized.

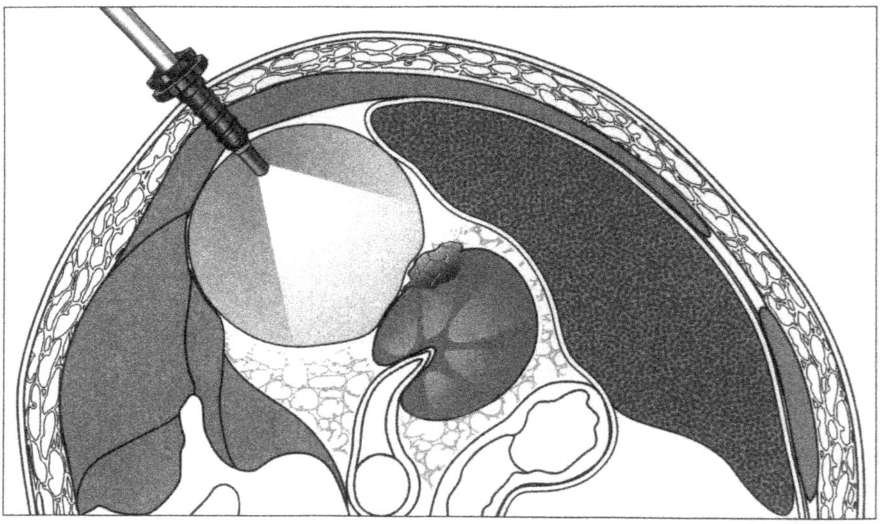

Fig. 1. Creation of retroperitoneal working space with balloon dilation between the kidney and psoas muscle. The kidney and Gerota's fascia are displaced anteromedially without violation of the peritoneal cavity (schematic illustration)

Table 1. Potential advantages of retroperitoneal/extraperitoneal laparoscopy

By avoiding violation of peritoneal cavity
- Minimal risk of intraperitoneal infection or seeding
- Reduced risk of intraperitoneal organ injury
- Bypass of prior intraperitoneal surgical adhesions
- Reduced postoperative ileus
- Shorter hospital stay
Direct access to renal artery and vein
Reduced morbidity in obese patients
Reduced morbidity in the elderly

These potential advantages are the author bias, given that no prospective randomized study comparing transperitoneal and retroperitoneal laparoscopic renal surgery have been reported to date.

In patients with previous abdominal operations, intraperitoneal adhesions can be avoided by selecting the retroperitoneal/extraperitoneal approach. This constitutes, in fact, an important reason for considering the retroperitoneal technique as a helpful adjunct to any urologic laparoscopist, since patients with multiple prior abdominal surgeries could still benefit from a minimally invasive treatment for many urologic disorders. Although previous retroperitoneal open or laparoscopic surgery should be considered a contraindication of the technique, a past history of percutaneous renal procedures (including percutaneous nephrolithotomy and renal biopsy) has not precluded efficacious retroperitoneoscopic access.

Finally, although no prospective, randomized comparison with transperitoneal renal laparoscopy has been reported to date, it is our impression that a shorter hospital stay may be associated with avoidance of the peritoneal cavity. The peritoneal distension due to intraoperative pneumoperitoneum and colonic mobilization during the transperitoneal approach may result in more postoperative paralytic ileus, as demonstrated in a comparative study of extraperitoneal and transperitoneal laparoscopic pelvic lymph node dissection in 75 patients [10]. A retrospective analysis of these patients demonstrated the slight superiority of retroperitoneoscopy in terms of postoperative recovery. In McDougall's retrospective comparison of retroperitoneal versus transperitoneal nephrectomy, the retroperitoneoscopic approach demonstrated a slight trend towards superior patient comfort, decreased analgesic use (35 mg of morphine sulfate vs. 39 mg) and shorter hospital stay (3.5 vs. 4 days) [11]. Our group recently reported the retroperitoneoscopic radical nephrectomy experience at the Cleveland Clinic, with an average hospital stay of 1.6 days [12]. In comparison, two large series of transperitoneal laparoscopic radical nephrectomy reported a mean hospital stay of 3.4 days [13] and 4.4 days [14], respectively. We believe that the decreased postoperative ileus, the resultant enhanced patient comfort, and physician/nursing staff counseling about early ambulation are responsible for the short hospital stay in our patients. When compared to an open radical nephrectomy group, the retroperitoneoscopic approach was associated with a fourfold decrease in both blood loss and hospital stay, and a ninefold decrease in narcotic analgesic use. Differences were not observed, however, in a prospective study performed at our institution comparing transperitoneal adrenalectomy versus retroperitoneoscopic adrenalectomy. Possibly, the minimal colon mobilization and the less invasive needlescopic techniques utilized during transperitoneal adrenalectomy were two reasons as to why no differences were encountered between the two laparoscopic approaches. Both groups presented excellent outcome parameters and similar hospital stay (25 h vs. 27.5 h) for this specific procedure [15].

A primary advantage of the retroperitoneoscopic approach to radical nephrectomy is the direct and early access to the renal artery and vein, allowing early control of these vessels. The rapid control of the main renal vessels prior to any instrument mobilization of the cancerous kidney replicates the principles of oncologic open surgery and promotes operator confidence.

As our experience increased with retroperitoneal laparoscopic procedures, we began to prefer this approach for renal and adrenal surgery in obese patients [16].

The majority of abdominal wall obesity is located in the pannus, which in the flank position shifts away from the operative side due to gravity. The flank, in comparison, has somewhat lesser amounts of subcutaneous fat, allowing use of normal size laparoscopic ports and instruments. Although the excessive retroperitoneal fat expectedly increases the degree of technical difficulty, a standardized stepwise anatomical approach by the experienced urologic laparoscopist allows retroperitoneoscopy to be performed effectively even in the morbidly obese patient. Our data suggest that laparoscopic surgery (mostly retroperitoneoscopy) in this group of patients (Body Mass Index >30) favorably compares to open surgery in terms of recovery, decreased blood loss, and reduced hospital stay. As such, retroperitoneoscopy is currently the preferred approach when renal or adrenal laparoscopic surgery is contemplated at our institution. Nevertheless, we caution that this population has increased surgical risks regardless of the approach, and laparoscopic surgery should be attempted in markedly obese patients only after reasonable laparoscopic experience has been acquired.

A distinct advantage of retroperitoneal laparoscopy over open surgery was also observed in the elderly population. A specific study addressing this issue was recently published from our institution, where retroperitoneal radical nephrectomy and nephroureterectomy in 11 octogenarian and nonagenarian patients were retrospectively compared to an open surgery group [17]. Although median surgical times and blood loss were similar, the retroperitoneoscopic group had a significantly quicker resumption of oral intake (less than 1 day versus 4 days), decreased narcotic requirements (14 mg versus 326 mg of morphine sulfate), shorter hospital stay (2 vs. 6 days) and faster convalescence (14 vs. 42 days). Postoperative complications were similar (36% vs. 33%) and medical in nature in all cases. In fact, all 11 patients in the retroperitoneoscopic group were referred by local urologists or departmental colleagues for consideration for laparoscopic surgery in a brief period of time (1 year), as opposed to the only six consecutive octogenarians who had undergone open surgery during the prior 5 years at the same institution. This may reflect the hesitation in performing curative open radical nephrectomy in the elderly, when watchful waiting is strongly advised due to concerns regarding operative morbidity. The laparoscopic approach may be, in the hands of an experienced surgical team, an excellent minimally invasive alternative to selected elderly patients.

Special Considerations

Some of the standardized laparoscopic procedures in urology, described in detail in previous chapters, present specific advantages when performed by the retroperitoneal approach:

- Adrenalectomy: The retroperitoneal approach provides effective identification and control of the adrenal vein. During a retroperitoneoscopic left adrenalectomy, the main adrenal vein can be controlled without the need for prior mobilization of the spleen and colon as in the transperitoneal technique.

- Nephrectomy: Either during simple or radical retroperitoneoscopic nephrectomy, the immediate access to the renal hilum is a key advantage of the method. Elimination of the need for colonic mobilization and early ligation of renal vessels, according to the oncologic principles of vascular control, is noted.
- Nephroureterectomy: Since the laparoscopic technique for nephroureterectomy was developed, different ways of retrieval of the bladder/ureteral cuff have been described. Resection of the bladder cuff can be accomplished laparoscopically with the EndoGIA stapler following nephrectomy. Alternatively, our preference is to endoscopically circumscribe and detach the en bloc bladder cuff under direct vision, using the Collings knife through the resectoscope [18]. In both situations, or even when the cuff is obtained through a Gibson incision developed for specimen extraction, the retroperitoneoscopic approach during the nephrectomy has the advantage to restrict any intraoperative or postoperative bladder extravasation to the extraperitoneal space.
- Pyeloplasty: The easy and rapid access to the retroperitoneal space provided by retroperitoneoscopy allows direct identification and dissection of the ureteropelvic junction (UPJ). Especially in the situation of a crossing vessel, a UPJ obstruction can be corrected in a minimally invasive manner with this method, without violating the peritoneal cavity and avoiding the risk of a postoperative intraperitoneal urinoma or hematoma [19].
- Adult polycystic kidney disease: Even hugely enlarged kidneys due to polycystic disease can be approached retroperitoneally, and bilateral nephrectomies have been reported by a modified retroperitoneoscopic approach, with both enlarged kidneys being synchronously extracted through an extraperitoneal, lower midline incision in the same operative session [20].
- Ureterolithotomy: Although rarely performed, laparoscopic ureterolithotomy remains an alternative in cases of failure after extracorporeal shock-wave lithotripsy or endourological attempts. The extraperitoneal approach also seems logical for this procedure, due to the ureteral location and avoidance of peritoneal cavity.
- Live-donor nephrectomy : Laparoscopic live-donor nephrectomy is usually performed by the transperitoneal approach, with retrieval of the left kidney due to the longer length of the left renal vein. Nevertheless, when a right-sided live-donor nephrectomy is indicated, we consider the retroperitoneoscopic technique as our preferred approach. Retroperitoneoscopy provides direct retrocaval access to the right renal artery, ensuring a long length. Also, complete exposure of the shorter right renal vein as it enters the inferior vena cava enables us to obtain the longest possible length of this vessel. Nevertheless, the length of the harvested right renal vein is short, although adequate for purposes of renal transplantation after bench dissection. The donor kidney can be extracted extraperitoneally, through a 6- to 8-cm, modified Pfannenstiel incision. In our initial series of nine patients (including four patients for autotransplantation), mean warm ischemia time was 4.4 min and mean renal vein length was 2.75 cm. All kidneys functioned adequately following transplantation [21].

Problems During Retroperitoneal/Extraperitoneal Surgery

As in any laparoscopic approach, the retroperitoneoscopic technique has certain limitations related to instrumentation, compromised tactile sensation, and the two-dimensional view of the operative field. All these limitations can be satisfactorily overcome after acquiring skill and accumulating experience in laparoscopic surgery. A detailed listing of the complications encountered during 1043 retroperitoneal laparoscopic procedures performed at 36 centers worldwide is presented in Table 2 [1].

Table 2. Major complications in 49 (4.7%) of 1043 retroperitoneal/extraperitoneal laparoscopic procedures (36 institutions worldwide) (modified from [1])

Complication	Total (*n*)	etiology	Conversion to open(*n*)
Visceral (*n*=26; 2.5%)			
Pneumothorax	6	Nephrectomy (6)	2
Pneumomediastinum	4	Renal cystectomy (2), nephrectomy (1), pyeloplasty (1)	0
Bladder	4	Bladder neck suspension (4)	4
Ureter	3	Pelvic lymphadenectomy (2), ureterolithotomy (1)	3
Colon	3	Ureterolysis (1), nephrectomy (1), morcellation/nephrectomy (1)	2
Small bowel	2	Pelvic lymphadenectomy (1), unspecified (1)	2
Pancreas	2	Nephrectomy (1), left adrenalectomy (1)	2
Spleen	1	Left adrenalectomy (1)	1
Liver	1	Right adrenalectomy (1)	0
Total	26		16
Vascular (*n*=23; 2.2%)			
Renal vein	6	Nephrectomy (6)	4
Inferior vena cava	4	Adrenalectomy (3), unspecified (1)	2
Gonadal vein	3	Nephrectomy (2), pelvic lymphadenectomy (1)	0
Inferior epigastric vessel	3	Pelvic lymphadenectomy (2), unspecified (1)	0
External iliac artery	2	Pelvic lymphadenectomy (2), ureterectomy (1)	2
External iliac vein	2	Pelvic lymphadenectomy (2)	1
Unspecified bleeding	2	Unspecified (2)	2
Lumbar vessel	1	Pyeloplasty (1)	1
Total	23		12

Perhaps the most significant difficulty encountered with retroperitoneoscopy was a reduced working space, as pointed out during the first descriptions of renal surgery with the method [4]. Related to the smaller space was the reported crowding of ports and inability to dissect large kidneys in the initial cases. However, with increasing experience and use of balloon dilation, an adequate and comfortable working space is routinely achieved and has allowed us to perform radical nephrectomy of large kidney tumors, up to 14 cm. Whenever the initial working space is not completely satisfactory, its expansion is usually achieved successfully as the laparoscopic dissection progresses. For extraction of uncommonly large specimens, a monitored, intentional peritoneotomy can be performed at the end of the procedure for intraperitoneal Endocatch bag entrapment of the specimen.

Although the retroperitoneal space does not contain the well-defined anatomical landmarks encountered in the transperitoneal approach, immediate visualization of distinct structures after proper balloon dilation has been established: psoas muscle and Gerota's fascia (routinely), lateral peritoneal reflection (83% of the time), ureter and/or gonadal vein (61% of the time), and pulsations of the fat-covered renal artery (56% of the time), bilaterally. In addition, aortic pulsations (90% of the time) and inferior vena cava (25% of the time) can be visualized immediately following proper balloon dilation on the left and right sides, respectively [12]. Colonic mobilization is avoided, as is retraction of organs such as liver and spleen. In fact, the retroperitoneal approach and flank positioning of the patient are classically familiar to the urologist. According to the familiarity with the technique, it is our experience that the renal vessels can be identified and circumferentially dissected in an easier and quicker manner than with the transperitoneal route.

Previous reports suggested an increased carbon dioxide (CO_2) absorption associated with retroperitoneal laparoscopy and related postoperative morbidity, such as subcutaneous emphysema [22]. However, a prospective study revealed that retroperitoneoscopy is not associated with greater CO_2 absorption compared to transperitoneal laparoscopy, and patients with subcutaneous emphysema exhibited only transient increases in CO_2 absorption above control levels [23]. An effective adjunct to prevent the occurrence of subcutaneous emphysema intraoperatively is the use of a blunt-tip balloon trocar as the primary port obtained with the open Hasson technique. This cannula contains an internal fascial retention balloon along with an external, adjustable foam cuff, which secure the port in an airtight manner when cinched down [12] .

Future Perspectives

As the search for noninvasive treatment modalities continues, retroperitoneoscopy and pelvic extraperitoneal surgery constitute nowadays a promising and versatile approach for a variety of urologic disorders. Its increasing popularity and acceptance during the last few years reflect the number of expanding indications for this technique (Table 3). From live-donor nephrectomies to retroperi-

Table 3. Established and expanding indications for retroperitoneal/extraperitoneal laparoscopy

Established
Simple nephrectomy
Radical nephrectomy
Adrenalectomy
Ureteral procedures
Bladder neck suspension
Pelvic lymphadenectomy
Pyeloplasty
Expanding
Live-donor nephrectomy (especially for the right kidney)
Partial nephrectomy
Renal cryoablation
Specimen extraction via extraperitoneal lower abdominal incision
Radical prostatectomy
Robotic surgery

toneoscopic radical and partial nephrectomies, technical and technologic advancements have made it possible to extract intact specimens through a low Pfannenstiel incision following major retroperitoneoscopic procedures. Renal cryotherapy, still an experimental technique of renal tumor ablation, is preferentially performed via retroperitoneoscopy for postero-latero renal masses (Fig. 2). In these cases, the iceball remains covered by Gerota's fascia, with minimal risk of bowel complications. Only for completely anterior lesions is the transperitoneal

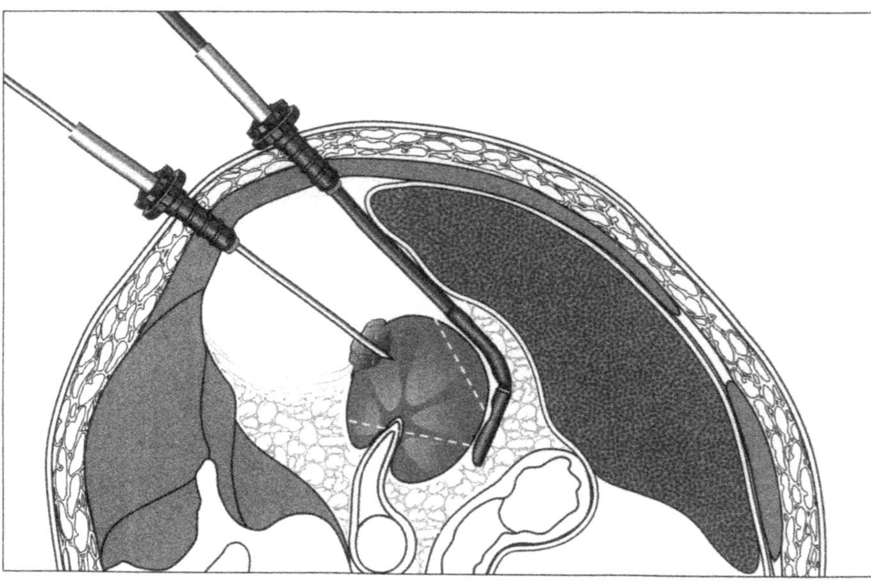

Fig. 2. Retroperitoneoscopic renal cryoablation under laparoscopic ultrasound monitoring (schematic illustration)

approach employed, with a potentially higher risk of intra-abdominal organ cryoinjury. Certainly, this and other forms of energy sources (radiofrequency thermal ablation, high-intensity focused ultrasound) will also be utilized percutaneously as technology advances.

As urologists become familiar with the method and improve their technical skills, newer indications will be described, such as retroperitoneal radical nephrectomy for tumors with level 1 renal vein thrombus [24]. The extraperitoneal technique for laparoscopic radical prostatectomy has been described recently [25] and may represent an attractive way to further reduce the morbidity of the existing transperitoneal approach. The previous experience with the extraperitoneal laparoscopic Bursch procedure for urinary incontinence and the growing acceptance of the totally extraperitoneal laparoscopic hernia repair indicate this as a natural route for other pelvic operations [26].

Lastly, of considerable enthusiasm and imminent clinical application is the concept of robotic surgery and single-surgeon operations. Use of the AESOP system robotic arm for camera control and telerobotic remote surgery [27], experimental models of robotic-assisted pyeloplasty [28], and completely robotic nephrectomy and adrenalectomy have already been reported [29]. Retroperitoneoscopy may become an excellent environment of study for robotic-assisted operations. Future incorporation of computed tomography or three-dimensional magnetic resonance imaging-generated images by newer software programs will become indispensable for surgical training. In videolaparoscopy simulators, the surgeon will be able to practice a specific procedure multiple times before being confronted with the real clinical situation. This will be equally useful during retroperitoneal surgery, where familiarity with the anatomy would be gained and confirmed prior to venturing into clinical application.

References

1. Gill IS, Clayman R, Albala D et al (1998) Retroperitoneal and pelvic extraperitoneal laparoscopy: an international perspective. Urology 52 (4):566-571
2. Bartel M (1969) Die Retroperitoneoscopie: eine endoskopische Methode zur Inspektion und bioptischen Untersuchung des retroperitonealen Raumes. Zentralbl Chir 94:377
3. Wickham JEA (1979) The surgical treatment of renal lithiasis. In: Wickham JEA (ed) Urinary calculus disease. Churchill Livingstone, New York, pp 145-198
4. Figenshau RS, Clayman RV, Kavoussi L et al (1991) Retroperitoneal laparoscopic nephrectomy: laboratory and initial clinical experience. J Endourol 5:S130, abstract PXIII-15
5. Gaur DD (1992) Laparoscopic operative retroperitoneoscopy: use of a new device. J Urol 148:1137
6. Gill IS, Grune M, Munch LC (1996) Access technique for retroperitoneoscopy. J Urol 156:1120-1124
7. Rassweiler JJ, Seemann O, Frede T et al (1998) Retroperitoneoscopy: experience with 200 cases. J Urol 160:1265-1269
8. Abbou CC, Cicco A, Gasman D et al (1999) Retroperitoneal laparoscopic versus open radical nephrectomy. J Urol 161:1776
9. Gill IS (1998) Retroperitoneal laparoscopic nephrectomy. Urol Clin North Am 25:343-360

10. Gill IS, Clayman RV, McDougall EM (1995) Advances in urological laparoscopy. J Urol 154:1275-1294
11. McDougall EM, Clayman RV, Fadden PA (1994) Retroperitoneoscopy: The Washington University Medical School experience. Urology 43: 446
12. Gill IS, Schweizer D, Hobart M et al (2000) Retroperitoneal laparoscopic radical nephrectomy: The Cleveland Clinic experience. J Urol 164:1665-1670
13. Dunn M, Portis AJ, Shalhav A et al (2000) Laparoscopic versus open radical nephrectomy: a 9-year experience. J Urol 164:1153-1159
14. Barret PH, Fentie D, Taranger LA (1998) Laparoscopic radical nephrectomy with morcellation for renal cell carcinoma: the Saskatoon experience. Urology 52:23
15. Sung GT, Gill IS, Hobart M et al (1999) Laparoscopic adrenalectomy: a prospective, randomized comparison of transperitoneal vs. retroperitoneal approaches. J Urol Suppl (abstract 69) AUA
16. Fazeli-Matin S, Gill IS, Hsu TH et al (1999) Laparoscopic renal and adrenal surgery in obese patients: comparison to open surgery. J Urol 162:665-660
17. Hsu TH, Gill IS, Fazeli-Matin S et al (1999) Radical nephrectomy and nephroureterectomy in the octogenarian and nonagenarian: comparison of laparoscopic and open approaches. Urology 53:1121-1125
18. Gill IS, Sung GT, Hobart M et al (2000) Laparoscopic radical nephroureterectomy for upper tract transitional cell carcinoma: the Cleveland Clinic experience. J Urol 164(5):1513-1522
19. Slama B, Salomon L, Hoznek A et al (2000) Extraperitoneal laparoscopic repair of ureteropelvic junction obstruction: initial experience in 15 cases. J Urol 56:45-48
20. Kaouk J, Gill IS, Hobart M et al (2002) Bilateral synchronous laparoscopic nephrectomy for adult polycystic kidney disease. J Urol (in press)
21. Gill IS, Uzzo RG, Hobart MG et al (2000) Laparoscopic retroperitoneal live-donor right nephrectomy for purposes of allotransplantation and autotransplantation. J Urol 164(5):1500-1504
22. Wolf JS, Monk TG, McDougall EM et al (1995) The extraperitoneal approach and subcutaneous emphysema are associated with greater absorption of carbon dioxide during laparoscopic renal surgery. J Urol 154:959
23. Ng C, Gill IS, Sung GT et al (1999) Retroperitoneoscopic surgery is not associated with increased carbon dioxide absorption. J Urol 162(4):1268-1272
24. Savage S, Gill IS (2000) Laparoscopic radical nephrectomy for renal cell carcinoma in a patient with level 1 renal vein tumor thrombus. J Urol 163:1243-1244
25. Bollens R, Bossche MV, Roumeguere T et al (2000) The extraperitoneal laparoscopic radical prostatectomy: a new approach. J Urol 163 [Suppl] :357 (abstract V56) AUA
26. Quilici P, Greaney Jr E, Quilicy J et al (2000) Laparoscopic inguinal hernia repair: optimal technical variations and results in 1700 cases. Am Surg 66:848-852
27. Kavoussi L, Moore RG, Partin JB et al (1995) Comparison of robotic versus human laparoscopic camera control. J Urol 54:2134
28. Sung GT, Gill IS, Hsu TH (1999) Robotic-assisted laparoscopic pyeloplasty: a pilot study. Urology 53(6):1099-1103
29. Gill IS, Sung GT, Meraney (2002) A. Remote tele-robotic laparoscopic nephrectomy and adrenalectomy: the initial experience. J Urol (in press)

Chapter 21

Limits and Controversies

Oscar Eduardo Fugita, Louis Raphael Kavoussi

The extraperitoneal location of the upper urinary tract makes the retroperitoneal laparoscopic approach an attractive option to the transperitoneal route. Almost all open surgical procedures of the kidney and ureter have been performed retroperitoneoscopically [1-7], with more complex operations such as pediatric nephrectomy [8], treatment of caliceal diverticula [9], adrenalectomy [10-12], and donor nephrectomy [13, 14] being reported. However, some characteristics of the retroperitoneoscopic technique may limit its indication.

The initial difficulty that the laparoscopist faces when performing retroperitoneoscopy is the relative unfamiliarity with external landmarks to help in the placement of trocars. Most surgeons utilize the ribs and iliac crest as starting points to initiate access. Some use Petit's triangle, formed by the intersection of the latissimus dorsi and external oblique muscles at the iliac crest, as an anatomical landmark for retroperitoneum access [15]. However, in some patients, particularly obese ones, palpation of landmarks may be difficult and visible anatomical landmarks such as the axillary lines must be used [16] or those found under ultrasound guidance.

The surgical technique for access to the retroperitoneum is also evolving. Although most of the surgeons use open technique for balloon insertion and dissection as well as primary port placement [17, 18], which allows development of the retroperitoneal space by digital manipulation [19], some prefer the closed (Veress needle) technique for obtaining pneumoretroperitoneum. Anatomical studies have demonstrated that the peritoneal reflection is consistently anterior to the posterior axillary line and that in lateral decubitus positioning the peritoneal contents fall anteriorly, increasing the diameter of the retroperitoneal space twofold [16]. If so, a needle placed posterior to the posterior axillary line should consistently enter the retroperitoneum. Unfortunately, inadvertent placement of the needle into the peritoneal cavity [18] or into the muscles of the posterior abdominal wall [16] may occur with this technique. Although both complications may require converting to open technique, a peritoneal opening does not necessarily lead to open surgery [11, 20] or a transperitoneal approach.

A modified open technique [21] using the tip of a cannula or a telescope to develop a retroperitoneal space has been described in order to prevent the leakage of gas, which sometimes occurs when making the incision for open placement of the first trocar. The disadvantage of this technique is that it does not allow a digital exploration of the retroperitoneal space. Some laparoscopists create the extraperitoneal space using the laparoscope with a combination of blunt and sharp dissection. The tendency of the lenses to become blurred and the interference of the laparoscope with the surgeon's visual field [22] are limitations of this technique.

The smaller working space of the retroperitoneal space is one of the main disadvantages of this approach. The use of balloon dilators and devices to lift the abdominal wall may not be satisfactory, particularly when approaching large tumors [23] or organs [22].

The use of hand-made or commercially available balloons is preferred by many of surgeons in order to create a retroperitoneal working space [21, 24]. However, placement is a blind procedure and, despite some technical modifications [25], it is still uncertain that the balloon has been positioned in the preferred area.

Optimal placement of the balloon is controversial; in simple nephrectomies, some surgeons advocate balloon placement under Gerota's fascia instead of outside [26]. Moreover, the balloons can rupture [10, 27], resulting in the distribution of latex fragments, particularly in obese patients. The use of two insufflators in order to maintain pneumoretroperitoneum in these patients has already been reported [28].

Mechanical retraction systems have been proposed in order to maintain a reasonable operative space without the use of carbon dioxide. With these devices (Laprofit/ Laparofan, Laparotenser) the abdominal wall is lifted by retractors attached to the operating table and inserted into the abdominal wall. However, only small series [29] have been reported and asymmetrical spaces with inadequate exposure [30-32] limit the use of these devices to very selected cases [29, 33].

The effect of insufflation of carbon dioxide on pulmonary and cardiovascular functions [31, 34-38] has been well described. Although it seems reasonable that the greater absorptive capacity of the peritoneal membrane associated with a larger space would result in greater systemic absorption of carbon dioxide in the transperitoneal laparoscopy [39], prolonged insufflation time and operative manipulation of the retroperitoneum may predispose to higher absorption of carbon dioxide [40, 41].

The limited skin area available for trocar placement, in combination with the few anatomical external landmarks, represents another technical challenge [22, 39]. The proximity of the trocars limits the maneuverability of the instruments and adds a higher level of difficulty to the procedure. Development of an adequate retropneumoperitoneum is essential for positioning the trocars further from each other.

Obliteration of the retroperitoneum space by previous surgeries or inflammatory processes may cause difficulties in creating adequate working space and in dissection [22].

The primary disadvantage of the retroperitoneal approach is poor visualization. It is difficult for the surgeon to keep his orientation in the retroperitoneum because there are fewer visual anatomical landmarks [18]. The surgeon's perspective is altered [42], and the abundant and sometimes adherent retroperitoneal fat limits the creation of an adequate working space and identification of structures [10].

These shortcomings make for a significant learning curve for retroperitoneal approach [42, 43]. In an analysis of 200 patients treated with retroperitoneoscopy for different pathological conditions, the overall complication rate — including conversion and re-intervention — decreased from 28% in the first 50 patients to 4% in the last 50 patients [27]. Of note, the theoretical advantages of the retroperitoneal approach, in regards to lower risk of visceral injury, easier intestinal retraction, no prolonged ileus, less frequent herniation of internal organs, and quicker access to the kidney and adrenal gland [18], did not lead to clinical improvements in terms of operative time [22, 27], morbidity rate [11,44-46], and rate of conversion [11, 43]. This may be explained by the small series of patients; however, the indications are expanding to more complex cases such as renal tuberculosis [47], massive hydronephrosis [26], infiltrating retroperitoneal lymphadenopathy [48], and tumor [49], and vascular reconstruction [50, 51].

In terms of costs, the same instruments are used for retroperitoneoscopy as for transperitoneal laparoscopy, except for the insufflation balloon. To avoid the added expense, some surgeons prefer the use of hand-made balloons [26, 46] that provide adequate expansion of the retroperitoneal space. Hospital stay and time to return to normal activities, which could also have impact on final surgical costs, are similar in the two approaches [10, 26, 27].

In conclusion, retroperitoneoscopy is an accepted approach to treat upper tract pathologies; however, it also has limitations. A close supervision by experienced laparoscopists comfortable with the retroperitoneal approach is advisable for beginners. Retroperitoneal laparoscopy should not be conducted until the surgeon has mastered the transperitoneal approach.

References

1. Gill IS, Clayman RV, McDougall EM (1995) Advances in urological laparoscopy. J Urol 154 (4): 1275-1294
2. Fahlekamp D, Rassweiler J, Fornara P, Frede T, Loening S (1999) Complications of laparoscopic procedures in urology: experience with 2,407 procedures at 4 German centers. J Urol 163 (3-I): 765-770

Subject Index

GPSR Compliance
The European Union's (EU) General Product Safety Regulation (GPSR) is a set of rules that requires consumer products to be safe and our obligations to ensure this.

If you have any concerns about our products, you can contact us on

ProductSafety@springernature.com

In case Publisher is established outside the EU, the EU authorized representative is:

Springer Nature Customer Service Center GmbH
Europaplatz 3
69115 Heidelberg, Germany

www.ingramcontent.com/pod-product-compliance
Lightning Source LLC
Chambersburg PA
CBHW071438230926
51846CB00001B/278
* 9 7 8 8 8 4 7 0 2 9 2 5 5 *